Cytotoxic Drug Resistance Mechanisms

METHODS IN MOLECULAR MEDICINE™

John M. Walker, Series Editor

29. **DNA Vaccines,** edited by *Douglas B. Lowrie and Robert Whalen,* 1999
28. **Cytotoxic Drug Resistance Mechanisms,** edited by *Robert Brown and Uta Böger-Brown,* 1999
27. **Clinical Applications of Capillary Electrophoresis,** edited by *Stephen M. Palfrey,* 1999
26. **Quantitative PCR Protocols,** edited by *Bernd Kochanowski and and Udo Reischl,* 1999
25. **Drug Targeting,** edited by *G. E. Francis and Cristina Delgado,* 1999
24. **Antiviral Chemotherapy Protocols,** edited by *Derek Kinchington and Raymond F. Schinazi, 1998*
23. **Peptidomimetics Protocols,** edited by *Wieslaw M. Kazmierski,* 1998
22. **Neurodegeneration Methods and Protocols,** edited by *Jean Harry and Hugh A. Tilson,* 1998
21. **Adenovirus Methods and Protocols,** edited by *William S. M. Wold,* 1998
20. **Sexually Transmitted Diseases Protocols,** edited by *Rosanna Peeling and P. Frederick Sparling,* 1998
19. **Hepatitis C Protocols,** edited by *Johnson Y. N. Lau,* 1998
18. **Tissue Engineering,** edited by *Jeffrey R. Morgan and Martin Yarmush,* 1998
17. **HIV Protocols,** edited by *Nelson Michael and Jerome H. Kim,* 1998
16. **Clinical Applications of PCR,** edited by *Y. M. Dennis Lo,* 1998
15. **Molecular Bacteriology:** *Protocols and Clinical Applications,* edited by *Neil Woodford and Alan P. Johnson,* 1998
14. **Tumor Marker Protocols,** edited by *Margaret Hanausek and Zbigniew Walaszek,* 1998
13. **Molecular Diagnosis of Infectious Diseases,** edited by *Udo Reischl,* 1998
12. **Diagnostic Virology Protocols,** edited by *John R. Stephenson and Alan Warnes,* 1998
11. **Therapeutic Applications of Ribozymes,** edited by *Kevin J. Scanlon,* 1998
10. **Herpes Simplex Virus Protocols,** edited by *S. Moira Brown and Alasdair R. MacLean,* 1998
9. **Lectin Methods and Protocols,** edited by *Jonathan M. Rhodes and Jeremy D. Milton,* 1998
8. ***Helicobacter pylori* Protocols,** edited by *Christopher L. Clayton and Harry L. T. Mobley,* 1997
7. **Gene Therapy Protocols,** edited by *Paul D. Robbins,* 1997
6. **Molecular Diagnosis of Cancer,** edited by *Finbarr E. Cotter,* 1996
5. **Molecular Diagnosis of Genetic Diseases,** edited by *Rob Elles,* 1996
4. **Vaccine Protocols,** edited by *Andrew Robinson, Graham H. Farrar, and Christopher N. Wiblin,* 1996
3. **Prion Diseases,** edited by *Harry F. Baker and Rosalind M. Ridley,* 1996
2. **Human Cell Culture Protocols,** edited by *Gareth E. Jones,* 1996
1. **Antisense Therapeutics,** edited by *Sudhir Agrawal,* 1996

METHODS IN MOLECULAR MEDICINE™

Cytotoxic Drug Resistance Mechanisms

Edited by

Robert Brown

University of Glasgow, Glasgow, UK

and

Uta Böger-Brown

BioMedEx, Killearn, UK

Humana Press ✱ **Totowa, New Jersey**

999 Riverview Drive, Suite 208
Totowa, New Jersey 07512

This publication is printed on acid-free paper. ∞
ANSI Z39.48-1984 (American Standards Institute) Permanence of Paper for Printed Library Materials.

Cover illustration: Fig. 1 from Chapter 17, "Analysis of the p53 Status of Tumors: *An Overview of Methods*," by Jonas Bergh.

Cover design by Patricia F. Cleary.

For additional copies, pricing for bulk purchases, and/or information about other Humana titles, contact Humana at the above address or at any of the following numbers: Tel.:973-256-1699; Fax: 973-256-8341; E-mail: humana@humanapr.com; Website: http://humanapress.com

Printed in the United States of America. 10 9 8 7 6 5 4 3 2 1

Library of Congress Cataloging in Publication Data

Main entry under title:

Methods in molecular medicine™.

Cytotoxic Drug Resistance Mechanisms / edited by Robert Brown and Uta Böger-Brown.
p. cm. — (Methods in molecular medicine™ ; 28)
Includes index.
ISBN 978-1-61737-093-9 e-ISBN 978-1-59259-687-4
1. Drug resistance in cancer cells—Research—Methodology.
I. Brown, Robert , 1956 Jan. 8– II. Böger-Brown, Uta. III. Series.
[DNLM: 1. Drug Resistance, Neoplasm. 2. Antineoplastic Agents—Pharmacology.
3. DNA Damage. 4. Genetic Techniques. QZ 267 C9975 1999]
RC271.C5C97 1999
616.99'4061—dc21
DNLM/DLC
for Library of Congress 98-43528
CIP

Preface

There is now a range of cytotoxic drugs that have considerable clinical usefulness in producing responses in tumors and even, in a small proportion of cases, cure. However, the acquisition of drug resistance is a major clinical problem and is perhaps the main limiting factor in successful treatment of cancer. Thus, a tumor initially sensitive to chemotherapy will, in the majority of cases, eventually recur as a resistant tumor, which will then progress. Much of our understanding of drug resistance mechanisms comes from the study of tumor cell lines grown in tissue culture. We now understand many of the molecular mechanisms that can lead to a cell acquiring resistance to anticancer drugs; however, we still do not know which mechanism(s) are those most relevant to the problem of clinical drug resistance. Indeed, given that many of the cytotoxic anticancer drugs were discovered by random screening, it is unclear what features give a clinically useful anticancer drug a sufficient therapeutic index to be of value.

The aim of *Cytotoxic Drug Resistance Mechanisms* is to provide protocols that are appropriate for examining the mechanisms of cellular resistance to anticancer cytotoxics in human tumor samples. Tumor cell lines have been enormously useful as experimental models of drug resistance mechanisms, however they have limitations and we need to address the relevance of such mechanisms in patients' tumors. Examining drug resistance in tumors is much more problematic than in cell lines. Not least, because it is difficult to define the cellular sensitivity or resistance of a tumor sample. A number of assays of in vitro sensitivity have been developed to address this question. Since the realization that many anticancer cytotoxics kill cells by an apoptotic process, these cell sensitivity assays have come to include in vitro and in vivo measures of apoptosis.

To an outside observer, drug resistance is often taken as being synonymous with the Multi-Drug Resistance Phenotype, conferred by *MDR1*/P-glycoprotein and related genes. This has been an intensively studied mechanism of resistance and is of clear clinical relevance. A large number of studies in this field have now led to a consensus on how *MDR1*/Pgp should be measured in tumor samples; this consensus should be a role model for future studies on other resistance mechanisms. Though P-glycoprotein-mediated drug efflux is important, it is clearly not the only mechanism of relevance to clinical drug resistance. A number of studies would suggest that *MDR1*/Pgp is not the reason for the acquired drug resistance of many solid tumors.

There is a large body of circumstantial evidence for most of the cytotoxics described in *Cytotoxic Drug Resistance Mechanisms*, all of which supports DNA as the crucial target. Delivering sufficient drug to the chemotherapeutic target is obviously important. Although the methods presented here do not deal with pharmacological resistance, means of measuring the amount of DNA damage induced by various cytotoxics are described. Undoubtedly the most exciting emerging area in drug resistance during the last five years has been the role of drug-induced apoptosis. A number of genes have now been implicated in modulating the ability of a cell to undergo drug-induced apoptosis, including DNA repair proteins, p53-dependent pathways, and the *bcl2* gene family. Such mechanisms modulate resistance in a manner that will be entirely independent of the amount of drug delivered. The relevance of these apoptosis-modulating mechanisms to clinical resistance will be an important research area over the next years.

Drug resistance can be clinically defined as a tumor's lack of response to therapy. It is possible that there are yet unknown mechanisms of clinical resistance still to be identified in experimental models. Therefore examining genetic alterations in clinical samples without prior assumption may prove invaluable. Molecular cytogenetics may prove to be one such approach that will provide important information.

For each of the methods described in *Cytotoxic Drug Resistance Mechanisms*, the most important ingredient is the effective admixture of clinical and laboratory scientists that allows correlations between molecular and biochemical data and the clinical responses of patients to be identified. With that in mind, I would like to thank all the surgeons, pathologists, biologists, medical oncologists, and other colleagues who have contributed their correct ingredients to the elucidation of drug resistance phenomena.

Robert Brown and Uta Böger-Brown

Contents

Contributors

D. Alan Anthoney • *CRC Department of Medical Oncology, Beatson Laboratories, University of Glasgow, Glasgow, UK*
Philip J. Beale • *CRC Centre for Cancer Therapeutics, The Institute of Cancer Research, Sutton, Surrey, UK*
Susan E. Bates • *Medicine Branch, National Cancer Institute, National Institutes of Health, Bethesda, MD*
Jonas Bergh • *Department of Oncology, University Hospital, Uppsala, Sweden*
Henk J. Broxterman • *Department of Medical Oncology, Free University Hospital, Amsterdam, The Netherlands*
Philip J. Coates • *Department of Molecular and Cellular Pathology, University of Dundee, Dundee, UK*
Caroline Dive • *Molecular and Cellular Pharmacology Group, University of Manchester, School of Biological Sciences, Manchester, UK*
Adrian J. Frank • *Leukaemia Research Fund Laboratory, University of Newcastle Upon Tyne, Medical School, Newcastle Upon Tyne, UK*
Erick Gamelin • *Medicine Branch, National Cancer Institute, National Institutes of Health, Bethesda, MD*
Andrew G. Hall •*Paediatric Oncology Laboratory, Cancer Research Unit, University of Newcastle upon Tyne, Medical School, Newcastle upon Tyne, UK*
Peter A. Hall • *Department of Molecular and Cellular Pathology, University of Dundee, Dundee, UK*
Janet M. Hartley • *CRC Drug-DNA Interactions Research Group, Department of Oncology, University College London Medical School, London, UK*
John A. Hartley • *CRC Drug-DNA Interactions Research Group, Department of Oncology, University College London Medical School, London, UK*
Gillian L. Hirst • *CRC Department of Medical Oncology, Beatson Laboratories, University of Glasgow, Glasgow, UK*
Linda A. Hogarth • *Paediatric Oncology Laboratory, Cancer Research Unit, University of Newcastle Upon Tyne, Medical School, Newcastle Upon Tyne, UK*

Stephen J. Johnston • *Department of Medicine and Therapeutics, Institute of Medical Sciences, University of Aberdeen, Foresterhill, Aberdeen, UK*

Neil A. Jones • *Molecular and Cellular Pharmacology Group, University of Manchester, School of Biological Sciences, Manchester, UK*

Stanley B. Kaye • *CRC Department of Medical Oncology, Beatson Laboratories, University of Glasgow, Glasgow, UK*

Pamela R. Kearns • *Paediatric Oncology Laboratory, Cancer Research Unit, University of Newcastle Upon Tyne, Medical School, Newcastle Upon Tyne, UK*

W. Nicol Keith • *CRC Department of Medical Oncology, Beatson Laboratories, University of Glasgow, Glasgow, UK*

Lloyd R. Kelland • *CRC Centre for Cancer Therapeutics, The Institute of Cancer Research, Sutton, Surrey, UK*

Glenda Kohlhagen • *Laboratory of Molecular Pharmacology, National Cancer Institute, National Institutes of Health, Bethesda, MD*

Geoffrey P. Margison • *Department of Carcinogenesis, Paterson Institute for Cancer Research, Christie Hospital NHS Trust, Manchester, UK*

Howard L. McLeod • *Department of Medicine and Therapeutics, Institute of Medical Sciences, University of Aberdeen, Foresterhill, Aberdeen, UK*

Lesley H. Milne • *CRC Department of Medical Oncology, Beatson Laboratories, University of Glasgow, Glasgow, UK*

Jane A Plumb • *CRC Department of Medical Oncology, Beatson Laboratories, University of Glasgow, Glasgow, UK*

Yves Pommier • *Laboratory of Molecular Pharmacology, National Cancer Institute, National Institutes of Health, Bethesda, MD*

Philippe Pourquier • *Laboratory of Molecular Pharmacology, National Cancer Institute, National Institutes of Health, Bethesda, MD*

Vicki Save • *Department of Molecular and Cellular Pathology, University of Dundee, Dundee, UK*

Celia M. A. Rabello • *Paediatric Oncology Laboratory, Cancer Research Unit, University of Newcastle Upon Tyne, Medical School, Newcastle Upon Tyne, UK*

Joanna Regis • *Medicine Branch, National Cancer Institute, National Institutes of Health, Bethesda, MD*

Victoria J. Spanswick • *CRC Drug-DNA Interactions Research Group, Department of Oncology, University College London Medical School, London, UK*

Michael J. Tilby • *Cancer Research Unit, University of Newcastle upon Tyne, Medical School, Newcastle upon Tyne, UK*

Li-Ming Ueng • *Laboratory of Molecular Pharmacology, National Cancer Institute, National Institutes of Health, Bethesda, MD*

Timothy H. Ward • *Cell Culture Unit, Paterson Institute for Cancer Research, Christie Hospital NHS Trust, Manchester, UK*

Amanda J. Watson • *Department of Carcinogenesis, Paterson Institute for Cancer Research, Christie Hospital NHS Trust, Manchester, UK*

Zhirong Zhan • *Medicine Branch, National Cancer Institute, National Institutes of Health, Bethesda, MD*

1

Drug Resistance

The Clinical Perspective

D. Alan Anthoney and Stanley B. Kaye

1. Introduction

There are very few tumor types in which the use of chemotherapy can bring about prolonged survival, and possibly cure, for individual patients. The most common reason for this is the development of drug resistance within tumor cells. The laboratory study of resistance to anticancer drugs has resulted in the discovery of numerous mechanisms present within tumor cells that act to reduce their cytotoxic effects. However, the failure to translate this basic laboratory research into improved clinical outcome for patients remains one of the most pressing problems in contemporary cancer research.

Clinical drug resistance encompasses two broad categories of treatment failure. Innate drug resistance is observed when a patient's disease fails to respond to therapy initially. Acquired resistance arises with the development of tumor recurrence at some time after completion of initial treatment. The recurrent disease often displays resistance to anticancer agents to which it has had no prior exposure. Although cellular mechanisms of drug resistance play a significant part in the failure of cancer chemotherapy, other important factors influence the likelihood that a certain form of treatment will be effective. Problems in applying the results of in vitro studies on drug resistance to a clinical setting arise out of the complexities involved in analyzing patients as opposed to tumor cells in culture.

This chapter attempts to define some of the significant problems that influence the study of drug resistance in the clinical setting. It then presents an overview of current clinical studies on the detection and circumvention of drug resistance.

From: *Methods in Molecular Medicine, Vol. 28: Cytotoxic Drug Resistance Mechanisms*
Edited by: R. Brown and U. Böger-Brown © Humana Press Inc., Totowa, NJ

2. Problems in the Clinical Analysis of Drug Resistance

The vast majority of laboratory studies on drug resistance have made use of in vitro tumor cell lines in monolayer culture. Such cell lines are most often clonally derived, reducing the risk that differences in sensitivity to specific cytotoxic agents arise through variability between cells of the same line. The ability to control the in vitro environment enables all cells to be exposed to identical conditions, e.g., a specific concentration of cytotoxic agent. The use of clonogenic and nonclonogenic methods of determining drug sensitivity and resistance allows multiple repetitions of each assay. This improves the statistical significance of the values obtained. Analysis of cell lines with different sensitivities to specific cytotoxic agents has uncovered biochemical and molecular differences that may underlie the development of resistance.

In the clinical setting, a different situation pertains. The analytical unit of clinical studies is the patient, a complex multicellular organism. Many features of an individual patient and their environment can influence the effectiveness of a particular form of drug treatment. Control of the environment in which patients are studied is extremely difficult. Thus interpretation of drug resistance in the clinical setting requires consideration of many confounding factors that may have little to do with direct biochemical or molecular features of the tumor cell.

One problem with clinical studies of drug resistance is that several different endpoints are used to determine the response of a tumor to a particular treatment. During the administration of a course of treatment, response is measured by use of serial X-rays, computerized tomography (CT) scans, assessments of serum tumor markers, etc. Thus, one can make an approximate determination as to whether there is disease progression, stable disease, or a complete or partial response. However, the clinical (radiological) limit of detection is a tumor of about 1 cm, which represents 10^8–10^9 tumor cells *(1)*. Therefore, although there may be a good clinical response to treatment, a significant, but undetectable, number of tumor cells may remain that may represent resistant disease.

Clinical measurements, therefore, can be used to determine initial responsiveness or resistance to treatment in an individual patient, but can only provide a crude indication of the development of resistance over a period of time. Clinical studies on new cytotoxic drugs, or combinations of drugs, use different end-points to assess response. The most obvious determinant of successful treatment is patient survival. However, problems arise in that the length of survival may depend on many variables not directly related to the treatment regimen under study. For example, patients who relapse after a specific course of treatment will most likely receive other forms of therapy, with greater or lesser effect in each individual's case. Often, this is not taken into account in the analysis of the overall survival of patients and may result in an underestimation of the resistance to the regimen. Is measurement of the time to clinical relapse, the disease-free survival, a better determinant of resistance to a particular form of treatment, within a given population, than overall survival? Confounding factors can arise prior to or during treatment that may influence the time to disease relapse. These may not be directly related to the inherent sensitivity of the tumor cells to a specific form of chemotherapy. Thus, differences in the surgical debulking of tumor, and whether done by a general or specialist surgeon, can have a significant effect on the time to disease relapse between patients *(2)*. Variations in the actual dose intensity of chemotherapy received, as opposed to the planned dose intensity, can also significantly influence the time to disease relapse between patients. Often such data are not included in the analysis of the response of a particular tumor type to a particular regimen of chemotherapy.

There are many other factors that influence the likely response of an individual patient to a particular treatment. These include components of previous health, genetic determinants of drug metabolism, prior exposure to other treatment modalities, and so on. Although important in the individual case, such variation between patients, not observed in clonal populations of cells, can obscure the results of clinical trials of chemotherapy. This can be overcome by enrolling large numbers of patients into such studies, often with the choice of which treatment they receive being randomized. However, the logistical difficulties in performing such trials are significant and patient recruitment is often problematic. These studies do provide a very valuable resource for projects aimed at understanding the causes of clinical drug resistance, because they comprise a group of patients treated in a homogeneous fashion, for whom other relevant data are also available.

It is obvious, therefore, that the study of the development of resistance to anticancer drugs in the clinical setting is more complex than in the laboratory and that often resistance can only be measured indirectly. This is not to say that clinical studies of the importance of laboratory-derived drug resistance markers cannot be done. It may help to explain, however, why the results are often less than clear.

3. Clinical Studies of Drug Resistance

Resistance to anticancer drugs is viewed as one of the most significant barriers to the effective treatment of malignant tumors. It is therefore not surprising that despite the difficulties previously mentioned, many studies have been and continue to be performed to determine the clinical significance of specific drug-resistance mechanisms.

3.1. P-glycoprotein (Pgp)

One of the major mechanisms of multidrug resistance in cultured cancer cells has been shown to be caused by over-expression of a surface-membrane, energy-dependent transport protein, P-glycoprotein (Pgp) *(3)*. This protein can increase the efflux of natural product anticancer drugs from the cell, thus reducing the effective intracellular concentration. Pgp is normally expressed in detectable quantities in tissues such as colon, adrenal cortex, kidney, and liver. Tumors from these organs often display inherent resistance to a range of anticancer drugs. The *MDR-1* gene, which encodes Pgp, is expressed at levels thought to be physiologically significant in about 50% of human cancers *(4)*. However, does Pgp play a major part in the development of clinical drug resistance? To answer this question, many studies have tried to correlate expression of Pgp with established prognostic indicators or with determinants of treatment outcome.

To date, the greatest number of studies have been performed in the hematological malignancies. This obviously reflects the more readily accessible sources of tissue, i.e., bone marrow, available for study in these conditions. A number of different techniques have been used to determine the levels of expression of Pgp on blast cells in both acute lymphoblastic leukemia (ALL) and acute myelogenous leukemia (AML). Attempts have then been made to correlate these with response to treatment or clinical outcome. The methodology for detection of Pgp in these studies has developed with time from determination of *MDR-1* gene expression by Northern blotting or reverse transcriptase-polymerase chain reaction (RT-PCR; *see* Chapter 7) to immunocytochemical analysis of Pgp and measurement of its function (*see* Chapter 6). In de novo AML a number of papers have reported a correlation between detectable levels of Pgp and a poor response to treatment. Flow cytometry using the MRK16 monoclonal antibody (MAb) was used by Campos et al. to study 150 patients with newly diagnosed AML *(5)*. Patients with no detectable Pgp displayed a significantly better rate of complete response to treatment and overall survival. The same method was used by Ino et al. *(6)*, who determined that Pgp detected by flow cytometry correlated with functional Pgp by the Rhodamine 123 assay. In a study of 52 patients with AML, they showed that although presence of Pgp did not correlate with a reduced chance of achieving a complete response (CR) after chemotherapy, it was associated with an increased risk of relapse *(6)*. Ludescher et al. *(7)* proposed that Pgp function, as assessed by the Rhodamine 123 assay, might act as an independent prognostic indicator in AML. This was after finding a significant survival difference between patients whose blast cells did and did not display functional Pgp by this method. Not all such studies show evidence of a correlation between the presence of Pgp on blast cells in

AML and a failure to respond to, or relapse after, chemotherapy. However, the overall impression is that Pgp probably has a role in the development of resistance to chemotherapy in AML.

The situation in other forms of hematological malignancy is less clear. A number of studies in ALL have shown positive correlation between the presence of Pgp and relapse of disease after chemotherapy *(8,9)*. However several other groups have shown no clinical significance associated with the presence of Pgp on blast cells in ALL *(10)*. It has been proposed that this may result from the different methodology used in different studies and perhaps also the different populations of patients. Analysis of a large number of patients with myeloma *(11)* before and after therapy with vincristine and doxorubicin revealed that expression of Pgp was strongly correlated with prior exposure to these drugs. The design of the study did not allow a determination of whether this affected outcome.

Does the presence of detectable Pgp in cells from solid tumors act as a prognostic indicator? The greatest amount of data collected to date has been for adenocarcinoma of the breast *(12)*. A number of studies have looked at whether Pgp expression in breast carcinoma is associated with response to chemotherapy *(12)*. Although Pgp levels measured before chemotherapy do not significantly determine the likelihood of response to treatment a significant association between elevated Pgp and poor outcome was noted if levels were measured post-treatment. This may relate to selection for Pgp positive cells during chemotherapy, but could also arise as an epiphenomenon if selection for other determinants of poor prognosis during treatment, (e.g., mutant p53) was associated with induction of *MDR-1* expression *(13)*. The prognostic significance of detectable Pgp in breast cancer remains unclear as there is no uniform result from those investigations performed to date *(12)*.

The expression of Pgp, as detected by immunohistochemistry (IHC), has been shown to display a positive correlation with increased relapse rate in osteosarcoma *(14)*. This prognostic significance of Pgp was unrelated to other features of the tumor such as chemotherapy-induced necrosis, which is currently the most important predictor of disease-free survival. It is of interest that in this study the relationship between Pgp and tumor relapse after chemotherapy could not be linked to increased drug efflux from the tumor cells. The chemotherapy used was composed of drugs that are not normally considered to be substrates for Pgp. Therefore, at least in osteosarcoma and perhaps also in colon and breast cancer, the presence of Pgp may not simply be a marker of tumor chemosensitivity, but also a sign of tumor aggressiveness *(15)*.

As with breast cancer, a state of uncertainty exists as to the significance of Pgp studies in colorectal carcinoma in which there appears to be an even spread of positive and negative correlations *(16)*. Pgp expression may have prognostic significance in a subset of non-seminomatous germ cell tumors *(17)*, but not in non-small cell lung cancer or adrenocortical carcinoma from the data published to date *(18,19)*.

3.2. Pgp-Related Transporters

Over recent years, it has become obvious that Pgp is not the only membrane protein that is associated with MDR. This was shown in tumor cells that displayed an MDR phenotype but without detectable levels of Pgp. Two further drug-resistance related proteins have been described. MDR-associated protein (MRP) is a member of the ATP-binding cassette (ABC)-transporter superfamily that confers resistance to a similar, but not identical, spectrum of drugs as Pgp *(20,21)*. Lung resistance protein (LRP) was first identified in a lung-cancer cell line displaying MDR *(22)*. There is evidence to suggest that LRP is expressed more frequently in chemoresistant tumor types than in chemosensitive cancers *(23)*. Clinical studies have been performed in an attempt to determine the clinical significance of MRP and LRP expression in tumors. Expression of MRP was found to be higher in patients with relapsed AML as opposed to newly diagnosed cases *(24)*. A positive correlation between MRP and *MDR-1* gene overexpression was observed in these AML cases, and this was associated with a higher rate of emergence of clinical drug resistance. In cases which were MDR negative, drug resistance was more frequent in MRP positive cases than in MRP negative ones. Several other studies have also suggested that over-expression of MRP can be detected in up to 35% of AML patients and is associated with a tendency towards chemo-resistant disease *(24)*. However, it has also been shown that pre-treatment levels of MRP mRNA may lack prognostic value in AML.

Metastatic neuroblastoma has a poor prognosis attributable, in part, to MDR. The contribution of *MDR-1*/Pgp to neuroblastoma MDR is unclear, but evidence suggests that MRP may play a significant role. A study of 60 neuroblastoma cases correlated elevated expression of MRP with other known indicators of poor prognosis, e.g., increased N-myc expression. MRP expression was also associated with reduced overall survival, and this appeared to be independent of the status of other prognostic indicators in the tumor. MDR gene expression in these tumors showed no prognostic significance. The consequences of elevated MRP have also been analyzed in other solid tumor types. Ota et al. *(25)* reported that MRP-expressing squamous-cell lung cancer showed a significantly worse prognosis than MRP negative tumors, but that this was not so in adenocarcinoma of the lung. MRP expression has also been shown to be associated with increased resistance to certain anti-cancer drugs in vitro, as measured using gastric cancer biopsies. However, there was no association between MRP status and outcome in patients with gastric adenocarcinoma *(26)*.

Far fewer studies to date have looked at the role of LRP in clinical drug resistance. LRP has been shown to have prognostic significance in AML and epithelial ovarian cancer *(23)*. In the latter study, LRP was an independent determinant of response to treatment and overall survival, whereas Pgp and MRP were not. LRP levels were also shown to be increased post-chemotherapy in osteosarcoma and this was a poor prognostic sign *(27)*. LRP levels prior to chemotherapy did not show prognostic significance.

3.3. Glutathione and Glutathione Transferases

Mechanisms of drug resistance involving membrane-associated protein pumps, although the most thoroughly characterized, are not the only means by which drug resistance can arise within tumor cells. Clinical studies investigating these other drug-resistance mechanisms are fewer in number, but are no less important. The concentration of intracellular enzymes (both activating and detoxifying) involved in the metabolism of cytotoxic drugs have been measured to determine whether there is a relationship with response to treatment. The glutathione S-transferases (GST) are a group of detoxifying enzymes that are thought to play a role in the metabolism of drugs such as cisplatin, doxorubicin, melphalan, cyclophosphamide and the nitrosoureas *(28)*. GST-π is the predominant isoenzyme subtype found in ovarian carcinoma and several studies have been performed to determine whether levels of this enzyme have prognostic significance. Using immunohistochemistry on formalin fixed, paraffin-embedded tumor sections, Green et al. *(28)* found that increased levels of GST-π were correlated to a poor response to chemotherapy. GST-π levels also correlated to overall survival, independent of other prognostic indicators. Similar results were obtained by Hamada et al. *(29)*, who also found that levels of GST-π were higher in residual tumor after the completion of chemotherapy. Several other reports, however, using immunohistochemical and Western immunoblot analysis of glutathione and GST-π levels in ovarian carcinoma, have shown no evidence of independent prognostic significance *(30,31)*. Attempts to correlate GST levels and clinical outcome in urothelial tumors and in cancers of the head and neck has also been attempted, but without clear conclusions *(32,33)*.

3.4. DNA Repair

The involvement of DNA repair pathways in the development of drug resistance has become increasingly apparent over recent years from in vitro studies on tumor cell lines. Measurement of the expression of specific genes involved in DNA repair pathways in tumor samples has been used to assess the possible clinical significance of DNA repair. Elevated levels of p53 protein in tumors suggest mutation in the *p53* gene. As p53 protein is involved in regulation of cell-cycle checkpoints, DNA repair and apoptotic pathways mutations in the gene may be responsible for altering the sensitivity of tumor cells to cytotoxic drugs. This may result in drug resistance. Immunohistochemical detection of elevated levels of p53 has been associated with established features of aggressive phenotype and poor prognosis in a number of tumor types, including ovarian, breast, and bladder carcinomas ***(31,34,35)***. Increased tumor p53 in ovarian carcinoma has been associated with a poor response to chemotherapy (cisplatin-based) in a report by Righetti ***(36)***, although a number of others show no significant correlation ***(31,37)***. The association of elevated tumor p53 protein levels and the length of progression-free survival (PFS) after chemotherapy has also been studied, particularly in ovarian carcinoma. There have been no indications that elevated p53 levels correlate with shorter PFS except in specific tumor sub-types ***(31,38)***.

A number of small studies have attempted to correlate response to chemotherapy with the levels of other DNA repair genes in tumor specimens. Thus, the levels of expression of nucleotide-excision repair genes *ERCC1*, *ERCC2*, and *XPA* have been compared to the response to cisplatin chemotherapy in ovarian cancer, but without any significant association being determined ***(39,40)***. There have also been suggestions that levels of Bcl2 expression in ovarian tumors might influence the response to chemotherapy. Reports from two groups suggest that detection of Bcl2 by immunohistochemistry (IHC), along with lack of detectable p53, is associated with a better response to chemotherapy in all but the worst prognosis patients ***(41,42)***. Unfortunately, the small number of patients in these studies limits their significance

4. Clinical Importance of Specific Mechanisms of Drug Resistance

As can be seen from the evidence previously presented, the significance that specific drug-resistance mechanisms play in the clinical response of tumors to cytotoxic agents is unclear. In the majority of tumors, for every study that has shown a correlation between a marker of resistance and poor outcome, another study has shown no such association. Does different evidence exist that might help in determining the clinical importance of specific mechanisms of drug resistance?

If a tumor cell develops resistance by increasing the rate at which drug is exported from the intracellular compartment, then it would appear reasonable to assume that increasing the concentration of drug to which the cell is exposed will overcome the resistance to some extent. Thus if a cell with classical MDR is exposed to a higher concentration of cytotoxic agent, more drug will enter the intracellular space and, despite the activity of Pgp, will lead to cytotoxicity. This is easily observed in vitro as even highly resistant tumor cell lines can be killed by exposure to a sufficient concentration of cytotoxic drug. The situation in vivo is obviously different as the effects of cytotoxic agents on normal cells in the body limits the doses that can be given safely. However, the idea that increasing the total dose and/or the dose intensity of specific cytotoxic agents might improve outcome has led to many studies which have used "high-dose" chemotherapy (HDC) to treat recurrent or poor prognosis tumors. Do the results of such studies help in determining the clinical importance of classical MDR-type resistance? The use of HDC and bone marrow rescue was initially developed for the treatment of hematological malignancies and it is here that the evidence appears to be most clear. For example, patients with non-Hodgkins lymphoma (NHL) who fail to achieve a CR after conventional chemotherapy or with relapsed disease have shown an improved response rate and survival after treatment with HDC, as compared to standard dose-salvage regimens *(43,44)*. This data is compatible with the notion that some of the resistance observed in relapsed or poorly responsive NHL may be owing to classical MDR-type mechanisms.

The benefits of HDC in treatment of a wide range of solid tumors are much less certain. The treatment of metastatic and poor prognosis forms of breast cancer with HDC has been investigated most extensively. There would appear to be little doubt that the use of high-dose regimens delivers a higher response rate to treatment than standard-dose treatment. However, this has seldom resulted in improvements in overall duration of response and survival *(45)*. Often the data has been difficult to interpret owing to the lack of clinical trials in which HDC was directly compared to standard-dose regimens. One feature that did arise from such studies was that there appeared to be a threshold of drug dose, below which the response to treatment was definitely poorer. Thus, "less was worse," but more was not necessarily better. More recently a number of controlled trials have been performed. Although the data from these studies is not without potentially significant flaws, they suggest that in certain specific groups of patients with poor prognosis breast cancer, HDC may result in improved overall survival *(46)*. In other solid tumors, there is no convincing evidence as yet that HDC can overcome resistance resulting in improved survival *(47)*.

There exists a further body of evidence that helps clarify the clinical relevance of Pgp-mediated classical MDR resistance. With numerous in vitro studies showing that Pgp was important in the development of MDR cell lines, and some evidence that this might be significant in vivo, the idea of Pgp as a specific target for therapy arose. A range of compounds have been shown to reverse the classical MDR phenotype in vitro through competitive inhibition of drug efflux *(48)*. Some of these are drugs that have established therapeutic roles in other forms of illness, e.g., calcium channel antagonists, cyclosporines, antimalarials, and steroids. The potential for reversal of MDR with such compounds has also been observed in Pgp-expressing tumor xenograft models *(49)*.

A number of these drugs have been used in clinical trials in an attempt to overcome treatment resistance in tumors where Pgp commonly contributes to the resistance phenotype. Some of these trials have shown that addition of Pgp antagonists, such as Verapamil and cyclosporin A, in the treatment of resistant myeloma and lymphoma appears to result in further responses to treatment *(50,51)*. However, there have been criticisms of many of the MDR reversal studies performed to date. For example, addition of Pgp antagonists can also alter the pharmacokinetics of cytotoxic drugs used in the treatment regimen. This normally results in exposure of the tumor cells to a higher concentration of cytotoxic drug. It is unclear, therefore, whether any improvement in results with an MDR modulator is owing to direct blocking of Pgp or to pharmacokinetic interaction *(52)* as with cyclosporin analog, PSC833. The development of more specific inhibitors of Pgp, e.g., LY335979 *(53)*, which may not alter the pharmacokinetics of cytotoxic agents, may help to clarify this issue.

The problems inherent in many of the MDR reversal studies published to date mean that they do not, as yet, provide strong evidence for the importance of Pgp in the development of clinical drug resistance. Improvements in trial design and the development of more specific antagonists of Pgp may result in more significant results in the not-too-distant future.

5. Conclusions

The preceding review illustrates that determining the clinical relevance of drug-resistance mechanisms discovered in vitro is far from simple. Often it appears that a consensus has been reached with regard to the significance of a particular factor when the next study comes along with a contradictory conclusion. The reasons for this, as have already been indicated, are numerous, and often arise from the complexity of studying the human organism in its environment. However, much of the difficulty also arises from significant differences in the way in which studies are performed. Clinical studies are often limited by the numbers of patients that can be recruited.

Standardization of trial methods, therefore, could allow data to be accumulated from multiple small studies, improving the significance of results. Obviously, advances in molecular biology alter the sensitivity with which drug-resistance genes or proteins can be detected. The differences between results observed in clinical studies of Pgp in the late 1980s and in mid-1990s have been attributed to the use of the more recent and sensitive technique of immunohistochemistry *(12)*. Attempts have been made to standardize the methods used in studying drug-resistance markers. A recent workshop conference published guidelines as to what criteria should be used to determine whether a tumor is Pgp-positive *(54)*. Such measures may increase the information that can be obtained from diverse clinical studies.

A different approach to improving the clinical data on the significance of drug-resistance mechanisms might be to study the development of resistance in sequential biopsy samples from the same individual(s). Although this seems attractive in principle, the reality is that, for most patients, tissue samples are not easy to obtain. With hematological tumors, repeat samples of bone marrow or lymph node biopsies obtained pre- and post-chemotherapy are a possibility. However, with solid tumors it is often unfeasible, or unethical, to attempt to obtain tissue samples after chemotherapy or at relapse.

The chapters that follow present a range of state-of-the-art techniques for investigation of mechanisms of drug resistance. Although not specifically aimed at clinical studies, it is to be hoped that they will be of benefit in translational research with its aims of bringing discoveries from the laboratory into the clinical domain. It is hoped that with advances in laboratory techniques and materials, along with improved design of clinical drug-resistance studies, the significance of resistance mechanisms will become clearer. This should be a realistic goal because, to steal a quote from another field of investigation, "The truth is out there."

References

1. Tannoch, I. (1989) Principles of cell proliferation: cell kinetics, in *Cancer: Principles and Practice of Oncology*, 3rd ed. (de Vita, V. T., Hellman, S., and Rosenberg, S. A., eds.), J. B. Lippincott, Philadelphia, pp. 3–13.
2. Junor, E. J., Hole, D. J., and Gillis, C. R. (1994) Management of ovarian cancer: referral to a multidiciplinary team matters. *Br. J. Cancer* **70,** 363–370.
3. Kartner, N., Riordan, J. R., and Ling, V. (1983) Cell surface P-glycoprotein associated with multidrug resistance in mammalian cell lines. *Science* **221,** 1285–1288.
4. Goldstein, L. J., Galski, H., Fojo, A., Willingham, M., Lai, S. L., Gazdar, A., Pirker, R., Green, A., Crist, W., Brodeur, G. M., Lieber, M., Cossman, J., Gottesman, M. M., and Pastan, I. (1989) Expression of multidrug resistance gene in human cancer. *J. Natl. Cancer Inst.* **81,** 116–124.
5. Campos, L., Guyotat, D., Archimbaud, E., Calmard-Oriol, P., Tsuruo, T., Troncy, J., Treille, D., and Fiere, D. (1992) Clinical significance of multidrug resistance P-glycoprotein expression on acute nonlymphoblastic leukaemic cells. *Blood* **79,** 473–476.
6. Ino, T., Miyazaki, H., Isogai, M., Nomura, T., Tsuzuki, M., Tsuruo, T., Ezaki, K., and Hirano, M. (1994) Expression of P-glycoprotein in de-novo acute myelogenous leukaemia at initial diagnosis: results of molecular and functional assays, and correlation with treatment outcome. *Leukaemia* **8,** 1492–1497.
7. Ludescher, C., Eisterer, W., Hilbe, W., Gotwald, M., Hofmann, J., Zabernigg, A., Cianfriglia, M., and Thaler, J. (1995) Low frequency of activity of P-glycoprotein (P-170) in acute lymphoblastic leukaemia compared to acute myeloid leukaemia. *Leukaemia* **9,** 350–356.
8. Goasguen, J. E., Dossot, J., Fardel, O., LeMee, F., LeGall, E., Leblay, R., LePrise, P. Y., Chaperon, J., and Fauchet, R. (1993) Expression of the multidrug resis-

tance-associated P-glycoprotein (P-170) in 59 cases of de novo acute lymphoblastic leukaemia: prognostic implications. *Blood* **81,** 2394–2398.

9. Savignano, C., Geromin, A., Michieli, M., Damiani, D., Michelutti, A., Melli, C., Fanin, R., and Baccarani, M. (1993) The expression of the multidrug resistance-related glycoprotein in adult acute lymphoblastic leukaemia. *Haematologica* **78,** 261–263.
10. Wattel, E., Leppelley, P., Merlat, A., Sartiaux, C., Bauters, F., Jouet, J. P., and Fenaux, P. (1995) Expression of the multidrug resistance P-glycoprotein in newly diagnosed adult acute lymphoblastic leukaemia: absence of correlation with response to treatment. *Leukaemia* **9,** 1870–1874.
11. Grogan, T. M., Spier, C. M., Salmon, S. E., Matzner, M., Rybski, J., Weinstein, R. S., Scheper, R. J., and Dalton, W. S. (1993) P-glycoprotein expression in human plasma cell myeloma: correlation with prior chemotherapy. *Blood* **81,** 490–495.
12. Trock, B. J., Leonessa, F., and Clarke, R. (1997) Multidrug resistance in breast cancer: Meta-analysis of MDR1/gp170 expression and its possible functional significance. *J. Natl. Cancer Inst.* **89,** 917–931.
13. Kaye, S. B. (1997) Multidrug resistance in breast cancer—is the jury in yet? *J. Natl. Cancer Inst.* **89,** 902,903.
14. Baldini, N., Scotlandi, K., Barbanti-Brodano, G., Manara, M. C., Maurici, D., Bacci, G., Bertoni, F., Picci, P., Sottili, S., Campanacci, M., and Serra, M. (1995) Expression of P-Glycoprotein in high-grade osteosarcomas in relation to clinical outcome. *N. Engl. J. Med.* **333,** 1380–1385.
15. Pinedo, H. M. and Giaccone, G. (1995) P-Glycoprotein—A marker of cancer-cell behavior. *N. Engl. J. Med.* **333,** 1417–1419.
16. Linn, S. C. and Giaccone, G. (1995) MDR1/P-glycoprotein expression in colorectal cancer. *Eur. J. Cancer* **31A,** 1291–1294.
17. Eid, H., Bodrogi, I., Csokay, B., Olah, E., and Bak, M. (1996) Multidrug resistance of testis cancer: the study of clinical relevance of P-glycoprotein expression. *Anticancer Res.* **16,** 3447–3452.
18. Oka, M., Fukuda, M., Sakamoto, A., Takatani, H., Soda, H., and Kohno, S. (1997) The clinical role of MDR1 gene expression in human lung cancer. *Anticancer Res.* **17,** 721–724.
19. Haak, H. R., van Seters, A. P., Moolenaar, A. J., and Fleuren, G. J. (1993) Expression of P-glycoprotein in relation to clinical manifestation, treatment and prognosis of adrenocortical cancer. *Eur. J. Cancer* **29A,** 1036–1038.
20. Cole, S. P. C., Bhardwaj, G., Gerlach, J. H., Mackie, J. E., Grant, C. E., Almquist, K. C., Stewart, A. J., Kurz, E. U., Duncan, A. M. V., and Deeley, R. G. (1992) Overexpression of a transporter gene in a multidrug-resistant human lung cancer cell line. *Science* **258,** 1650–1654.
21. Grant, C. E., Valdimarssan, G., Hipfner, D. R., Almquist, K. C., Cole, S. P. C., and Dudley, R. G. (1994) Overexpression of multidrug resistance-associated protein (MRP) increases resistance to natural product drugs. *Cancer Res.* **54,** 357–361.
22. Scheper, R. J., Broxterman, H. J., and Scheffer, G. L. (1995) Overexpression of a M(r) 110,000 vesicular protein in non-P-glycoprotein-mediated multidrug resistance. *Cancer Res.* **53,** 1475–1479.

23. Izquierdo, M. A., van der Zee, A. G. J., Vermorken, J. B., van der Valk, P., Belien, J. A. M., Giaccone, G., Scheffer, G. L., Flens, M. J., Pinedo, H. M., Kenemans, P., Meijer, C. J. L. M., de Vries, E. G. E., and Scheper, R. J. (1997) Drug resistance-associated marker Lrp for prediction of response to chemotherapy and prognoses in advanced ovarian carcinoma. *J. Natl. Cancer Inst.* **87,** 1230–1237.
24. Zhou, D., Zittoun, R., and Marie, J. (1995) Expression of multidrug resistance-associated protein (MRP) and multidrug resistance (MDR1) genes in acute myeloid leukaemia. *Leukaemia* **9,** 1661–1666.
25. Ota, E., Abe, Y., Oshika, Y., Ozeki, Y., Iwasaki, M., Inoue, M., Yamazaki, H., Ueyama, Y., Takazi, K., Ogata, T., Tamaoki, N., and Nakamura, M. (1995) Expression of the multidrug resistance-related protein (MRP) gene in non-small cell lung cancer. *Br. J. Cancer* **72,** 550–554.
26. Endo, K., Maehara, Y., Ichiyoshi, Y., Kusumoto, T., Sakaguchi, Y., Ohno, S., and Sugimachi, K. (1996) Multidrug resistance-associated protein expression in clinical gastric carcinoma. *Cancer* **77,** 1681–1687.
27. Uozaki, H., Horiuchi, H., Ishida, T., Lijima, T., Imamura, T., and Machinami, R. (1997) Overexpression of resistance-related proteins (metallothioneins, glutathione-S-transferase, heat shock protein 27, and lung resistance-related protein) in osteosarcoma. *Cancer* **79,** 2336–2344.
28. Green, J. A., Robertson, L. J., and Clark, A. H. (1993) Glutathione-S-transferase expression in benign and malignant ovarian tumours. *Br. J. Cancer* **68,** 235–239.
29. Hamada, S., Kamada, M., Furumoto, H., Hirao, T., and Aono, T. (1994) Expression of glutathione S-transferase pi in human ovarian cancer as an indicator of resistance to chemotherapy. *Gynecol. Oncol.* **52,** 313–319.
30. Tanner, B., Hengstler, J. G., Dietrich, B., Henrich, M., Steinberg, P., Weikel, W., Meinert, R., Kaina, B., Oesch, F., and Knapstein, P. G. (1997) Glutathione, glutathione-S-transferase alpha and pi, and aldehyde dehydrogenase content in relationship to drug resistance in ovarian cancer. *Gynecol. Oncol.* **65,** 54–62.
31. van der Zee, A. G. J., Hollema, H., Suurmeijer, A. J. H., Krans, M., Sluiter, W. J., Willemse, P. H. B., Aadlers, J. G., and de Vries, E. G. E. (1995) Value of P-glycoprotein, glutathione-S-transferase ppi, c-erbB-2, and p53 as prognostic factors in ovarian carcinomas. *J. Clin. Oncol.* **13,** 70–78.
32. Kim, W. J., Kakehi, Y., Wu, W. J., Fukumoto, M., and Yoshida, O. (1996) Expression of multidrug resistance-related genes (mdr1, MRP, GST-pi and DNA topoisomerase II) in urothelial cancers. *Br. J. Urol.* **78,** 361–368.
33. Mulder, T. P., Manni, J. J., Roelofs, H. M., Peters, W. H., and Wiersma, A. (1995) Glutathione S-transferases and glutathione in human head and neck cancer. *Carcinogenesis* **16,** 619–624.
34. Eissa, S., Khalifa, A., el-Gharib, A., Salah, N., and Mohamed, N. K. (1997) Multivariate analysis of DNA ploidy, p53, c-erbB-2 proteins, EGFR, and steroid hormone receptors for prediction of poor short term prognosis in breast cancer. *Anticancer Res.* **17,** 1417–1423.
35. Lacombe, L., Dalbagni, G., Zhang, Z., Cardon-Cordo, C., Fair, W. R., Herr, H. W., and Reuter, V. E. (1996) Overexpression of p53 protein in a high risk popula-

tion of patients with superficial bladder cancer before and after bacillus Calmette-Guerin therapy: correlation to clinical outcome. *J. Clin. Oncol.* **14,** 2646–2652.
36. Righetti, S. C., Torre, G. D., Pilotti, S., Menard, S., Ottone, F., Colnaghi, M. I., Pierotti, M. A., Lavarino, C., Cornarotti, M., Oriana, S., Bohm, S., Bresciani, G. L., Spatti, G., and Zunino, F. (1996) a comparative study of p53 gene mutations, protein accumulation and response to cisplatin-based chemotherapy in advanced ovarian carcinoma. *Cancer Res.* **56,** 689–693.
37. Hartmann, L. C., Podratz, K. C., Keeney, G. L., Kamel, N. A., Edmonson, J. H., Grill, J. P., Su, J. Q., Katzmann, J. A., and Roche, P. C. (1994) Prognostic significance of p53 immunostaining in epithelial ovarian cancer. *J. Clin. Oncol.* **12,** 64–69.
38. Levesque, M. A., Katsaros, D., Yu, H., Zola, P., Sismondi, P., Giardina, G., and Diamandis, E. P. (1995) Mutant p53 protein overexpression is associated with poor outcome in patients with well or moderately differentiated ovarian carcinoma. *Cancer* **75,** 1327,1328.
39. Dabholkar, M., Bostick-Bruton, F., Weber, C., Bohr, V. A., Egwuagu, C., and Reed, E. (1992) ERCC1 and ERCC2 expression in malignant tissues from ovarian cancer patients. *J. Natl. Cancer Inst.* **84,** 1512–1517.
40. Yu, J. J., Dabholkar, M., Bennett, W. P., Welsh, J. A., Mu, C. J., Bostick-Bruton, F., and Reed, E. (1996) Platinum-sensitive and platinum-resistant ovarian cancer tissues show differences in the relationships between m-RNA levels of p53, ERCC1 and XPA. *Intl. J. Cancer* **8,** 313–317.
41. Diebold, J., Baretton, G., Felchner, M., Meier, W., Dopfer, K., Schmidt, M., and Lohrs, U. (1996) bcl-2 expression, p53 accumulation, and apoptosis in ovarian carcinomas. *Am. J. Clin. Pathol.* **105,** 341–349.
42. Herod, J. J. O., Eliopoulos, A. G., Warwick, J., Neidobiteck, G., Young, L. S., and Kerr, D. J. (1996) The prognostic significance of Bcl-2 and p53 expression in ovarian carcinoma. *Cancer Res.* **56,** 2178–2184.
43. Philip, T., Guglielmi, C., Hagenbeek, A., Somers, R., van der Lelie, H., and Bron, D. (1995) Autologous bone marrow transplantation as compared with salvage chemotherapy in relapses of chemotherapy-sensitive Non-Hodgkin's lymphoma. *N. Engl. J. Med.* **333,** 1540–1545.
44. Mills, W., Chopra, R., McMillan, A., Pearce, R., Linch, D. C., and Goldstone, A. H. (1995) BEAM chemotherapy and autologous bone marrow transplantation for patients with relapsed or refractory Non-Hodgkin's lymphoma. *J. Clin. Oncol.* **13,** 588–595.
45. Eddy, D. M. (1992) High-dose chemotherapy with autologous bone marrow transplantation for the treatment of metastatic breast cancer. *J. Clin. Oncol.* **10,** 657–670.
46. Bezwoda, W. R., Seymour, L., and Dansey, R. D. (1995) High-dose chemotherapy with hematopoietic rescue as primary treatment for metastatic breast cancer: a randomised trial. *J. Clin. Oncol.* **13,** 2483–2489.
47. Hornedo, J. and Cortes-Funes, H. (1996) The role of high dose chemotherapy in adult solid tumours other than breast cancer. *Ann. Oncol.* **7,** 23–30.
48. Raederer, M. and Scheithauer, W. (1993) Clinical trials of agents that reverse multidrug resistance—a literature review. *Cancer* **72,** 3553–3563.

49. Sikic, B. I. (1993) Modulation of MDR: at the threshold. *J. Clin. Oncol.* **11,** 1629–1635.
50. Miller, T. P., Grogan, T. M., Dalton, W. S., Spier, C. M., Scheper, R. J., and Salmon, S. E. (1991) P-glycoprotein expression in malignant lymphomas and reversal of clinical drug resistance with chemotherapy plus high-dose verapamil. *J. Clin. Oncol.* **9,** 17–24.
51. Sonneveld, P., Durie, B. G. M., Lokhorst, H. M., Marie, J. P., Solbu, G., Suciu, S., Zittoun, R., Lowenberg, B., and Nooter, K. (1992) Modulation of multidrug-resistant multiple myeloma by cyclosporin. *Lancet* **340,** 255–259.
52. McLeod, H. L. (1994) Clinical reversal of the MDR phenotype: true tumour modulation or pharmacokinetic interaction? *Eur. J. Cancer* **30A,** 2039–2041.
53. Dantzig, A. H., Shepard, R. L., Cao, J., Law, K. L., Ehlhardt, W. J., Baughman, T. M., Bumol, T. F., and Starling, J. J. (1996) Reversal of P-glycoprotein-mediated multidrug resistance by a potent cyclopropyldibenzosuberane modulator, LY335979. *Cancer Res.* **56,** 4171–4179.
54. Beck, W. T., Grogan, T. M., Willman, C. L., Cardon-Cordo, C., Parham, D. M., Kuttesch, J. F., Andreeff, M., Bates, S. E., and Berard, C. W. (1996) Methods to detect P-glycoprotein-associated multidrug resistance in patients' tumours: consensus recommendations. *Cancer Res.* **56,** 3010–3020.

2

Cell Sensitivity Assays

Clonogenic Assay

Jane A. Plumb

1. Introduction

The use of cell culture systems to assess the toxicity of anticancer agents began over 50 years ago following the observation of the antineoplastic effects of nitrogen mustard *(1)*. There are a wide variety of assays designed to evaluate cellular drug sensitivity described in the literature. These assays essentially fall into two groups; those that measure cell survival and those that measure cytotoxicity. Cytotoxicity assays include methods such as trypan blue dye exclusion, ^{51}Cr release and ^{3}H-thymidine incorporation *(2–4)* and these assays assess the structural integrity and metabolic function of the cells following drug exposure. In contrast, cell survival assays measure the end result of these effects on the cell which can be either cell death or recovery. A cell survival assay thus requires a measure of the ability of cells to proliferate and this is usually an estimate of the ability of individual cells to form colonies. However, cytotoxicity assays can also measure the ability of cells to proliferate if the cells are allowed a period of growth following drug exposure. This recovery time is comparable to the time taken for formation of colonies in a clonogenic assay.

Clonogenic assays are commonly regarded as the "gold standard" cellular sensitivity assay. This idea originates from the early 1960s when radiobiologists were comparing the radiosensitivities of tumour cell lines in vitro. This involved estimation of multiple logs of cell kill and it was thought that only a clonogenic assay would have sufficient sensitivity to be able to assess cell kill at low percentage survivals (<1%). However, the results obtained with a cell growth assay were similar to those obtained with a clonogenic assay *(5)*. Nevertheless, the

From: *Methods in Molecular Medicine, Vol. 28: Cytotoxic Drug Resistance Mechanisms*
Edited by: R. Brown and U. Böger-Brown © Humana Press Inc., Totowa, NJ

clonogenic assay has retained its superior status *(6)*. Many factors influence cellular drug sensitivity and no one assay can take account of all these variables.

The human tumour stem cell assay has been widely used in attempts to predict the response of tumors to chemotherapeutic agents *(7)*. In order to distinguish between normal and tumour cells present within a biopsy the assay measures the ability of cells to undergo substrate independent proliferation in agar. Overall, the ability of the assay to predict treatment response is good but only about 30% of biopsies processed resulted in sufficient colony numbers to allow evaluation *(8)*. This is a major problem with the assay and many human tumour cell lines show a very poor cloning efficiency in agar (<1%) whereas the cloning efficiency on tissue culture treated plastic can be greater than 50%. The clonogenic assay described is based on monolayer cloning which is widely applicable to continuous cell lines.

In the standard clonogenic assay cells in the exponential phase of growth are exposed to a cytotoxic drug. The drug exposure time depends on a number of factors. If the drug is cell cycle specific (i.e., specific for cycling as opposed to noncycling cells) a short exposure may be sufficient and this can be related to the estimated duration of exposure in the clinic. In contrast, if the drug is phase specific it may be necessary to extend the exposure period to the take account of the cell doubling time. Cells are normally exposed to drug in the exponential phase of growth since the majority of cytotoxic drugs are active against cycling cells. However, the assay can be used equally well with confluent noncycling cells provided that they will re-enter the cell cycle on subculture. Following drug exposure the cells are disaggregated to form a single cell suspension and are plated out at low density to allow colony formation. The colonies are fixed, stained and counted. Each colony is assumed to be derived from a single cell and thus the colony count is an estimate of the number of cells that survived the drug treatment.

The number of cells within each colony depends on the number of cell doublings and can be used as an estimate of the effects, if any, of the drug on the cell doubling time. A clonogenic assay can thus discriminate between cytotoxic (cell kill) and cytostatic (decreased growth rate) effects. Because a cytostatic effect may be lost upon removal of the drug a cytotoxicity assay based on colony formation is also described since this allows continuous drug exposure.

2. Materials

1. Petri dishes (6 cm, tissue-culture grade).
2. Tissue-culture flasks (25 cm^2).
3. Universal containers (30 mL).
4. Plastic box.
5. Wash bottles.

6. Growth medium.
7. Phosphate buffered saline (PBS, Dulbecco's A).
8. 0.25% Trypsin in PBS.
9. Methanol.
10. 1% Crystal Violet in water (Merck).

3. Methods

3.1. A Standard Clonogenic Assay

1. Trypsinise a sub-confluent monolayer culture and collect cells in growth medium containing serum. Centrifuge the suspension (200*g*, 5 min) to pellet cells and resuspend in fresh growth medium. Use a haemocytometer to count the cells and ensure that a single cell suspension is obtained (*see* **Note 1**). Dilute cells to a density of 8×10^4 cells/mL (*see* **Note 2**) in a total volume of 10 mL. Add 4 mL of culture medium to each of 9 tissue culture flasks (25 cm^2) and transfer 1 mL of the cell suspension to each flask (*see* **Note 3**). Equilibrate with CO_2 and incubate cells at 37°C for 2–3 d such that cells are in the exponential phase of growth for drug addition.
2. Prepare a serial five-fold dilution of the cytotoxic drug in growth medium to give eight concentrations (*see* **Note 4**). Pipet 6 mL of growth medium in to each of seven universal containers (30 mL). Prepare 10 mL of the highest concentration of the drug and transfer 1.5 mL of this solution to the first universal container. Mix and then transfer 1.5 mL to the next universal. Continue until the seventh universal is reached. The concentrations should be chosen such that the highest concentration kills most of the cells and the lowest kills none of the cells (*see* **Note 5**).
3. Label the nine flasks with one for each of the eight drug concentrations and one as a control. Remove the medium from the flasks of cells. Add 5 mL of growth medium to the control flask and 5 mL of the appropriate drug solution to the other eight. Equilibrate the flasks with CO_2 and incubate at 37°C for 24 h (*see* **Note 6**).
4. Remove the medium from the nine flasks, add 1 mL of trypsin solution and incubate at 37°C. While waiting for the cells to detach, label the Petri dishes on the side of the base (*see* **Note 7**). Use three dishes for the control and for each drug concentration. When the cells have detached add 4 mL of growth medium to each flask. Disperse the cells by repeat pipeting to give a single cell suspension and transfer the flask contents to a universal container (30 mL). Count the cells from the control flask only and dilute to give a density of 10^3 cells/mL and a total volume of 4 mL (*see* **Note 8**). Follow exactly the same dilution steps for the cell suspensions from each of the drug treated flasks (*see* **Note 9**). Transfer 1 mL of the control cell suspension to each of the three labeled Petri dishes. Repeat for each of the drug treatments. Finally, add 4 mL of growth medium to each Petri dish (*see* **Note 10**). Place the Petri dishes in a plastic box and incubate for 10 days in a humidified atmosphere at 37°C (*see* **Note 11**).

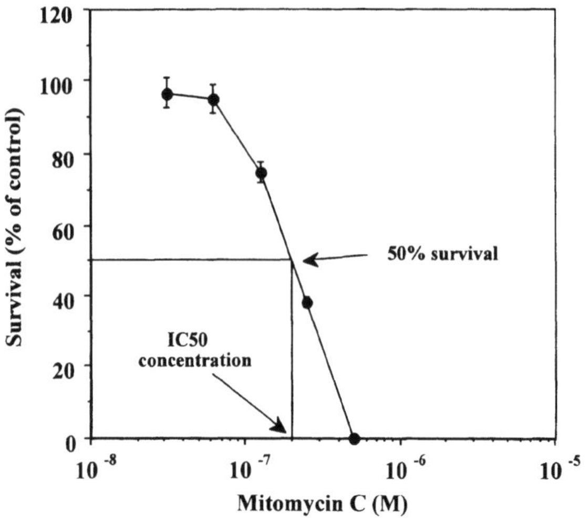

Fig. 1. A typical dose response curve obtained by clonogenic assay. The human colon tumor cell line HT29 in exponential growth was exposed to mitomycin C for 3 h and then plated out at a density of 500 cells/6 cm Petri dish. The mean colony count in the control dishes was 281, which is a cloning efficiency of 56%. Three flasks of cells were used at each dose level and each point is the mean ± standard error of the mean of the three estimates. Estimation of the IC_{50} value (the drug concentration required to kill 50% of the cells) is shown by the straight lines.

4. Fill a wash bottle with PBS and a second with methanol. Remove and discard the lids from the Petri dishes. Pour the medium from the Petri dish into a container for disposal and carefully add about 5 mL of PBS to wash off the remaining medium. Pour off the PBS and add about 5 mL of methanol and leave for 5 min. Repeat for all dishes. After 5 min pour off the methanol and add another 5 mL of methanol to each dish and leave for 5 min. Pour off the methanol and allow dishes to dry.
5. Add 5 mL of crystal violet to each Petri dish and leave for 5 min. Pour off the stain and rinse the dish under running tap water to remove excess dye. Invert dishes and leave to dry.
6. Count the colonies in each Petri dish (*see* **Note 12**). If the drug has a cytostatic effect this will be seen as a reduction in the size of the colonies and should be apparent to the naked eye. In this case, as well as counting the total number of colonies per dish, the number of cells per colony should also be counted (*see* **Note 13**).
7. Calculate the mean colony count for each of the treatments. Divide the number of colonies in the drug treated dishes by the number of colonies in the control dishes and express as a percentage. Plot a graph of percent survival (y axis) against drug concentration (x axis). Results are usually expressed as the IC_{50} value which is the drug concentration required to kill 50% of the cells or as in this assay to reduce the number of colonies to 50% of that in the control untreated dishes (*see* **Fig. 1**). Values for the IC_{10} and IC_{90} can be determined in the same manner. The

shape of the survival curve depends on a number of factors. For a cycle specific drug and a homogeneous cell population the curve can be very steep such that only a small increment of drug is required to go from 0–100% cell kill. Sometimes a tail is seen on the curve such that cell kill does not reach 100% even at high drug concentrations. This can be due to the presence of a resistant subpopulation. It can also occur when a phase specific drug, such as camptothecin, is used and the duration of drug exposure is less than the cell doubling time. In this case the tail should not be apparent if the drug exposure time is increased.

3.2. A Cytotoxicity Assay Based on Colony Formation

1. Trypsinise a sub-confluent monolayer culture and collect cells in growth medium containing serum. Centrifuge the suspension (200*g*, 5 min) to pellet cells, resuspend in growth medium and count cells. Dilute cells to a density of 10^3 cells/mL (*see* **Note 7**). Label Petri dishes (6 cm), allowing three per treatment, and add 1 mL of cell suspension to each dish. Add 3 mL of medium to the dishes and place in a plastic box. Incubate in a humidified atmosphere at 37°C for 4 h to allow cell to adhere (*see* **Note 14**).
2. Prepare a range of concentrations of the cytotoxic drug in growth medium (*see* **Notes 4** and **5**). The drug is diluted five-fold when added to the Petri dishes, so these solutions should be prepared at five times the required final concentration.
3. Add 1 mL of the drug solution to the 4 mL of medium in each of the three Petri dishes. Incubate for 10 d in an humidified atmosphere at 37°C (*see* **Notes 11** and **15**).
4. Fix and stain the colonies and evaluate as for the standard clonogenic assay.

4. Notes

1. It is essential that a single cell suspension is plated out and it may be necessary to adjust the trypsin concentration or duration of exposure to achieve this.
2. A density of 8×10^4 cells/25cm^2 culture flask is a suggested density for cells with a doubling time of about 24 h and a plating efficiency of around 60%. Clearly the density may need to be increased or decreased depending on the cell line used. The aim is to obtain a sub-confluent culture of cells in the exponential phase of growth for drug treatment.
3. An experimental design based on one control and eight drug treatments is a suggested starting point and it should be noted that this does not include replicates. The number of flasks that can be set up in one experiment is limited by the time required to carry out **step 4**.
4. The drug solution should be prepared just before use and should be sterile. Many cytotoxic drug are insoluble in water. Any diluent used to solubilize the drug should be included as a separate control, usually at the highest concentration to be used. DMSO can be used and since this is self sterile it avoids possible loss of drug owing to binding to the filter. Most cells will tolerate up to 1% DMSO in culture medium.
5. If the cytotoxicity of the drug is not known a serial dilution with a starting concentration of 10^{-5} *M* can be used. Once the cytotoxicity is known the drug concentration range can be reduced to cover the area of interest.

6. The drug exposure period can be varied. As a rule cytotoxicity increases with increasing drug exposure. The most marked effects are seen during the first 24 h and sensitivity usually shows a plateau by 72 h. Factors to take into account are the mechanism of action of the drug such that if it is S-phase specific the exposure period should allow for all cells to have passed through S-phase. The stability of the drug in culture medium should also be taken in to account. For drug exposure periods of greater than 24 h, it is recommended that the drug is replaced at 24 h intervals.
7. Do not label the lids, because these are removed when the colonies are fixed. Make sure that the marker pen used is resistant to methanol.
8. Accuracy of the dilution is important and it is recommended that individual dilution steps are no greater than 1 in 10 and that the volume of cell suspension used is greater than 200 µL. A density of 10^3 cells/mL is a suggested density assuming a plating efficiency for the cell line of about 50%. This would give 500 colonies in the control dishes. The aim is to retain separated colonies in the control dishes at the end of the experiment but to still have a sufficient number of colonies in the drug treated dishes to allow accurate estimation of survival at the higher drug concentrations. It is possible to compensate for the low survival at higher drug concentrations by increasing the number of cells plated out for these concentrations. To do this either increase the volume of cell suspension used or reduce the dilution factor.
9. It is not necessary to count the cells in the drug treated flasks because all flasks contained the same number of cells at the start of the experiment. Any difference in cell counts between the flasks at this stage is due to the effects of the drug and is thus part of the experiment. Remember to resuspend the cells well before diluting.
10. Care must be taken to ensure an even distribution of cells in the Petri dish. This is achieved if the cells are added first and then the bulk of the medium added. Do not be tempted to swirl the dishes to mix the cells because this results in the cells accumulating in the centre of the dish and forming one large colony.
11. The incubation time will vary depending on the doubling time of the cell line used but is usually between 8–12 d. This allows for about 10 doubling times. It is advisable to check the dishes after about 8 d and colonies should be clearly visible to the naked eye.
12. Following drug treatment some cells will plate and undergo a few cell divisions before the damage is expressed. This leads to the formation of small colonies that fail to develop further. These cells are not viable and the colonies should not be counted. This is usually avoided by limiting the counts to those colonies that have undergone more that five cell doublings, i.e., those containing more than 50 cells.
13. A cytostatic effect will result in a reduction in the number of cell doublings in a given time and thus a reduction in the number of cells within a colony. There are several ways of quantifying a cytostatic effect. The most direct method is to count the number of cells in 50 representative colonies per dish. Alternatively, it can be estimated by measuring the diameter of the colony and thus calculating the area of the colony. This method assumes that there is no change in cell size.

14. For most continuous cell lines, 4 h is sufficient for adherence to plastic. The time can be increased, but it should not exceed the doubling time for the cell line because the assay relies on colonies originating from single cells. In some protocols the cells and drug are added together. The disadvantage of this approach is that the drug may have an effect *per se* on the plating of the cells separate from effects on cell survival.
15. This assay protocol is best suited to continuous drug exposure but it is possible to limit the drug exposure time by replacing the medium. However, as explained in **Note 14** the total time for plating and drug exposure should not exceed the doubling time for the cell line.

References

1. Dendy, P. P. and Hill, B. T. (1983) *Human Tumour Drug Sensitivity Testing in Vitro: Techniques and Clinical Applications.* Academic, London.
2. Wilson, A. P., Ford, C. H. J., Newman, C. E., and Howell, A. (1984) A comparison of three assays used for the in vitro chemosensitivity testing of human tumours. *Br. J. Cancer* **49,** 57–63.
3. Weisenthal, L. M. (1981) In vitro assays in preclinical antineoplastic drug screening. *Seminars Oncol.* **8,** 362–376.
4. Weisenthal, L. M., Dill, P. L., Kurnick, N. B., and Lippman, M. E. (1983) Comparison of dye exclusion assays with a clonogenic assay in the determination of drug-induced cytotoxicity. *Cancer Res.* **43,** 258–264.
5. Nias, A. H. W. and Fox, M. (1968) Minimum clone size for estimating normal reproductive activity of cultured cells. *Br. J. Radiol.* **41,** 468–474.
6. Weisenthal, L. M. and Lippman, M. E. (1985) Clonogenic and nonclonogenic in vitro chemosensitivity assays. *Cancer Treat. Rep.* **69,** 615–632.
7. Salmon, S. E. (1980) *Cloning of Human Tumour Stem Cells.* Liss, New York, NY.
8. Von Hoff, D. D. (1990) He's not going to talk about in vitro predictive assays again, is he? *J. Natl. Cancer Inst.* **82,** 96–101.

3

Cell Sensitivity Assays

The MTT Assay

Jane A. Plumb

1. Introduction

The clonogenic assay described in Chapter 2 is not suitable for all cell lines. Many adherent cell lines do not form colonies and clearly it is not applicable to non-adherent cell lines. Furthermore, it is slow and time consuming. This chapter describes an alternative cytotoxicity assay that has a number of advantages when compared with a clonogenic assay. It is quick and easy and allows a large number of assays to be carried out in one batch. This is an important consideration when making comparisons between cell lines, between cytotoxic agents, or when evaluating combinations of drugs. No one cytotoxicity assay is ideal and it is always advisable to support results with those from alternative assays where possible.

Cytotoxicity assays are widely used particularly in the field of new drug development. Clonogenic assays are not amenable to automation and centers such as the American National Cancer Institute and the Pharmaceutical Industry have developed rapid throughput microtitration assays to use as a screen for new cytotoxic agents. These assays measure the effect of a drug on the growth of a population of cells and the endpoint is an estimate of cell number. Use of a tetrazolium dye (MTT) as an indirect measure of cell number was first reported in the early eighties *(1)*. The NCI evaluated MTT-dye reduction as a possible endpoint in a rapid screening assay *(2)* and this stimulated interest in the wider scientific community. At that time a major limitation of microtiter assays was that the endpoint tended to involve the use of a radioisotope.

Cells in exponential phase of growth are exposed to a cytotoxic drug. The duration of exposure is usually determined as the time required for maximal

From: *Methods in Molecular Medicine, Vol. 28: Cytotoxic Drug Resistance Mechanisms*
Edited by: R. Brown and U. Böger-Brown © Humana Press Inc., Totowa, NJ

damage to occur but is also influenced by the stability of the drug. After removal of drug the cells are allowed to proliferate for two to three doubling times in order to distinguish between cells which remain viable and are capable of proliferation and those which remain viable but cannot proliferate. Surviving cell numbers are then determined indirectly by MTT dye reduction. MTT is a yellow water soluble tetrazolium dye that is reduced by live but not dead cells *(3)* to a purple formazan product that is insoluble in aqueous solutions. The amount of MTT-formazan produced can be determined spectrophotometrically once solubilized in a suitable solvent. A drawback of the assay is that it does not *per se* distinguish between a cytotoxic (cell kill) and a cytostatic (reduced growth rate) effect. However, it should be noted that cytostatic effects are not usually seen with cytotoxic drugs.

There is no such thing as "The MTT assay." Many laboratories use cytotoxicity assays that are based on MTT dye reduction but the assay protocols differ markedly. Many factors affect the reduction of MTT. The cells require an adequate energy supply from the culture medium and reduction is inhibited by some cytotoxic drugs. For these reasons the NCI chose not to use MTT reduction in their screening assay *(4)*. The assay described here has been optimized such that it has been shown to give the same results as are obtained with a standard clonogenic assay *(5)*. An important feature of the assay is the inclusion of a growth period after removal of the drug. This allows cells to recover from the effects of the drug, or to die, and also avoids possible interference of drug in the reduction of MTT.

2. Materials

1. Microtiter plates (Corning).
2. Multichannel pipette (Costar).
3. Tip box, autoclavable (ICN Flow).
4. Pipette tips (ICN-Flow).
5. Hypodermic needles (18G, 24G).
6. Petri dishes, 5 cm and 10 cm (Sterilin).
7. Universal containers, 30 mL and 100 mL (Sterilin).
8. Plastic box.
9. Growth medium.
10. Phosphate buffered saline (PBS, Dulbecco's A).
11. 0.25% Trypsin, 1 m*M* EDTA in PBS.
12. 3-(4,5-dimethylthiazol-2-yl)-2,5-diphenyltetrazolium bromide (MTT, Sigma) prepared at a concentration of 5 mg/mL in PBS. This is filter-sterilized, which also removes any reduced MTT, and can be stored at 4°C in the dark for 1 mo.
13 Sorensen's glycine buffer : 0.1 *M* glycine, 0.1 *M* NaCl adjusted to pH 10.5 with 1 *M* NaOH.
14. Dimethysulphoxide (DMSO).

15. ELISA plate reader (Molecular Devices).
16. Plate carriers for centrifuge (for nonadherent cell lines).

3. Methods

3.1. Adherent Cell Lines

1. Trypsinise a sub-confluent monolayer culture and collect cells in growth medium containing serum. Centrifuge the suspension (200*g*, 5 min) to pellet cells, resuspend in growth medium and count cells. Dilute cells to a density of 5×10^3 cells/mL (*see* **Note 1**) allowing 60 mL of cell suspension for 3 microtiter plates. Transfer cell suspension to a 10 cm Petri dish and with a multichannel pipet add 200 µL to each well of the central 10 columns of a flat bottomed 96-well plate (80 wells/plate) starting with column 2 and ending with column 11 (*see* **Note 2**). Add 200 µL of growth medium to the eight wells in columns 1 and 12. Put plates in a plastic box and incubate in a humidified atmosphere at 37°C for 2–3 d such that cells are in the exponential phase of growth for drug addition.
2. Prepare a serial five-fold dilution of the cytotoxic drug in growth medium to give eight concentrations (*see* **Note 3**). Pipet 6 mL of growth medium in to each of seven universal containers (30 mL). Prepare 10 mL of the highest concentration of the drug and transfer 1.5 mL of this solution to the first universal container. Mix and then transfer 1.5 mL to the next universal. Continue until the seventh universal is reached. The concentrations should be chosen such that the highest concentration kills most of the cells and the lowest kills none of the cells (*see* **Note 4**). Normally, three plates are used for each drug to give triplicate determinations within one experiment.
3. The medium is removed from all the wells in columns 2–11. This can be achieved with a hypodermic needle attached to a suction line. The cells in the eight wells in columns 2 and 11 are fed with 200 µL of fresh growth medium. The drug solutions are transferred to 10 cm Petri dishes and 200 µL added to all eight wells of a column. For ease of analysis, arrange the drug solutions in order so that the highest is in column 3 down to the lowest in column 10. Plates are returned to the plastic box and incubated for 24 h (*see* **Note 5**).
4. At the end of the drug-exposure period the medium is removed from all wells containing cells and the cells fed with 200 µL of fresh medium.
5. Plates are fed daily for two more days.
6. Plates are fed with 200 µL of fresh medium and 50 µL of the MTT solution (5 mg/mL in PBS) is added to all wells in columns 1 to 11. Plates are wrapped in aluminium foil and incubated for 4 h in a humidified atmosphere at 37°C (*see* **Note 6**).
7. The medium and MTT are then removed from the wells and the purple MTT-formazan crystals dissolved by addition of 200 µL of DMSO to all wells in columns 1 to 11 (*see* **Note 7**). Glycine buffer is added (25 µL/well) to all wells containing DMSO (*see* **Note 8**).
8. Absorbance is recorded at 570 nm with the wells in column 1, which contained medium, MTT but no cells used as a blank.

9. A graph is plotted of absorbance (y axis) against drug concentration (x axis). The mean absorbance reading from the wells in columns 2 and 11 is used as the control absorbance and the IC_{50} concentration is determined as the drug concentration required to reduce the absorbance to half that of the control. IC_{10} or IC_{90} values can be determined in the same manner (*see* **Note 9**).

3.2. Nonadherent Cells

1. Prepare a cell suspension in fresh growth medium from a flask of cells in exponential growth and count cells. Dilute cells to density of 10^4 cells /mL (*see* **Note 1**) allowing 30 mL of cell suspension for 3 plates. Transfer the cell suspension to a 10 cm Petri dish and with a multichannel pipet add 100 µL to the central 10 columns of a round bottomed microtitre plate. Add 200 µL of growth medium to the wells in columns 1 and 12. Put plates in a plastic box and incubate in a humidified atmosphere at 37°C while drug solutions are prepared.
2. Eight drug dilutions are prepared essentially as for adherent cells except that the solutions are prepared at twice the desired final concentration.
3. Growth medium (100 µL) is added to the wells in columns 2 and 11. The drug solutions are added as for the adherent cells but only 100 µL is added to the 100 µL of cells already in the wells. Plates are placed in the plastic box and incubated for 24 h.
4. Plates are centrifuged (200*g*, 5 min) to pellet cells before removal of the medium and a fine gauge needle (24G) is used to prevent removal of the cell pellet. Cells are fed with 200 µL of growth medium.
5. Plates are processed as for the adherent cells except that they are centrifuged each time the medium is removed.

4. Notes

1. A cell density of 10^3 cells/well is suggested as a starting point and is usually suitable for cell lines with a doubling time of around 24 h. The aim is for the cells to remain in exponential growth throughout the assay. If cells in the control wells (i.e., those not exposed to drug) become confluent they will stop dividing whilst the drug treated cells will continue growth. As a result, drug sensitivity will be underestimated since the control absorbance will be lower than it should be. The initial cell density can range between 5×10^2 to 10^4 cells/well depending on the cell line. An easy way to determine the optimum density is to plate out cells at a range of densities in a microtiter plate and feed daily for the duration of the assay. Incubate the plates with MTT and select the density that gives an absorbance value of around 1. Remember to prepare a cell suspension at five times the density required per well since only 200 µL is added to the well (10 times for non-adherent cells).
2. Microtiter plates vary in their overall plating efficiency and in the variablity of plating between wells. The assay requires that all wells are replicates and the choice of plates is therefore a compromise between the optimum overall plating efficiency and the reproducibility between wells. A detailed statistical evaluation of microtitre plates showed Corning to be suitable. Furthermore, these plates do not demonstrate the so called "edge effect" where plating is noticeably reduced

in the outer wells. Cells are not plated in columns 1 and 12 because these are used as a blank for the plate reader to allow for the absorbance of the residual medium and MTT in the wells.

3. The drug solution should be prepared just before use and should be sterile. Many cytotoxic drug are insoluble in water. Any diluent used to solubilize the drug should be included as a separate control, usually at the highest concentration to be used, and added in medium to the cells in column 11. DMSO can be used and since this is self sterile it avoids possible loss of drug due to binding to the filter. Most cells will tolerate up to 1% DMSO in culture medium.
4. If the cytotoxicity of the drug is not known a serial dilution with a starting concentration of 10^{-5} *M* can be used. Once the cytotoxicity is known the drug concentration range can be reduced to cover the area of interest.
5. The drug exposure period can be varied. As a rule, cytotoxicity increases with increasing drug exposure. The most marked effects are seen during the first 24 h and sensitivity usually shows a plateau by 72 h. Factors to take in to account are the mechanism of action of the drug such that if it is S-phase specific the exposure period should allow for all cells to have passed through S-phase. The stability of the drug in culture medium should also be taken in to account. For drug-exposure periods of greater than 24 h it is recommended that the drug is replaced at 24 h intervals. Regardless of the drug exposure period the cells must be allowed to undergo two to three cell doubling times after removal of the drug.

   It is not necessary to use eight wells for each drug concentration. Reproducible results can be obtained from 4 wells/concentration and it is practical to divide the plate such that one drug is used in rows A–D and a second in rows E–H.
6. MTT supplied by Sigma has a variable amount of the reduced formazan present. This is insoluble in PBS and can be filtered out when the solution is prepared. The solution can be stored, but if it is not sterile or is exposed to light the MTT will undergo reduction. Check that the solution is bright yellow and if not refilter. Plates are wrapped in foil to minimize the reduction of MTT by light. The 4-h incubation period is the time required for maximal MTT reduction. For convenience plates can be incubated for up to 6 h without loss of accuracy.
7. DMSO can damage some multichannel pipets. Costar pipettes are essentially resistant, but DMSO should still be dispensed with caution.
8. MTT reduction is used to estimate cell numbers at the end of the assay. The validity of the endpoint depends on a linear relationship between MTT reduction and cell number. The absorption spectrum of MTT-formazan is pH dependent and the pH of the MTT-formazan solution in DMSO depends on the cell density in the well. Glycine buffer is added to shift the pH of all wells to pH 10.5. At this pH the spectrum shows a single peak with an absorption maximum at about 570 nm. In contrast, at pH 7 the spectrum shows two absorption maxima, at 500 nm and 570 nm and measurement at a single wavelength underestimated the amount of MTT-formazan present.

9. Microtiter plate readers were developed for ELISA techniques and this is reflected in the computer software available. The Molecular Devices reader is recommended since the software (Softmax™) was developed for diverse applications and contains a curve fitting facility that is ideal for analysis of survival curves.

References

1. Mosman, T. (1983) Rapid colorimetric assay for cellular growth and survival: application to proliferation and cytotoxicity assays. *J. Immunol. Methods* **65,** 55–63.
2. Alley, M. C., Scudiero, D. A., Monks, A., Hursey, M. L., Czerwinski, M. J., Fine, D. L., Abbott, B. J., Mayo, J. G., Shoemaker, R. H., and Boyd, M. R. (1988) Feasibility of drug screening with panels of human tumour cell lines using a microculture tetrazolium assay. *Cancer Res.* **48,** 589–601.
3. Liu, Y., Peterson, D. A., Kimura, H., and Schubert, D. (1997) Mechanism of cellular 3-(4,5-dimethylthiazol-2-yl)-2,5-diphenyltetrazolium bromide (MTT) reduction. *J. Neurochem.* **69,** 581–593.
4. Vistica, D. T., Skehan, P., Scudiero, D., Monks, A., Pittman, A., and Boyd, M. R. (1991) Tetrazolium-based assays for cellular viability: A critical examination of selected parameters affecting formazan production. *Cancer Res.* **51,** 2515–2520.
5. Plumb, J. A., Milroy, R., and Kaye, S. B. (1989) Effects of the pH dependence of 3-(4,5-dimethylthiazol-2-yl)-2,5-diphenyltetrazolium bromide-formazan absorption on chemosensitivity determined by a novel tetrazolium-based assay. *Cancer Res.* **49,** 4435–4440.

4

Cell Sensitivity Assays

Detection of Apoptotic Cells In Vitro Using the TUNEL Assay

Neil A. Jones and Caroline Dive

1. Introduction

1.1. Principles of Flow Cytometry

Flow cytometry allows rapid multiparameter analyses of individual cells. Cells are illuminated with incident laser light of a specific wavelength. Resultant light scatter signals and fluorescence-emission signals from fluorochromes contained at the surface of the cell or within it are detected by an array of photomultiplier tubes. For example, fluorochrome-conjugated antibodies and DNA interchelating dyes can be used to acquire information on protein expression and DNA ploidy (via fluorescence signals) together with information on cell size and structure (via light-scatter signals).

1.2. Chromatin Changes During Apoptosis

Apoptosis is a process whereby cells die via an ordered cellular program and is therefore often referred to as programmed cell death. Apoptosis is important in the maintenance of tissue homeostasis and during animal development *(1,2)*. Many currently used cytotoxic drugs kill tumor cells because of their ability to induce apoptosis *(3)*, and apoptosis is increasingly being studied in the context of drug resistance. Despite the wide variety of stimuli that can induce apoptosis, most cells undergoing the process exhibit a similar series of changes, suggesting that these signals converge to engage a common pathway that is required for the execution of cell death. One of the most widely studied biochemical process that occurs during apoptosis is the nonrandom cleavage of genomic DNA. This cleavage is owing to the activation of specific endogenous endonucleases and results in the formation of a large numbers of DNA strand

From: *Methods in Molecular Medicine, Vol. 28: Cytotoxic Drug Resistance Mechanisms*
Edited by: R. Brown and U. Böger-Brown © Humana Press Inc., Totowa, NJ

breaks *(4)*. The separation of DNA from these apoptotic cells by agarose gel electrophoresis and subsequent visualization using ethidium bromide reveals a characteristic 'ladder' pattern *(4)*. Such 'ladders' consist of multiples of ~200 base pairs, and occur as a result of cleavage of DNA between nucleosome histone complexes (or bundles). In some cells, such nucleosomal DNA laddering is not seen, and in these cases high molecular weight (50 or 300 kbp) DNA fragments may be produced *(5–7)*. These high molecular weight DNA fragments are thought to arise as a result of the release of chromatin from the nuclear matrix. The identification of such DNA fragmentation by agarose gel electrophoresis, although indicative of apoptosis, cannot be used as a quantitative assay. In addition, apoptosis of mammalian cells in culture, although regulated, is often asynchronous, and therefore accurate determination of levels and rates of apoptosis is difficult using the aforementioned assay.

An alternative methodology that can be used to rapidly detect and quantitate DNA strand breaks in individual cells undergoing apoptosis utilizes flow cytometry *(8)*. This has the advantage of simultaneous detection of the DNA strand breaks and cell-cycle distribution in individual cells. In addition this methodology has been used to detect DNA strand breaks in clinical samples before and after treatment with cytotoxic drugs *(8,9)*.

During cell death there is an alteration in the ability of cells to scatter light at a forward angle, reflecting cell size, and at 90°, reflecting cell granularity. These changes can be detected using flow cytometry. Such changes can be used to discriminate between live cells, dead cells, and cells that are undergoing apoptosis *(10)*. As mentioned above apoptotic cells characteristically exhibit DNA strand breaks and these can be detected using terminal deoxynucleotidyl transferase (TdT)-mediated dUTP Nick End Labeling (TUNEL) and flow cytometry *(8)*. Exogenous terminal deoxynucleotidyl transferase is used to incorporate either bromodeoxyuridine triphosphate (BrdUTP) or biotinylated deoxyuridine triphosphate (dUTP) to the 3' end of single-stranded DNA. Fragmented DNA can then be detected by using fluorescein isothiocyanate (FITC)-conjugated antibody or FITC-labeled avidin to reveal the incorporation of labeled nucleotide. By counterstaining with propidium iodide information on cell cycle distribution can also be obtained within the same cell. We shall outline the methodology, which can be used to label strand breaks in suspension or adherent tissue-culture cells induced to undergo apoptosis, using both of these deoxynucleotides.

2. Materials (*see* Note 6)

1. Phosphate-buffered saline (PBS): 10X PBS tablets can be obtained from Oxoid. 1X PBS is made by dissolving 1 tablet in every 100 mL of dH_2O. PBS should be made weekly and kept at 4°C.

2. Fixatives:
   a. 1% (v/v) formaldehyde in PBS: formaldehyde is normally supplied as a 20% or 40% solution and should therefore be diluted freshly for each experiment and kept on ice. The formaldehyde should be methanol-free and can be purchased from Polysciences Inc. (Warrington, PA).
   b. 100% ethanol and PBS should be prechilled on ice.
3. Terminal deoxynucleotidyl transferase (TdT): can be purchased from Boehringer Mannheim (Mannheim, Germany) and is supplied as 25 units/µL and stored at –20°C.
4. TdT reaction buffer: supplied with the TdT enzyme as a 5X concentrated solution (5X concentrated= 1 *M* potassium cacodylate, 125 m*M* Tris-HCl, pH 6.6, 1.25 mg/mL bovine serum albumin [BSA]) and stored at –20°C.
5. Cobalt Chloride ($CoCl_2$): supplied as a 25 m*M* solution with the enzyme and is stored at –20°C.
6. 20X Sodium chloride-sodium citrate (SSC): Dissolve 17.5g NaCl and 8.8g Tri sodium citrate in 80 mL dH_2O. pH to 7.0 and make up to 100 mL with dH_2O. This should be autoclaved and then stored at room temperature.
7. BrdUTP solution: brdUTP powder (Sigma, St. Louis, MO) is prepared as a 2 m*M* solution in 50 m*M* Tris-HCl, pH 7.5, and stored at –20°C.
8. Biotin-16-dUTP (bt-dUTP) solution: obtained from Boehringer Mannheim as a 50 nM solution and stored at –20°C.
9. Fluorescein isothiocyanate (FITC)-conjugated anti-BrdU antibody: purchased from Becton Dickinson, Rutherford, NJ.
10. FITC-conjugated anti-BrdU antibody staining solution: Make a solution of PBS + 0.1% Triton X-100 + 1% BSA + 0.1 µg/mL FITC-conjugated anti-BrdU antibody. This is made up freshly for each experiment and kept on ice.
11. Avidin-FITC stock (1000X): obtained from Sigma. Made as a 5 mg/mL solution in PBS. This stock solution should be aliquoted and stored at –20°C. Working stock solutions can be stored at 4°C but should be used within 1 mo and should only be diluted to a working dilution when required.
12. Avidin-FITC solution: 4X SSC (diluted from 20X SSC using dH_2O) + 0.1% (v/v) Triton X-100 and 5% (w/v) fat-free dried skimmed milk (Marvel, Premier Beverages, Stafford, UK) +5 µg/mL avidin-FITC (purchased from Sigma). Makeup fresh for each experiment.
13. Washing solution: PBS + 0.1% (v/v) Triton X-100 + 5 mg/mL BSA, make fresh for each experiment.
14. Propidium iodide (PI) staining solution: PBS + 5 µg/mL PI (Molecular Probes, Eugene, OK) + 200 µg/mL DNase-free RNase (Sigma) make up fresh immediately before use. The RNase can be made as a stock of 20 mg/mL in H_2O and stored in aliquots at –20°C.

    Flow cytometer: We use a Becton Dickinson FACS Vantage instrument. Whatever flow cytometer to which you have access, the machine must be set up appropriately; because dual-color detection will be used, the machine may require color compensation adjustment (*see* **Subheading 3.3.**). It is important, therefore, that control reactions are included in each experiment (*see* **Note 5**). It is wise to use

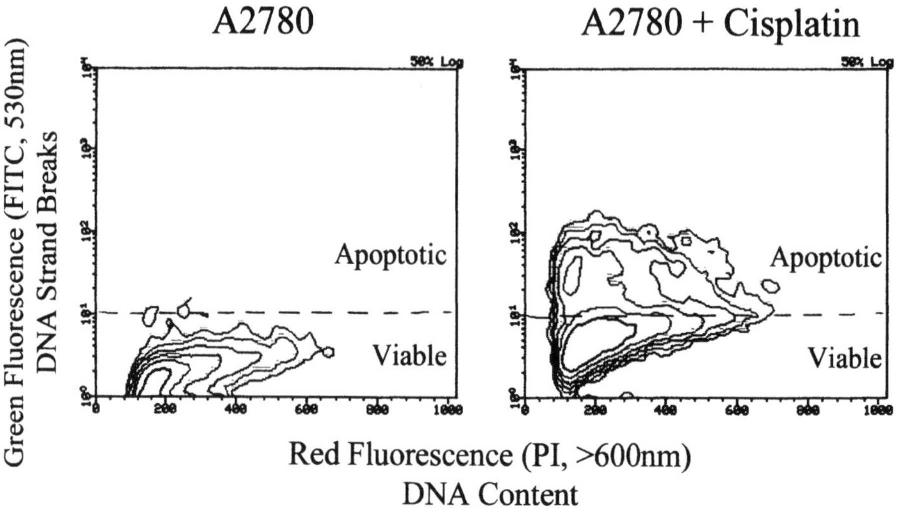

Fig. 1. Incorporation of bt-dUTP by exogenous TdT into the DNA of human ovarian carcinoma cells exposed to the DNA damaging agent cisplatin. Two-dimensional frequency contour plots of red fluorescence (x-axis; PI stained DNA) vs green fluorescence (y-axis, bt-dUTP labeled with avidin-FITC). Untreated human A2780 ovarian carcinoma cells; these cells were exposed to 20 μ*M* cisplatin for 1 h and then incubated for 96 h at 37°C. They were then processed using Method B. Cells with green fluorescence above the dotted line are considered to be positive for incorporation of labeled nucleotide by exogenous TdT and therefore undergoing apoptosis.

an experienced flow-cytometry user to undertake such adjustments, unless you know what you are doing. The data analysis shown in **Fig. 1** was obtained using Lysis II software supplied with instrument.

3. Methods

We will describe the two basic methodologies of the TdT assay that can be used to detect DNA strand breaks in cells undergoing apoptosis (*see* **Note 1**). Both methods are essentially identical, except that Method A utilizes brdUTP to label DNA ends whereas Method B uses biotinylated nucleotide (biotin-16-dUTP; bt-dUTP). Incorporation of both the nucleotides is obtained using exogenous TdT. Detection of incorporation of these nucleotides is achieved using a FITC-conjugated BrdU antibody or FITC-labeled avidin (avidin binds to the biotin conjugated onto the nucleotide). Control reactions must also be carried out, in addition to experimental samples. These are used to determine nonspecific binding of detection reagents and allow the flow cytometer to be adjusted to compensate for such binding. These control reactions are highlighted in the notes section (*see* **Note 5**).

3.1. Method A: Using BrdUTP to Label the DNA Strand Breaks

1. Harvest cells and count using a hemocytometer (*see* **Note 2**). Place aliquots of 1×10^6 cells into flow cytometer tubes. Wash once in ice-cold PBS and pour off the PBS, leaving the pellet with a small amount of fluid. Cells are pelleted at 200*g* for 5 min.
2. Vortex the cell pellet while adding 1 mL of the formaldehyde fixative solution (*see* **Note 3**). Vortexing at the same time as adding the fixative will reduce cell clumping, which could block the flow cytometer. Leave the cells to fix on ice for 15 min.
3. Pellet cells and wash once with 2 mL PBS. Resuspend the pellet in 300 µL ice-cold PBS. Add 700 µL ice-cold ethanol, again while the cells are being vortexed. The cells can now be stored in the refrigerator for up to 2 wk; if the cells are to be used immediately, they must be in this ethanol fixative for at least 30 min on ice. The ability to keep the fixed cells for a period of time means that time-course experiments can be undertaken and the samples then processed for end-labeling at the same time.
4. On the day of the end-labeling experiment, spin the cells down and remove the ethanol solution. The cells should then be rehydrated in 1 mL PBS for 15 min. It is a good idea at this stage to look at the cells by microscopy to make sure there are no large clumps of cells.
5. Spin cells down (*see* **Note 4**) and resuspend the pellets in 50 µL of 1X TdT reaction buffer (the 5X concentrated stock is diluted to 1X with dH_2O). Add 1 µL TdT (5 units; the enzyme is supplied at 25 U/µL and should be diluted to 5 U/µL with 1X reaction buffer) and 2 µL brdUTP. Incubate at 37°C for 40 min.
6. Add 2 mL of washing buffer to each tube and spin down (*see* **Note 4**).
7. Resuspend the pellet in 50 µL of the FITC-conjugated BrdU antibody solution and incubate at room temperature for 30 min in the dark.
8. Add 2 mL of washing buffer to each tube and spin down.
9. Resuspend the cell pellet in 1 mL of PI staining solution and incubate for 30 min at room temperature again in the dark.
10. Analyze the cells by flow cytometry (*see* **Note 5**).

3.2. Method B: Using Biotin-16-dUTP to Label the Strand Breaks

1. Harvest cells and count using a hemocytometer (*see* **Note 2**). Place aliquots of 1×10^6 cells into flow cytometer tubes. Wash once in ice-cold PBS, then pour off the PBS, leaving the pellet with a small amount of fluid. Cells are pelleted at 200*g* for 5 min.
2. Vortex the cell pellet while adding 1 mL of the formaldehyde fixative (*see* **Note 3**). Vortexing at the same time as adding the fixative will reduce cell clumping, which may block the flow cytometer. Leave the cells to fix on ice for 15 min.
3. Pellet cells and wash once with 2 mL PBS. Resuspend the pellet in 300 µL ice cold PBS. Add 700 µL ice-cold ethanol, again while the cells are being vortexed. The cells can now be stored in the refrigerator for up to 2 wk; if the cells are to be used immediately, they must be in this ethanol fixative for a minimum of 30 min on ice.

4. On the day of the labeling experiment, spin the cells down and remove the ethanol solution. The cells should then be rehydrated in 1 mL PBS for 15 min. Look at the cells now by microscopy to make sure there are no large clumps of cells.
5. Spin cells down (*see* **Note 4**) and resuspend the pellets in 50 µL of TdT reaction buffer (the 5X concentrated stock is diluted to 1X with H_2O). Add 1 µL TdT (5 units; (the enzyme is supplied at 25 U/µL and should be diluted to 5 U/µL with 1X reaction buffer) and 0.5 µL of bt-dUTP (0.5 nM final concentration). Incubate at 37°C for 40 min.
6. Add 2 mL of washing buffer to each tube and spin down (*see* **Note 4**).
7. Resuspend the pellet in 50 µL of the avidin-FITC solution containing 5 µg/mL avidin-FITC (1 in 1000 dilution of the stock solution). Incubate in the dark at room temperature for 30 min.
8. Add 2 mL of washing buffer to each tube and spin down.
9. Resuspend the cell pellet in 1 mL of PI staining solution and incubate for 30 min at room temperature again in the dark.
10. Analyze the cells by flow cytometry (*see* **Note 5**).

3.3. Data Analysis

Light-scatter properties are used to discriminate large cell clumps and cellular debris by placement of an electronic gate around intact fixed cells on a scatter plot prior to analysis of DNA fragmentation. Such gating should be done when running the control samples (*see* **Subheading 3.** and **Note 5**). To measure the binding of FITC-labeled antibody to incorporated nucleotide at the same time as cell-cycle distribution via PI binding to DNA, the following laser wavelengths should be used:

1. The samples should be illuminated with a 488 nm laser line. 10,000 cells are analyzed/sample with a flow rate of 300–500 cells/s.
2. Green fluorescence of the FITC is detected using a 530 nm ± 20 nm band pass filter. Red fluorescence of the PI bound to DNA is measured at 630 ± 22 nm band pass filter. The green and red fluorescence should be separated using a 560 nm short pass dichroic filter. Check to see whether color compensation is required by analysis of green only, and then red only fluorescing cells. Two cells in G_1 phase of the cell cycle passing the laser together can be discriminated from a single cell in G_2 using pulse width analysis (*see* ***11***).

A typical two-dimensional profile of green and red fluorescence is shown in **Fig. 1**. For each cell that passes in single file through the laser, both red fluorescence and green fluorescence are measured. The amount of PI binding to DNA which indicates phase of cell cycle is plotted on the x axis. The y axis shows the amount of green fluorescence displayed by the cells and therefore indicates the extent of incorporation of the labeled nucleotide. Elevated green fluorescence exhibited by the cells is taken as a measure of the number of strand breaks and therefore the extent of apoptosis in the cells. The percentage of cells exhibiting high green fluorescence is determined using a gate positioned above the green fluorescence levels observed in control samples.

4. Notes

1. In our experience quantification of apoptosis using this assay in apoptotic cells that fail to 200bp ladder, but that do produce 30 and 500 kb DNA fragments, is quite difficult, although not impossible *(12)*. This is because there are fewer DNA strand breaks and therefore fewer free DNA ends with which to label. It is therefore worthwhile to determine if your chosen cell type does undergo nucleosomal DNA laddering when they apoptose, this can be determined using conventional agarose gel electrophoresis.
2. All samples should contain equal cell numbers (1×10^6 or more is ideal because of the inevitable loss of cells during the washing steps) to ensure that the reagents are not limiting for efficient labeling of the DNA.
3. Cell fixation using cross-linking agents is essential. This prevents loss of small DNA fragments during the labeling and detection reactions and after the washes. Vortexing of the cells when adding the fixatives is vital, particularly when using cells that normally grow as adherent monolayers in vitro, this reduces cell clumping that, if high, would block the flow of sample in the flow cytometer. It is therefore worthwhile to check by microscopy that the cell suspension contains single cells and not clumps before running the samples through the flow cytometer. Very fragile cells may not survive these procedures and therefore this may not be an ideal method with which to measure apoptosis; empirical determination of the suitability of this method to detect strand breaks for different cell types must be carried out. (Alternatively, try the Annexin V binding assay on fixed cells *[13]*, or the Hoeschst assay on unfixed cells *[14]*.)
4. During washes, make sure the wash buffer is completely removed and that the pelleted cells are as dry as possible. The small reaction volumes used mean that any wash buffer that does remain with the pellets after washing will dilute the enzyme or antibody reaction mixes, which may therefore reduce the efficiency of incorporation of nucleotides into the strand breaks and their subsequent detection.
5. As highlighted in **Subheading 3.**, it is essential that control reactions are included in every experiment, this allows the flow cytometer to be set up and adjusted as necessary. The following samples are needed in addition to the experimental samples you want to run:

   Using control healthy cells with no strand breaks:

   a. blank (just cells).
   b. TdT only (no BrdU antibody or avidin-FITC or PI).
   c. BrdU antibody or avidin-FITC only (no TdT enzyme or PI).
   d. TdT and BrdU antibody or avidin-FITC (no PI).
   e. PI only (no TdT or BrdU antibody or avidin-FITC).

   Dying cells with strand breaks

   f. TdT and BrdU antibody or avidin-FITC.
   g. PI only.

6. There are now a number of commercially available kits with which to undertake this assay; they can be obtained, for example, from Appligene Oncor (Illkirch, France), Boehringer Mannheim, Pharmingen (San Diego, CA), or Promega (Madison, WI).

References

1. Raff, M. C. (1992) Social controls on cell survival and cell death. *Nature* **356,** 397–399.
2. Williams, G. T. and Smith, C. A. (1993) Molecular recognition of apoptosis: genetic controls on cell death. *Cell* **74,** 777–779.
3. Hickman, J. A. (1992) Apoptosis induced by anticancer drugs. *Cancer Metastasis Rev.* **11,** 121–139.
4. Wyllie, A. H. (1994) Apoptosis: death gets a break. *Nature* **369,** 272–273.
5. Anthoney, D. A., McIlwrath, A. J., Gallagher, W. M., Edlin, A. R. M., and Brown, R. (1996) Microsatellite instability, apoptosis and loss of p53 function in drug-resistant tumour cells. *Cancer Res.* **56,** 1374–1381.
6. Ormerod, M. G., O'Neill, C. F., Robertson, D., and Harrap, K. (1994) Cisplatin induced apoptosis in a human ovarian carcinoma cell line without concomitant internucleosomal degradation of DNA. *Exp. Cell Res.* **211,** 231–237.
7. Oberhammer, F., Wilson, J. W., Dive, C., Morris, I. D., Hickman, J. A., Wakeling, A. E., Walker, P. R., and Sikorski, M. (1993) Apoptotic death in epithelial cells: cleavage of D. N.,A to 300 and/or 50kb fragments prior to or in the absence of internucleosomal fragmentation. *EMBO J.* **12,** 3679–3684.
8. Gorczyca, W., Gong, J., and Darzynkiewicz, Z. (1993) Detection of DNA strand breaks in individual apoptotic cells by the in situ terminal deoxynucleotidyl transferase and nick translation assays. *Cancer Res.* **53,** 1945–1951.
9. Gorczyca W., Bigman K., Mitterman A., Ahmed T., Gong J., Melamed A. R., and Darzynkiewicz Z (1993) Induction of DNA strand breaks associated with apoptosis during the treatment of leukaemias. *Leukaemia* **7,** 659–670.
10. Gregory, C. D., Dive, C., Henderson, S., Smith, C. A., Williams, G. T., Gordon, J., and Rickinson, A. B. (1991) Activation of Epstein Barr Virus latent genes protects human B cells from death by Apoptosis. *Nature* **249,** 612–614.
11. Ormerod, M. G., ed. (1990) *Flow Cytometry: A Practical Approach.* IRL Press, Oxford, UK.
12. Chapman, R. S., Chresta, C. M., Herberg, A. A., Beere, H. M., Heer, S., Whetton, A. D., Hickman, J. A., and Dive, C. (1995) Further characterisation of the in situ terminal deoxynucleotidyl transferase (TdT) assay for the flow cytometric analysis of apoptosis in drug resistant and drug sensitive leukaemic cells. *Cytometry* **20,** 245–256.
13. Vermes, I., Haanen, C., and Reutelingsperger, C. (1995) A novel assay for apoptosis based upon flow cytometric detection of phosphatidylserine on the cell surface with use of FITC-labelled annexin V. *Clin. Chem.* **41,** 91.
14. Dive, C., Gregory, C. D., Phipps, D. J., Evans, D. L., Milner, A. E., and Wyllie, A. H. (1992) Analysis and discrimination of necrosis and apoptosis (programmed cell death) by multi parameter flow cytometry. *Biochim. Biophys. Acta.* **1133,** 275–285.

5

Analysis of Apoptosis in Tissue Sections

Vicki Save, Philip J. Coates, and Peter A. Hall

1. Introduction

The recognition over the past decade that apoptosis represents a critical element in cell number control in physiological and pathological situations has been well-reviewed *(1–4)*. In addition there is increasing recognition that many of the effects of chemo- and radiotherapeutic agents are mediated by apoptosis *(5–7)*. The seminal work of Kerr, Wyllie, and Currie *(8)*, building upon the earlier observations of Glucksmann *(9)* and Saunders *(10)*, should be read by those interested in assaying apoptosis because of the excellent photomicrographs that document the morphological features of the process. This is important, because despite considerable progress in the understanding of the mechanistic basis of apoptosis, morphological analysis remains unquestionably the "gold standard" for its assessment and quantitation.

Apoptosis is a regulated and active process. Although a diverse range of insults and physiological events can lead to apoptosis, the process is remarkably stereotyped, with a program of activities leading to the final morphological events that are similar throughout phylogeny and may be recapitulated in most (if not all) cell types. Mounting data indicate that much of the machinery for the implementation of the apoptotic response is "hard-wired" in cells, being present all the time but kept in an "off" state, and rapidly recruited into an "on" state if needed. Consequently, and despite much effort, there remain few biochemical markers of the apoptotic process that are specific for this complex regulated process. Similarly, although many potential regulators of apoptosis are described, critical examination of the available data indicates that there is little consensus on their value as markers of apoptosis.

A critical point for the quantitation of apoptosis is that, irrespective of the initiating insult, the time course of apoptosis is very fast *(11,12)*. Moreover,

From: *Methods in Molecular Medicine, Vol. 28: Cytotoxic Drug Resistance Mechanisms*
Edited by: R. Brown and U. Böger-Brown © Humana Press Inc., Totowa, NJ

the clearance of the resultant debris (either by professional phagocytes or bystander [amateur] phagocytes) is, rapid. Coles et al. ***(13)*** suggested that clearance times of less than 1 h were typical. The rapid nature of apoptosis means that in any static analysis, a very small number of apoptotic cells observed at a given instant might, in fact, reflect a very considerable contribution to cell turnover. Dramatic evidence for this came from studies of the physiological contribution of apoptosis in renal development ***(13)*** and in the steady-state regulation of intestinal epithelial populations ***(14)***. Although the process of apoptosis and its clearance is (as far as we can tell) always rapid, there may be some variation between cell types or in relation to different insults. This has important implications for the quantitation of apoptosis, as highlighted by Potten ***(15)***.

Given its contribution to cell turnover in physiological, pathological, and toxicological situations, it is important to be able to identify and quantitate the process of apoptosis in cells and in tissues. Ideally, one would like a technique that is sensitive and highly selective for apoptosis, as well as being easily applicable to routinely prepared tissue sections. Here, we review the various options that can be used to identify and quantitate apoptosis, concentrating on those methods applicable to tissues sections. A detailed method for the identification of apoptosis using *in situ* end-labeling of DNA fragments (*In situ* end-labeling techniques [ISEL]/terminal deoxynucleotidyl transferase-mediated UTP nick-end labeling [TUNEL]) is given.

2. Materials

1. Tissues and cells: *in situ* end-labeling techniques can be applied to cells grown in culture, to frozen tissue sections, or to formalin-fixed, paraffin-embedded material, such as that found in surgical pathology archives.
2. Frozen material or tissue culture cells may be fixed by immersion for 10 min in 50% methanol/50% acetone at –20°C, followed by air drying. Alternatively, a 4% solution of paraformaldehyde can be prepared by dissolving 4 g of paraformaldehyde powder in 80 mL of water with gentle heating and the addition of 1 *M* NaOH until the powder dissolves. The solution is made up to 90 mL with distilled water, and 10 mL of a 10X PBS solution added.
3. Proteinase K: A stock solution of proteinase K (Sigma, Poole, Dorset, UK; P2308) is prepared by dissolving 10 mg of enzyme in 1 mL of water, to give a 10 mg/mL concentration. The enzyme is aliquoted and stored frozen. The aliquots should not be thawed and re-frozen more than twice. For use, 5 mL of the stock solution is diluted into 5 mL of sterile 50 m*M* Tris-HCl, pH 8.0, 1 m*M* ethylenediaminetetraacetic acid (EDTA).
4. In Situ End-Labeling Buffer: 0.01 m*M* of each of biotin-dATP, dCTP, dGTP, and dTTP, in 50 m*M* Tris-HCl, pH 7.5, 5 m*M* MgCl2, 10 m*M* 2-Mercaptoethanol, 0.005% bovine serum dibumin (BSA) (molecular biology grade, e.g., Sigma

B2518), and 5 units/mL Klenow fragment of DNA polymerase I. The labeling solution without polymerase can be prepared in bulk and stored frozen in aliquots, but the DNA polymerase must be added immediately prior to use. The biotinylated nucleotide can be obtained from Life Technologies Ltd. (Paisley, Scotland; cat. no. 19534-016). Deoxynucleotide triphosphates can be purchased as a set from Boehringer Mannheim UK, East Sussex, UK; cat. no. 1277 049 (*see* **Notes 4**, **5**, and **7**).

5. Horseradish peroxidase-conjugated avidin (Dako Ltd., Bucks, UK; P364) is made freshly by diluting 5 mL into 1 mL of phosphate-buffered saline (PBS) containing 1% BSA (Sigma, A9647).
6. 70, 90, and 95% alcohol (analytical grade).

3. Methods

3.1. Demonstration of Apoptosis: Comparison of Methods

3.1.1. Morphology

The phenomenon of apoptosis is defined by a series of morphological changes ***(8,16,17)***. The classical features are best seen by electron microscopy, but can be observed at the light microscopic level using nucleic acid-binding dyes, such as haematoxylin, acridine orange, or propidium iodide (PI) ***(8,13,16,18)***. The first signs of apoptotic cell death are a condensation of the nuclear material, with a marked accumulation of densely stained chromatin, typically at the edge of the nucleus. This is accompanied by cell shrinkage. Cytoplasmic blebs appear on the cell surface, best seen by time-lapse video-microscopy ***(19)***, and the cell detaches from its neighbors. The nuclear outline often becomes highly folded and the nucleus breaks up, with discrete fragments dispersing throughout the cytoplasm. Eventually, the cells themselves fragment, with the formation of a number of membrane-bound apoptotic bodies. Apoptotic bodies are generally phagocytosed by surrounding cells, which are not necessarily derived from the mononuclear phagocytic system. Therefore, the most common sign of apoptosis in a tissue section is the presence of apoptotic bodies, which may be seen as extracellular bodies, or, after phagocytosis, inside other cells. Apoptotic bodies have a diverse appearance, particularly in regard to their size. They are generally oval or round in shape, and are most easily recognized when they contain large amounts of homogeneous, condensed chromatin. The morphological features of apoptosis have been extensively reviewed, and plentiful illustrations of both the light and electron microscopic appearances are provided in these publications ***(8,16,17,20,21)***.

3.1.2. DNA Laddering

A characteristic feature of apoptosis is DNA fragmentation. Wyllie ***(22)*** described, in association with apoptosis, nucleosomal fragmentation which can be seen by agarose electrophoresis with a ladder of DNA bands representing multiples of 180–200 base pairs. This DNA "ladder" correlates with the early morphological signs of apoptosis ***(23)***, and so this technique has been widely used as a distinctive marker of the process ***(24–28)***. DNA laddering is not seen in cells that have undergone necrosis, which show a random fragmentation pattern, leading to smears on agarose electrophoresis ***(22)***. However, the method is not easily quantified and cannot be applied (in this form) to tissue sections. Moreover, although it is clear that DNA degradation is a common feature of apoptosis, it is also evident that not all cells which undergo apoptosis show the formation of a nucleosomal-sized ladder of DNA. In some cases, DNA fragmentation appears to be delayed ***(29)***, although other researchers reported a complete lack of DNA laddering ***(30)***. It has recently been shown that cells undergoing apoptosis may show only very limited DNA degradation, with the formation of 300 or 50 kilobase fragments ***(31)***. These fragments are thought to represent the release of loops of chromatin from their attachment points on the nuclear scaffold. These changes cannot be seen on conventional electrophoresis, but require the use of pulsed field gel electrophoresis (PFGE) to allow the separation of large DNA fragments.

3.1.3. ISEL or TUNEL

The property of DNA fragmentation in apoptosis can be utilized to identify cells undergoing this process ***(32–36)*** because certain enzymes can add labeled nucleotides to the DNA ends. The labeled nucleotides can then be identified by immunological methods akin to immunohistochemistry. Such methods were originally termed TUNEL (terminal deoxynucleotidyl transferase mediated UTP nick end labeling) but are also referred to as ISEL (*In Situ* end-labeling techniques). Strictly, the different names relate to the different enzymes employed, and while there are theoretical and some practical differences, the similarity of technique and result make the names essentially interchangeable. A comparison of the methodologies employing terminal deoxynucleotidyl transferase (TdT) (TUNEL) and Klenow fragment of DNA polymerase (ISEL) was reported by Mundle et al. ***(37)***, who demonstrated that TUNEL appeared more sensitive than ISEL. This is because TdT can label 3' recessed, 5' recessed, or blunt ends of DNA, whereas ISEL labels only those with 3' recessed ends. All three types of DNA end are seen in apoptosis, and thus, in principle, TdT-based methods should be more sensitive than Klenow polymerase methods. Despite this, in practice ISEL and TUNEL appear functionally interchangeable.

Irrespective of the enzyme employed a variety of labels could be used, including radioactive nucleotide triphosphates. However, methods based on the use of nonisotopic labels have been developed and are superior for a variety of reasons, including ease of use, stability, simplicity, and speed of detection, and the increased resolution obtained. Using this approach, it has been clearly shown that the amount and distribution of labeled cells is closely correlated with the amount and distribution of cells known to be undergoing apoptosis using other methods ***(33–36)***. The method can be modified for fluorescence detection *in situ* or by flow cytometry or detection at the light or ultrastructural levels ***(36,38)***. In addition, the use of immunocytochemistry for cell-surface antigens in combination with TUNEL/ISEL allows the identification of the particular cell types undergoing apoptosis, and could also be used to measure phenotypic changes in apoptotic cells ***(36,39)*** and with *in-situ* hybridization methods ***(40)***.

The protocol for TUNEL/ISEL is given in **Subheading 3.3.**, based upon our experience ***(14,35,41,42)***. A number of variables must be considered when performing the technique. The staining results depend on a variety of factors, including the rapidity and extent of fixation, the extent and nature of proteolytic digestion, the specificity of the DNA polymerase, the extent of incorporation of labeled nucleotide triphosphate and the sensitivity of detection of the label.

3.2. Fixation

Frozen material or tissue-culture cells may be fixed by immersion for 10 min in 50% methanol/50% acetone at –20°C, followed by air drying. Alternatively, a 4% solution of paraformaldehyde can be prepared by dissolving 4 g of paraformaldehyde powder in 80 mL of water with gentle heating and the addition of 1 *M* NaOH until the powder dissolves. The solution is made up to 90 mL with distilled water, and 10 mL of a 10X PBS solution added. Fixation is for 10 min at 4°C, and slides are then rinsed in PBS. Tissues or cells which are to be used for TUNEL/ISEL should be fixed as quickly as possible, because delay causes significant artifacts.

Importantly, it has been shown that TUNEL/ISEL can be performed on sections of archival tissues after formalin fixation and storage as wax blocks. When using tissue sections that have been fixed in formaldehyde, it is necessary to use a protease in order to break some of the cross- links formed between proteins, and thereby allow access of the reagents to the degraded DNA. Either pepsin or proteinase K can be used for this step, and the extent of digestion varies with the extent of fixation. In general, too much digestion leads to some nonspecific staining, whereas too little digestion results in a decrease in the intensity of staining of apoptotic cells. Proteolytic digestion is not required when using frozen cells or tissue sections fixed in acetone/methanol.

3.3. ISEL

1. 3–4 mm paraffin sections are mounted on silane-coated glass slides and allowed to dry.
2. Sections are dewaxed, rinsed in alcohol, and air-dried.

3. Digest with 10 mg/mL of proteinase K (Sigma, P2308) diluted in sterile buffer (50 m*M* Tris-HCl, pH 8.0, 1 m*M* EDTA) for 30 minutes at 37°C (*see* **Notes 2** and **3**).
4. Wash in sterile distilled water three times, rinse in 70, 90, and 95% alcohol and air-dry.
5. Prepare 40–60 mL ISEL buffer for each section and keep on ice (*see* **Notes 4**, **5**, and **7**).
6. Carefully pipet the mixture over the tissue section, and place a cleaned glass coverslip over the section to prevent evaporation.
7. Incubate at 37°C for 1 h in a moist chamber.
8. Terminate the reaction by washing sections in distilled water three times, being careful not to scratch the tissue surface when removing the coverslip.
9. Block endogenous peroxidase activity with methanol containing 0.5% H_2O_2 (100 volumes) for 30 min (*see* **Note 6**). Wash three times in distilled water and rinse in PBS, pH 7.4.
10. Incubate with diluted horseradish peroxidase-conjugated avidin (*see* **Notes 5** and **6**).
11. Wash in PBS three times (5 min each) and develop in diaminobenzidine-H_2O_2. Lightly counterstain with hematoxylin and mount in resin.
12. View under a light microscope, where apoptotic nuclei are stained brown and nonapoptotic cell nuclei appear blue (*see* **Notes 8**, **9**, **10**).

4. Notes

1. A number of kits are available and work very well and have good documentation. For example, the ApopTag Plus Kit marketed by Oncor (Appligene), the *in situ* cell-death detection kits (Boehringer Mannheim), or the FragEL kits (Calbiochem/Oncogene Research). However, these kits can be expensive and there is no reason why the component parts cannot be purchased from other competitive suppliers and incorporated into the methods. The ability to undertake these methods is critically based on having good basic histological and immunohistological skills. If you do not have these, go to a lab that has them, in order to learn.
2. Proteinase K should not be used if preparations have been fixed in methanol/acetone.
3. The conditions for proteolytic digestion may need to be varied, and it is advisable in the first instance to perform a series of digestions, varying the concentration of proteinase K from 1–20 mg/mL. In principle, any enzyme with proteolytic activity can be used, but remember that enzyme preparations may be contaminated with nuclease activities which could give false positive results. For this reason, pepsin or proteinase K are good choices, because the former is used at low pH where nucleases would not be active, and the latter is supplied in a highly purified form and is effectively free of nuclease activity.
4. To avoid contamination by DNases, it is advisable to sterilize the solutions used in the TUNEL/ISEL procedure, particularly the labeling buffer, and to use sterile pipet tips and microcentrifuge tubes.
5. Digoxigenin-11-dUTP (Boehringer Mannheim) can be substituted for the biotinylated dATP at the same concentration (but note that the unlabeled nucleotides should then be dATP, dCTP, and dGTP). In this case, the reaction is

detected by incubation with antidigoxigenin antibodies (e.g., peroxidase conjugated antidigoxigenin, cat. no. 1207733, diluted 1:200). Nucleotide triphosphates labeled with fluorescent markers are also available.

6. This method uses detection of biotinylated sites with peroxidase and is highly suited for assessment of paraffin sections. The protocol should be amended if a different label has been used, or if a different detection system is preferred (e.g., fluorescent detection).
7. A variety of enzymes can be used for incorporation of the label. Klenow fragment of DNA polymerase I is preferable to the DNA polymerase I holoenzyme because it has the identical polymerase activity, but lacks the exonuclease activity that could cause artifactual labeling ***(43)***. Alternatively one can use TdT ***(33)***, which adds on long tails of nucleotides to the 3' hydroxyl ends of DNA without the need for a template strand ***(43)***. It is extremely important to use the correct concentration of enzyme, as increased amounts will lead to nonspecific staining of morphologically normal nuclei ***(34,35)***. Obviously, insufficient enzyme will lead to a reduction in the staining of apoptotic nuclei.
8. Modifications of the basic method for are well documented for flow cytometry (*see* Chapter 4) ***(36)***, and Kits are also sold by Oncor, Appligene, and Boehringer Mannheim.
9. Controls: As with any technique it is essential to perform a number of controls. A positive control section should be included with each batch, to test for variations; in the intensity of staining from day to day. For each test section, an appropriate immunohistochemical control should be performed to test for the presence of endogenous enzyme activities and/or nonspecific binding of the detection reagents. This is most easily achieved by the exclusion of the enzyme or the labeled nucleotide from the TUNEL/ISEL reaction mixture.
10. Staining Patterns and their Interpretation: Irrespective of the enzyme or label employed, not all apoptotic bodies are intensely stained, and in particular, it is not uncommon to see that the extremely condensed nuclei are relatively unstained. This may be owing to problems with penetration of the reagents into these nuclei. The nuclei of nonapoptotic cells should be unstained by the technique, if the enzyme digestion has been performed correctly. A generalized staining of all or many apparently normal nuclei suggests that proteolytic digestion has been too harsh—a similar effect is seen if a DNAase treatment is used as a positive control ***(34,35)***. Necrotic cells are also stained by the method ***(41)*** and there are a number of situations in which staining can be seen in morphologically normal nuclei, for example in spermatogonia ***(35)*** and after exposure to some DNA damaging agents ***(44)***. DNA breaks could be present as the result of fixation and processing procedures, which result in the accumulation of lower molecular-weight DNA. In addition, the action of section cutting and various pretreatments, such as exposure to hydrogen peroxide to block endogenous peroxidase activity, might also cause DNA breaks in cells. In practice, this means that a range of concentrations of enzyme may need to be tested, particularly when using the technique for the first time.

11. Specificity: TUNEL/ISEL can by no means be said to be specific for apoptosis. Fortunately, the discrimination between large numbers of stained cells in an area of necrosis, and the presence of scattered cells undergoing apoptosis should not pose a great problem to a trained histologist. However, of course, the effects of speed of fixation, and the penetration rates of fixative may also influence the staining characteristics of the tissue. For instance, if a large piece of tissue is immersed in fixative, there will be a significant delay before cells in the center of the tissue are fixed, with the possible result of autolysis. For most purposes, the TUNEL/ISEL technique can be considered a selective (rather than a specific) technique for the identification of apoptosis in histological material. The technique assists with the identification and quantitation of apoptosis, but must be employed in conjunction with simple morphological examination in order to exclude artefactual staining caused by technical aspects, and staining as a result of demonstrating DNA strand breaks, resulting from other physiological or pathological processes.
12. Immunohistochemical methods. In recent years, a large number of antibodies have been marketed for apoptosis research. The vast majority of these recognize proteins that can influence apoptosis in certain instances, but are neither universal nor specific. Indeed, because apoptosis is a consequence of the activation of pre-existing mechanisms within a cell, there has been relatively little progress in the identification and use of antigens whose expression is correlated with this form of cell death. Immunohistological detection of the expression of regulatory proteins (e.g., Bcl-2 or BAX) has been reported (*see* also Chapter 18), but the utility of this approach as a marker of apoptosis is unsubstantiated. Moreover, there have been significant problems with the specificity of some reagents purported to be, apoptosis specific and the authors urge extreme caution (*see*, for example, the caveat on BAX staining in ref. ***45***). A novel approach recently reported is the detection of Annexin IV expression in apopotic cells as a consequence of membrane changes ***(46,47)***. Unfortunately, this method requires the use of unfixed cells and cannot be applied (at present) to histological material. The use of antibodies to clusterin (also known as TRPM-2, or SOP-2) has also been correlated with apoptosis in certain situations, although this protein is not a universal marker, nor is it specific for apoptosis ***(48)***. Perhaps the most widely used immunhistochemical marker of apoptosis is the identification of tissue transglutaminase (tTG) ***(49,50)***, although even here recent data suggests that TG is not always induced during apoptosis ***(51)*** Finally, apoptosis can also be demonstrated by *in situ* hybridization ***(52)*** although the utility of this method also remains to be established.
13. Flow Cytometry (*see* also Chapter 4). The detection of fragmented nuclei by flow cytometry is now a widely used and accepted method for the detection and quantitation of apoptosis ***(28,53)***. The methods rely on the use of DNA binding dye (usually PI), which intercalates stoichiometrically with DNA and allows the quantitation of DNA content. A sub-G1 peak is reliably found to be indicative of apoptosis (because of the DNA fragmentation) and the peak size reflects the amount of apoptosis in the sample. The method is easily applied to cell suspen-

sions and can also be applied to material derived from histological samples, although this is associated with higher 'background levels' and, of course, results in the loss of potentially important spatial and micro-anatomical information. The appearance of phosphatidylserine on the cell surface can also be measured by fluorescence activated cell sorter (FACS), through binding of fluorescein isothiocyanate (FITC)-tagged annexin V. Simultaneous staining with PI aids with the identification of the apoptotic cell population.

14. A variety of enzyme-linked immunosorbent assay (ELISA)-based methods for the quantitation of apoptosis that are limited to cell culture systems have recently been developed and marketed (Boehringer Mannheim; Calbiochem, for example). These assays utilize the release of usually insoluble nuclear molecules into the cytoplasm of dying cells, and kits are available for the measurement of nucleosomes or nuclear matrix proteins. In addition, a western blot method has also been proposed, based on the cleavage of the 113kDa poly(ADP-ribose) polymerase into 89kDa and 24kDa fragments by members of the interleukin converting enzyme (ICE)-like proteases, which are activated during apoptosis ***(54)***.
15. Quantitation of apoptosis: comparison of methods: *This is a real problem!* Much of the currently available literature on apoptosis is problematic because of inadequate quantitation procedures. The application of stereological and morphometric principles to quantitation in histology is difficult: many authors get around this problem by ignoring it. Moreover, many texts on the subject are at best impenetrable. The use of flow cytometric methods (*see* Chapter 4) does lend to the problem the advantages of objective assessment of large numbers of events ($>10^4$ typically): those wishing to use *in situ* techniques will not be easily able to match that, but will obtain valuable information relating to micro-anatomical variation, which may be of fundamental biological importance. It is worth restating that the ability of cells to proliferate, differentiate, and die by apoptosis is regulated by position (anatomical and within cellular hierarchies) ***(15)***.

    The critical issues are simply stated:
    a. The confidence that can be placed on the data depends upon the effort and rigor invested in its generation.
    b. Where the levels of apoptosis are low (the usual state of affairs), very large numbers of events must be quantitated for accuracy.
    c. Methods based on semiquantitative approaches, the use of high-power fields as denominator, the failure to define reproducibility of assessment, and methods that do not consider the heterogeneity implicit in biological samples are to be deprecated.

4.1. Given This, What Can Be Done?

4.1.1. What to Count?

ISEL- or TUNEL-stained samples will make the microscopic assessment easier and perhaps more objective, particularly if the observer is not an experienced microscopist. On the other hand, these methods may underestimate the true number of apoptotic bodies and may be influenced by artefacts (owing to fixation *(14)* or nonapoptotic processes *(35,44)*]. The former may not matter, because the 'error' will be systematic and the same in all samples. The latter is significant, but can be minimized by careful control of sample handling. In the hands of an experienced microscopist then, fluorescent dye-based assays *(13)*, or even simple hematoxylin, will be useful *(14)*. Double labeling may be useful in very specialized circumstances *(14)* and ISEL methods can be combined with both immunocytochemical techniques (*see,* for example, ref. ***39***) and with *in situ* hybridization methods (*see,* for example, ref. ***40***) to good effect.

4.1.2. How Many Events to Count?

Pragmatism must be the key word, and there must be a compromise between the quality of the data, the time taken to generate that data, and the importance of the question. Although statistical approaches can be employed to determine how many events must be assessed (*see* ref. ***55*** for a discussion), the authors favor an experimental approach based on the generation of a 'wandering mean' in a small number of representative examples from the population of cases to be studied. To generate this data the following procedure should be undertaken. Count the number of events (TUNEL/ISEL-positive or apoptotic bodies) and total number of relevant cells in the first microscopic field. This will give the first score (A1 based on N1 cells). In the second field, the process is repeated and running scores recorded to give a running mean (A2 based on N2 cells). This process is repeated to give multiple running averages (A3, N3 . . . An, Nn). If these are plotted, the mean will be seen to wander and eventually oscillate about a mean value, and as N increases, this will become less. This procedure can then define experimentally the number of events to be assessed to produce a given quality of data.

5. Conclusions

Although we have a burgeoning knowledge of the mechanistic basis of apoptosis and an increasing recognition of its contribution to both physiological and pathological processes, the ability to quantitate objectively this process remains poorly developed. It is the view of these authors that if apoptosis is to be assessed in histological material, then there is no escape from meticulous and painstaking microscopy coupled with rigorous and meticulous quantitation. Whether this is the quantitation of morphologically defined events ('the gold standard'), or of TUNEL/ISEL-defined events, is in our view a relatively unimportant issue; they will correlate very well, but both have inherent problems. Arguably, the morphological approach is perhaps more satisfactory, but, curiously, the additional complexity of TUNEL/ISEL attracts some workers! In the end, the choice of method will depend on the experience of the researcher in histological analysis and microscopy.

Acknowledgment

Dr. Save is supported by a research contract awarded to Peter A. Hall from the Department of Health. Dr. Coates has been supported by the Association for International Cancer Research. Research in the laboratory is also supported by the Association for International Cancer Research, the Commission of the European Community, the Cancer Research Campaign, and the Pathological Society of Great Britain and Ireland.

References

1. Korsmeyer, S. J. (1995) Regulators of cell death. *Trends Genet.* **11,** 101–105.
2. Wyllie, A. H. (1995) The genetic regulation of apoptosis. *Curr. Opin. Gen. Dev.* **5,** 97–104.
3. White, E. (1996) Life, death and the pursuit of apoptosis. *Genes Dev.* **10,** 1–15.
4. Kroemer, G. (1997) The proto-oncogene Bc1-2 and its role in regulating apoptosis. *Nature Med.* **3,** 614–620.
5. Eastman, A. (1990) Activation of programmed cell death by anti-cancer agents: cisplatin as a model system. *Cancer Cells* **2,** 275–280.
6. Dive, C. and Hickman, J. A. (1991) Drug-target interactions: only the first step in the commitment to a programmed cell death? *Br. J. Cancer* **64,** 192–196.
7. Hickman, J. A. (1992) Apoptosis induced by anticancer drugs. *Cancer Metastasis Rev.* **11,** 121 139.
8. Kerr, J. F. R., Wyllie, A. H., and Currie, A. R. (1972) Apoptosis: a basic biological phenomenon with wide ranging implications in tissue kinetics. *Br. J. Cancer* **26,** 239–257.
9. Glucksman, A. (1951) Cell deaths in normal vertebrate ontogeny. *Biol. Rev.* **26,** 59–86.
10. Saunders, J. W. (1966) Death in embryonic systems. *Science* **154,** 604–612.
11. Sanderson, C. J. (1976) The mechanism of T-cell mediated cytotoxicity II. Morphological studies of cell death by time-lapse microcinematography. *Proc. Roy. Soc. Lond. B.* **192,** 241–255.
12. Matter, A. (1979) Microcinematographic and electron microscopic analysis of target cell lysis induced by cytotoxic T lymphocytes. *Immunology.* **36,** 179–190.
13. Coles, H. S. R., Burne, J. F., and Raff, M. C. (1993) Large-scale normal cell death in the developing rat kidney and its reduction by epidermal growth factor. *Development.* **118,** 777–784.
14. Hall, P. A., Coates, P. J., Ansari, B., and Hopwood, D. (1994) Regulation of cell number in the mammalian gastrointestinal tract: the importance of apoptosis. *J. Cell Sci.* **107,** 3569–3577.
15. Potten, C. S. (1996) What is an apoptotic index measuring? A commentary. *Br. J. Cancer* **74,** 1743–1748.
16. Wyllie, A. H., Kerr, J. F. R., and Currie, A. R. (1980) Cell death: the significance of apoptosis. *Intl. Rev. Cytol.* **68,** 251–306.

17. Kerr, J. F. R., Searle, J., Harmon, B. V., and Bishop, C. J. (1987) Apoptosis, in *Perspectives on Mammalian Cell Death* (Potten, C. S., ed.), Oxford Science Publications, Oxford, UK, pp. 93–128.
18. Gregory, C. D., Dive, C., Henderson, S., Smith, C. Williams, G. T., Gordon, J., and Rickinson, A. B. (1991) Activation of Epstein-Barr virus latent genes protects human B cells from death by apoptosis. *Nature* **349,** 612–614.
19. Evan, G. I., Wyllie, A. H., Gilbert, C. S., Littlewood, T. D., Land, H., Brooks, M., Waters, C. M., Penn, L. Z., and Hancock, D. C. (1992) Induction of apoptosis in fibroblasts by c-myc protein. *Cell* **69,** 119–128.
20. Ucker, D. S. (1991) Death by suicide: One way to go in mammalian cellular development? *New Biol.* **3,** 103–109.
21. Schwartz, L. M. and Osborne, B. A. (1993) Programmed cell death, apoptosis and killer genes. *Immunol. Today* **14,** 582–590.
22. Wyllie, A. H. (1980) Glucocorticoid-induced thymocyte apoptosis is associated with endogenous endonuclease activation. *Nature* **284,** 555–556.
23. Wyllie, A. H., Morris, R. G., Smith, A. L., and Dunlop, D. (1984) Chromatin cleavage in apoptosis: association with condensed chromatin morphology and dependence on macromolecular synthesis. *J. Pathol.* **142,** 67–77.
24. Compton, M. M. and Cidlowski, J. A. (1986) Rapid *in vivo* effects of glucocorticoids on the integrity of rat genomic deoxyribonucleic acid. *Endocrinology* **118,** 38–45.
25. Cohen, J. J. and Duke, R. C. (1984) Glucocorticoid activation of a calcium dependent endonuclease in thymocyte nuclei leads to cell death. *J. Immunol.* **132,** 38–42.
26. McConkey, D. J., Hartzell, P., Duddy, S. K., Hakansson, H., and Orrenius, S. (1988) 2,3,7,8-Tetrachlordibenzo-p-dioxin kills immature thymocytes by Ca^{2+}-mediated endonuclease activation. *Science* **242,** 256–258.
27. Takano, Y. S., Harmon, B. V., and Kerr, J. F. R. (1991) Apoptosis induced by mild hyperthermia in human and murine cell lines: a study using electron microscopy and DNA gel electrophoresis. *J. Pathol.* **163,** 329–336.
28. Compton, M. M. (1992) A biochemical hallmark of apoptosis: internucleosomal degradation of the genome. *Cancer Metastasis Rev.* **11,** 105–119.
29. Zakeri, Z. F., Quaglino, D., Latham, T., and Lockshin, R. A. (1993) Delayed internucleosomal DNA fragmentation in programmed cell death. *FASEB J.* **7,** 470–478.
30. Schwartz, L. M., Smith, S. W., Jones, M. E., and Osborne, B. A. (1993) Do all programmed cell deaths occur via apoptosis? *Proc. Natl. Acad. Sci. USA* **90,** 980–984.
31. Walker, P. R., Smith, C., Youdale, T., Leblanc, J., Whitfield, J. F., and Sikorska, M. (1991) Topoisomerase II-reactive chemotherapeutic drugs induce apoptosis in thymocytes. *Cancer Res.* **51,** 1078–1085.
32. Fehsel. K., Kolb-Bachofen, V., and Kolb, H. (1991) Analysis of TNF alpha-induced DNA strand breaks at the single cell level. *Am. J. Pathol.* **139,** 251–254.
33. Gavrieli, Y., Sherman, Y., and Ben-Sasson, S. A. (1992) Identification of programmed cell death in situ via specific labelling of nuclear DNA fragmentation. *J. Cell Biol.* **119,** 493–501.

34. Wijsman, J. H., Jonker, R. R., Keijzer, R., van de Velde, C. J. H., Cornelisse, C. J., and van Dierendonck, J. H. (1993) A new method to detect apoptosis in paraffin sections: in situ end-labelling of fragmented DNA. *J. Histochem. Cytochem.* **41,** 7–12.
35. Ansari, B., Coates, P. J., Greenstein, B. D., and Hall, P. A. (1993) In situ end-labelling detects DNA strand breaks in apoptosis and other physiological and pathological states. *J. Pathol.* **170,** 1–8.
36. Gold, R., Schmied, M., Rothe, G., Zischler, H., Breitschopf, H., Wekerle, H., and Laussmann, H. (1993) Detection of DNA fragmentation in apoptosis: application of in situ nick translation to cell culture systems and tissue sections. *J. Histochem. Cytochem.* **41,** 1023–1030.
37. Mundle, S. D., Gao, X. Z., Khan, S., Gregory, S. A., Preisler, H. D., and Raza, A. (1995) Two in situ end labelling techniques reveal different patterns of DNA firagmentation during spontaneous apoptosis in vivo and induced apoptosis in vitro. *Anticancer Res.* **15,** 1895–1904.
38. Migheli, A., Attanasio, A., and Schiffer, D. (1995) Ultrastructural detection of DNA strand breaks in apoptotic neural cells by in situ end-labelling techniques. *J. Pathol.* **176,** 27–35.
39. Kurrer, M. O., Pakala, S. V., Hanson, H. L., and Katz, J. D. (1997) Beta cell apoptosis in T cell-mediated autoimmune diabetes. *Proc. Natl. Acad. Sci. USA* **94,** 213–218.
40. Strater, J., Walczak, H., Krammer, P. H., and Moller, P. (1996) Simultaneous in situ detection of mRNA and apoptotic cells by combined hybridization and TUNEL. *J. Histochem. Cytochem.* **44,** 1497–1499.
41. Coates, P. J. (1994) Molecular methods for the identification of apoptosis in tissues. *J. Histotechnol.* **17,** 261–267.
42. Coates, P. J., Hales, S. A., and Hall, P. A. (1996) The association between cell proliferation and apoptosis: studies using the cell cycle associated proteins Ki-67 and DNA polymerase alpha. *J. Pathol.* **178,** 71–77.
43. Sambrook, J., Fritsch, E. F., and Maniatis, T. (eds.) (1989) *Molecular Cloning. A Laboratory Manual.* Cold Spring Harbor Laboratory Press, Cold Spring Harbor, NY.
44. Coates, P. J., Save, V., Ansari, B., and Hall, P. A. (1995) Demonstration of DNA damage/repair in individual cells using in situ end labelling: association of p53 with sites of DNA damage. *J. Pathol.* **176,** 19–26.
45. Coopersmith, C. M. and Gordon, J. I. (1997) Gamma-ray-induced apoptosis in transgenic mice with proliferative abnormalities in their intestinal epithelium: re-entry of villus enterocytes into the cell cycle does not affect their radioresistance but enhances the radiosensitivity of the crypt by inducing p53. *Oncogene* **15,** 131–141.
46. Martin, S. J. Reutelingsperger, C. P. M., McGahon, A. J., Rader, J. A., Vanschie, R. C. A., Laface, D. M., and Green, D. R. (1995) Early redistribution of plasma-membrane phosphatidylserine is a general feature of apoptosis regardless of the initiating stimulus—inhibition by overexpression of Bc1-2 and Abl. *J. Exp. Med.* **182,** 1545–1556.

47. Koopman, G., Reutlingsperger, C. P. M., Kuijten, G. A. M., Keehnen, R. M. J., Pals, S. T., and Vanders, M. H. J. (1994) Annexin-V for flow cytometric detection of phosphatidylserine expression on B cells undergoing apoptosis. *Blood* **84,** 1415–1420.
48. Garden, G. A., Bothwell, M., and Rubel, E. W. (1991) Lack of correspondence between mRNA expression for a putative cell death model (SGP-2) and neuronal cell death in the central nervous system. *J. Neurobiol.* **22,** 590–604.
49. Fesus, L., Thomazy, V., Autori, F., Ceru, M. P., Tarcsa, E., and Piacentini, M. (1989) Apoptotic hepatocytes become insoluble in detergents and chaotropic agents as a result of transglutaminase action. *FEBS Lett.* **245,** 150–154.
50. Cummings, M. (1996) Apoptosis of epithelial cells in vivo involves tissue transglutaminase upregulation. *J. Pathol.* **179,** 288–293.
51. Szondy, Z., Molnar, P., Nemes, Z., Boyiadzis, M, Kedei, N., Toth, R., and Fesus, L. (1997) Differential expression of tissue transglutaminase during in vivo apoptosis of thymocytes induced via distinct signalling pathways. *FEBS Lett.* **404,** 307–313.
52. Hilton, D. A., Love, S., and Barber, R. (1997) Demonstration of apoptotic cells in tissue sections by in situ hybridization using digoxigenin-labelled poly(A) oligonucleotide probes to detect thymidine-rich DNA sequences. *J. Histochem. Cytochem.* **45,** 13.
53. Nicoletti, I., Migliorati, G., Pagliacci, M. C., Grignani, F., and Riccardi, C. (1991) A rapid and simple method for measuring thymocyte apoptosis by propidium iodide staining and flow cytometry. *J. Immunol Meth.* **137,** 271–279.
54. Tewari, M., Quan, L. T., O'Rourke, K., Desnoyers, S., Zeng, Z., Beidler, D. R., Poirer, G., Salvesen G. S., and Dixit, V. M. (1995) CPP32b, a mammalian homolog of CED-3, is a Crm-A inhibitable protease that cleaves the death substrate poly(ADP-ribose) polymerase. *Cell* **81,** 801–809.
55. Aherne, W. A. and Dunnill, M. S. (1982) Morphometry. Edward Arnold, London, UK.

6

Measurement of P-glycoprotein Function

Henk J. Broxterman

1. Introduction

The *MDR*1-encoded P-glycoprotein (Pgp), when overexpressed in tumor cells, confers resistance to many clinically important classes of anticancer drugs. This phenomenon is called multidrug resistance (MDR). The finding that this gene was expressed in many types of human cancers has stimulated many studies into the relevance of this protein for clinical chemotherapy resistance *(1)*. Pgp is a protein that causes a net transport of substrate drug molecules over the plasma membrane of the cell, resulting in a lowered free cytosolic drug concentration. Therefore, the drug target(s) "feel" a lower drug concentration, resulting in less drug-induced damage and cell-kill. The measurement of the active (adenosine triphosphate [ATP]-dependent) drug transport or efflux function of Pgp is, therefore, a theoretically elegant way to quantify the number of active or "functional" Pgp molecules per cell *(2,3)*. Such assays are called functional assays in this chapter. One disadvantage is, however, that without additional data no unambiguous evidence of the molecular nature of the transport protein is obtained, the advantage is that the relevant biological feature is measured. The latter cannot be derived easily from the mRNA or protein expression levels, because a number of factors may influence the net effect of transporter proteins, such as other membrane properties specific to certain cells *(3,4)*. In practice, important criteria for the usefulness of any MDR assay are its specificity, sensitivity, and reproducibility. During an international workshop, it was found that functional Pgp assays performed better than other assays in the study of acute myelogenous leukemia (AML) *(5)*. This fits closely with the experience that functional Pgp assays are, in practice, limited to the study of "liquid" tumors, mainly leukemias *(6)*. In fact, the only limitation—albeit a serious one—of the functional assays is the need

From: *Methods in Molecular Medicine, Vol. 28: Cytotoxic Drug Resistance Mechanisms*
Edited by: R. Brown and U. Böger-Brown © Humana Press Inc., Totowa, NJ

of viable tumor-cell suspensions, which are difficult to obtain from many solid tumors. Because of the limited use of functional assays for solid tumor-derived cells, we describe here a protocol only for leukemias. If viable tumor cells from a solid tumor can be obtained, functional Pgp assays can be set up analogous to the assays for leukemias *(7,8)*. As mentioned, a functional assay for Pgp is a measure of the active efflux of a Pgp substrate over the plasma membrane. This requires detection of substrate molecules taken up by the cells after a certain time period of incubation of cells with the substrate. Alternatively, the substrate that is retained in the cells or effluxed into the medium after an efflux period in substrate-free medium is measured. Substrates initially used for these assays were the anthracyclines doxorubicin or daunorubicin. These can be conveniently measured because of their intrinsic fluorescence properties *(9)* or their availability in radiolabeled form *(10)*. The use of a flow cytometer with fluorescence detection has great advantage in routine detection in hematology; therefore, it is the method of choice.

An important improvement of these assays is the use of fluorescent Pgp substrates with a much higher sensitivity than the anthracyclines. Many of these are dyes that had other applications to monitor cellular functions, such as viability, mitochondrial potential, or pH. We and others have compared extensively many of these dyes for their sensitivity and specificity to detect Pgp function in tumor cell lines *(8,11)*, hematopoietic progenitor cells *(12)* and AMLs *(13)*. We have chosen to use rhodamine 123 as dye and have validated its use by direct comparison with radiolabeled daunorubicin and vincristine accumulation in AMLs *(14)*.

A second important and practical improvement is the use of a compound that blocks the efflux of the fluorescent substrate. The measurement of the ratio of fluorescent probe accumulating in the cell with and without a Pgp blocker makes the obtained data less dependent on a number of parameters that may cause variation between cells and samples. We have chosen to use the cyclosporin analog PSC 833 as Pgp inhibitor, which, at a concentration of 2 μM, completely blocks the Pgp-mediated efflux of probes such as daunorubicin or rhodamine 123 in cells with a clinically relevant Pgp content *(6,11,14)*. In addition, we have chosen to measure the practically more convenient cellular accumulation of probe instead of cellular retention after an efflux period, although the latter is theoretically more sensitive *(15)*. In our experience, the use of rhodamine 123 as Pgp probe, combined with PSC 833 as Pgp inhibitor, offers a sensitive and reproducible Pgp functional assay in AML. Although we prefer to use fresh cells, appropriately frozen and thawed cells can be used for this assay, as extensively discussed previously *(4,14)*.

A final, general point of attention when using a functional Pgp assay is the use of a control cell line. Although the use of fluorescent beads in flow cytometry is indicated in order to be able to monitor day-to-day (intra-laboratory) or inter-instrumental/laboratory variations, we have chosen to assay a cell line with no Pgp expression (KB3-1) ***(16)*** and one with a very low Pgp content (KB8) ***(16)*** in parallel to the experimental samples. This procedure allows us to control for performance of the probe, incubation procedures, and instrument. However, because a cell line in culture may continuously change its resistance pattern, it is not an absolute, stable control. Also, because a cell line also does not control for the very important quality of the experimental sample with regard to membrane permeability, metabolism, and so forth, great care and reproducibility in handling of the leukemic cells is of utmost importance.

2. Materials

1. Lymphoprep (Ficoll-Paque; Pharmacia Biotech, Uppsala, Sweden) or similar cell-separation medium. Storage according to manufacturer's recommendations.
2. A sterile, well-buffered medium, such as Dulbecco's minimal essential medium (DMEM) without phenol red or sodium bicarbonate, supplemented with 20 m*M* HEPES and set at pH = 7.4 at 37°C, (which is 7.58 at room temperature because of temperature coefficient of HEPES). Store sterile at 4°C.
3. Fetal calf serum (FCS) or another convenient protein supplement (for instance 4% bovine serum albumin [BSA] solution). Store sterile at 4°C or for periods longer than 1 mo at –20°C.
4. Dimethyl sulfoxide (DMSO), analytical grade.
5. Ethanol, analytical grade.
6. 1 mg/mL rhodamine 123 (Sigma, St. Louis, MO; Molecular Probes, Eugene, OR) in DMSO; store in polypropylene vials (Eppendorf) in aliquots protected from light at –20°C.
7. 4 m*M* daunorubicin hydrochloride (Sigma) in DMSO; store in polypropylene vials (Eppendorf) in aliquots protected from light at –20°C.
8. 5 m*M* PSC 833 (Novartis, Basel, Switzerland) in ethanol; store in aliquots in well-sealed, screw-cap polypropylene vials at –20°C.
9. Shaking waterbath at 37°C.
10. Centrifuge for Eppendorf vials.
11. Flow cytometer.

3. Methods

1. You will need mononuclear cells from peripheral blood or bone marrow collected in heparinized glass tubes and isolated on Ficoll-Paque as rapidly as possible. After collecting the interphase cells, they are washed and resuspended in the buffered medium supplemented with 10% FCS (= assay medium) and kept on melting ice until analysis. Alternatively, the cells are frozen in medium with 10% DSMO and at least 10% FCS in liquid nitrogen according to protocols for cryopreservation (*see* **Note 1**).

2. When frozen cells are used for the assay, they have to be thawed carefully. Pre-warm buffer with 40% FCS to 37°C. Rapidly thaw the vial from the liquid nitrogen by shaking in a 37°C waterbath and pipet the cell suspension without air bubbles in 10 volumes of the pre-warmed medium, mix gently to dilute the DMSO out rapidly, and spin the cells down. Resuspend the cells in pre-warmed assay medium and incubate the cells 1 h at 37°C for recovery of metabolic functions (*see* **Note 2**), then resuspend in assay medium (10% FCS) and record the viability of the cells with trypan blue, which is preferably >90%.
3. Dilute rhodamine 123 and optionally also daunorubicin (*see* **Note 3**) from the stock solutions shortly before use in assay medium to make a solution of 200 mg/mL (or 0.5 μ*M*) rhodamine 123 (4 μL of the stock into 20 mL) and 2 μ*M* daunorubicin (10 μL of stock into 20 mL). These solutions are divided in two parts and 4 μL of PSC 833 stock is added to 10 mL solution to make 2 μ*M* PSC 833 (*see* **Note 4**). Rapidly re-freeze the rest of the stocks or if vials are for one-time use (which is preferable) discard the remainder as chemical waste. These probes are light sensitive; therefore, incubations and samples stored until analysis should be protected from light. Brief handling of the solutions, such as diluting, centrifuging, and so on can be done at normal light.
4. Optional: if control cell lines are used in parallel to the leukemic sample these should have been cultured on previous days to have logarithmic growth. They are harvested, counted and suspended in assay medium (*see* **Note 5**).
5. The leukemic cells should be counted and 0.5–1 × 10^6 cells pipetted in Eppendorf vials. Control tumor cells from a cell line should be used at about 100,000 cells/vial. Cells are spun down in a table centrifuge, decanted, and the cells resuspended in 1 mL of probe solutions with or without PSC 833. Do all determinations in duplicate. Incubate the closed vials protected from light in a shaking waterbath for 75 min at 37°C and shake by hand every 15 min to avoid pelleting of the cells during the incubation (*see* **Note 6**). Spin the cells down in an Eppendorf centrifuge for 10 s and wash the cells once in ice-cold assay medium. Resuspend the cells in 1 mL of assay medium and keep the cells on ice protected from light until flow cytometric analysis (as soon as possible, however, the drug efflux is negligible for at least 1 h on ice). Blanks (singular) are parallel vials with cells to which 1 mL of the appropriate cold drug solution is added, which are then centrifuged immediately, washed, and resuspended similarly to the experimental vials. These blanks are used to determine the aspecific binding of dye to the cells. PSC 833 did not affect the background fluorescence under the present conditions (*see* **Note 7**).
6. The fluorescence distribution of the cells is determined on a flow cytometer for rhodamine 123 in the FL1 channel and for daunorubicin in the FL2 channel. Preferably, identical detector settings are used every day. The blanks are used to position the signal in the first decade. The leukemic blast population is selected based on scatter characteristics.
7. The Pgp function index is the effect of the Pgp inhibitor (PSC 833) on the mean fluorescence (F_{mean}) of the leukemic cell population and is calculated as the ratio

of the F_{mean} of the cells incubated with PSC 833 and without PSC 833: [F_{mean}(probe + PSC 833) – F_{mean}(blank)]: [F_{mean}(probe) – F_{mean}(blank)]. In addition, report the same parameter for a subpopulation, if present, and the percentage of cells in this subpopulation (*see* **Note 8**). Determined in this way, the maximal ratios found in primary untreated AMLs are about 1.5 for daunorubicin and about 5 for rhodamine 123, with a subpopulation with higher values found only occasionally ***(4,14)***.

8. It is recommended (at least when starting this assay) to determine the day-to-day reproducibility in the investigator's hands by running cell lines and/or frozen samples from a known Pgp- negative and a known Pgp-positive AML thawed on consecutive days.

4. Notes

1. Freezing in medium with a high protein content may preserve cells better. Up to 90% FCS with 10% DMSO has been used ***(13)***. In general, we recommend performing the assays as rapid as possible after collecting the blood or marrow from the patient (preferably within 2–6 h). During this period, we prefer to keep the cells on ice in protein rich-medium (i.e., the assay medium) for reproducibility of conditions. It may be possible to store the cells as whole blood or marrow at room temperature for a few hours, but—at least for the less sensitive probe (daunorubicin)—a good performance of those cells cannot be guaranteed ***(4)***. One study has reported in detail the consequences for the Pgp function of storage of AML samples under different conditions and found that, after overnight storage of whole blood at room temperature, the results were inferior ***(17)***. We have found similar results when using doxorubicin as probe ***(4)***. Although some studies use leukemic samples after overnight shipping at ambient temperature, such a procedure has not been validated, to my knowledge. Rather, it would be preferable to keep samples on ice or to freeze samples if a storage time longer than one working day is anticipated. Of course, especially in cases where the result of the test may have implications for the treatment of the patient, the fresh cell assay is indicated, and results can be obtained within a few hours.
2. For a highly sensitive probe such as rhodamine 123 ***(14)*** or 3,3'-diethyloxacarbocyanine iodide ($DiOC_2(3)$) ***(13)***, the performance of the assay with thawed cells seems to be good, which means that very similar—although not exactly the same—values are obtained as with the fresh cells ***(14)***. When a probe with less sensitivity is used, the assay is more likely to be subject to small variations in viability or membrane alterations of the cells that will occur after a freezing and thawing procedure. The optimal time for recovery of cells (as well as the exact events that occur during this "recovery" period) has not been extensively investigated for different probes, but, admittedly, seems to be partly intuitive. An incubation period substantially longer than 2 h, however, may not be advisable (*see* **Note 1** and ref. *17*).
3. We routinely use rhodamine 123 and daunorubicin, because the use of two different probes may give useful information. However, as noted in the Introduction

daunorubicin is not a sensitive probe when compared to rhodamine 123 (*see* also **Subheading 3.7.**). Recently we have identified a third probe with high sensitivity, namely SYTO® 16 (Molecular Probes). We strongly recommend using this in addition to, or instead of, daunorubicin, for those who wish to perform more extensive investigations (details for the use of this probe are described in ref. ***8***). Another very sensitive probe for the Pgp function, as described by others, is $DiOC_2(3)$, which can also be combined more easily with reagents used for double- or triple-labeling than rhodamine 123, because there is less spectral overlap with flow cytometry dyes such as fluorescein isothiocyantate (FITC) and phycoerythrin (PE) ***(12,13)***. Rhodamine 123 can be combined in a double-labeling procedure with PE, but extensive compensation is needed ***(12)***. As far as I know, methods for the combination of a functional Pgp test with the labeling of an antigen (Pgp or CD34) on the same cells have not yet been validated rigorously. However, this certainly is a clinically very relevant option for those laboratories that have the opportunity to do so (*see* ref. ***13***). Our preliminary data suggest that it is possible to combine a functional Pgp test with SYTO® 16 (± PSC 833; 45 min, 37°C) after washing the cells with anti-CD34 labeling (30 min, 0°C). Routinely, we run samples in parallel for the determination of Pgp expression by flow cytometry with the monoclonal antibody (MAb) MRK-16.

4. The choice of Pgp inhibitor is not without importance. When measuring fluorescence one always has to be aware of direct interactions with fluorescence of the dye not related to the Pgp function. This can be checked in Pgp-negative cell lines and AML samples. In addition, effects on other transporters than Pgp may theoretically occur, which are unwanted if one intends to have a Pgp-specific method. On the other hand, if one wishes to determine the effect of a certain drug on the cellular accumulation of a probe, whether or not related to one specific transporter, this is not an unwanted side-effect. For instance, Pgp modulators such as verapamil or cyclosporin A may be less Pgp-specific in combination with certain dyes. (For an extensive discussion of this matter *see* ref. ***4***.)
5. Unfortunately, no internationally agreed-upon standard cell lines are available from a central supplier as stocks cultured under identical conditions. Apart from the ketone bodies (KB) series of cell lines chosen by us ***(16)***, other series of cell lines have been proposed ***(5)***. Anyone who uses cell line controls should take care to use (at least) one *MDR*1/Pgp negative cell line and one cell line with a low Pgp expression, comparable to most clinical samples. In particular, the low Pgp-expressing cells may increase Pgp expression even when cultured with a constant concentration of the selecting drug.
6. An incubation time of 75 min was chosen because a steady-state for daunorubicin is reached, which is the preferred situation. It takes a (far) longer time to reach steady-state accumulation of rhodamine 123, depending on the cell type. For simplicity, the same time was chosen. For the novel probe SYTO 16, 45 min incubation is sufficient to reach steady-state ***(8)***.

7. Although, preferably, samples with a low viability count are discarded, one may wish to exclude dead cells from the analysis by adding propidium iodide (PI) (Sigma, 1 µg/mL) immediately before the analysis and gating them out. Also, DNAse I (0.005%) may be added to avoid the loss of viable cells in such samples by clumping during incubation and centrifugation.
8. The reporting of data of Pgp expression and function has been a matter of much debate ***(4,5,13)***. Many papers have reported the results exclusively as percentage "Pgp-positive" cells, whatever the detection method was. In our experience in all daunorubicin-labeled AMLs and in the great majority of rhodamine 123-labeled AMLs there is extensive overlap of the plus and minus PSC 833 populations, without clear indications of the presence of discrete subpopulation(s). This means that also the potential contamination of the blast gate with remaining normal cells apparently does not show up as a discrete population in the present Pgp function test. The ratio that we use to express the data (*see* **Subheading 3.7.**) has the advantage that this parameter can easily be interpreted as a percentage of increase in cellular drug uptake after inhibition of Pgp ***(14)***. Nevertheless, it may be recommended to use in addition to this ratio the Kolmogarov-Smirnov test (D-value) ***(18)*** to reveal in an objective, numerical way potential small differences between the two distributions as applied by some authors ***(13,19)***.

References

1. Fojo, A. T., Ueda, K., Slamon, D. J., Poplack, D. G., Gottesman, M. M., and Pastan, I. (1987) Expression of multidrug-resistance gene in human tumors and tissues. *Proc. Natl. Acad. Sci. USA 84,* 265–269.
2. Reizenstein, P. (1993) Resistance modifying agents are active in some patients with hematological malignancy. *Leukemia Res.* **17,** 295–298.
3. Chaudhary, P. M., Mechetner, E. B., and Roninson, I B. (1994) Response. *Blood* **83,** 329–330.
4. Broxterman, H. J., Lankelma, J., Pinedo, H. M., Eekman, C. A., Währer, D. C. R., Ossenkoppele, G. J., and Schuurhuis, G. J. (1997) Theoretical and practical considerations for the measurement of P-glycoprote in function in acute myeloid leukemia. *Leukemia* **11,** 1110–1118.
5. Beck, W. T., Grogan, T. M., Willman, C. L., Cordon-Cardo, C. L., Parham, D. M., Kuttesch, J. F., Andreeff, M., Bates, S. E., Berard, C. W., Boyett, J. M., Brophy, N. A., Broxterman, H. J., Chan, H. S. L., Dalton, W. S., Dietel, M., Fojo, A. T., Gascoyne, R. D., Head, D., Houghton, P. J., Srivastava, D. K., Lehnert, M., Leith, C. P., Paietta, E., Pavelic, Z. P., Kimsza, L., Roninson, I. B., Sikic, B. I., Twentyman, P. R., Warnke, R., and Weinstein, R. (1996) Methods to detect P-glycoprotein-associated multidrug resistance in patients' tumors: consensus recommendations. *Cancer Res.* **56,** 3010–3020.
6. Broxterman, H. J., Lankelma, J., and Pinedo, H. M. (1996) How to probe clinical tumour samples for P-glycoprotein and multidrug resistance-associated protein. *Eur. J. Cancer* **32A,** 1024–1033.

7. Broxterman, H. J., Feller, N., Kuiper, C. M., Boven, E., Versantvoort, C. H. M., Teerlink, T., Pinedo, H. M., and Lankelma, J. (1995) Correlation between functional and molecular analysis of mdrl P-glycoprotein in human solid tumor xenografts. *Int. J. Cancer* **61,** 880–886.
8. Broxterman, H. J., Schuurhuis, G. J., Lankelma, J., Oberink, J. W., Eekman, C. A., Claessen, A. M. E., Hoekman, K., Poot, M., and Pinedo, H. M. (1997) Highly sensitive and specific detection of P-glycoprotein function for hematological and solid tumor cells using a novel nucleic acid stain. *Br. J. Cancer* **76,** 1029–1034.
9. Nooter, K., Sonneveld, P., Oostrurn, R., Herweijer, H., Hagenbeek, T., and Valerio, D. (1990) Overexpression of the *mdr1* gene in blast cells from patients with acute myelocytic leukemia is associated with decreased anthracycline accumulation that can be restored by cyclosporin-A. *Int. J. Cancer* **45,** 263–268.
10. Schuurhuis, G. J., Broxterman, H. J., Ossenkoppele, G. J., Baak, J. P. A., Eekman, C. A., Kuiper, C. M., Feller, N., van Heyningen, T. H. M., Klumper, E., Pieters, R., Lankelma, J., and Pinedo, H. M. (1995) Functional multidrug resistance phenotype associated with combined overexpression of Pgp/MDR1 and MRP together with 1-β-D-arabinofuranosylcytosine sensitivity may predict clinical response in acute myeloid leukemia. *Clin. Cancer Res.* **1,** 81–93.
11. Feller, N., Kuiper, C. M., Lankelma, J., Ruhdal, J. K., Scheper, R. J., Pinedo, H. M., and Broxterman, H. J. *(1995)* Functional detection of *MDR*1/P170 and *MRP*/P190-mediated multidrug resistance in tumour cells by flow cytometry. *Br. J. Cancer* **72,** 543–549.
12. Chaudhary, P. M. and Roninson, I. B. (199 l) Expression and activity of P-glycoprotein, a multidrug efflux pump, in human hematopoietic stem cells. *Cell* **66,** 85–94.
13. Leith, C. P., Chen, I-M, Kopecky, K. J., Appelbaum, F. R., Head, D. R., Godwin, J. E., Weick, J. K., and Willman, C. L. (1995) Correlation of multidrug resistance (MDR1) protein expression with functional dye/drug efflux in acute myeloid leukemia by multiparameter flow cytometry: identification of discordant MDR^-/$efflux^+$ and MDR^+/$efflux^-$ cases. *Blood* **86,** 2329–2342.
14. Broxterman, H. J., Sonneveld, P., Feller, N., Ossenlcoppele, G. J., Wahrer, D. C. R., Eekman, C. A., Schoester, M., Lankelma, J., Pinedo, H. M., Löwenberg, B., and Schuurhuis, G. J. (1996) Quality control of multidrug resistance assays in adult acute leukemia: correlation between assays for P-glycoprotein expression and activity. *Blood* **87,** 4809–4816.
15. Ross, D. D., Wooten, P. J., Sridhara, R., Ordóñez, J. V., Lee, E. J., and Schiffer, C. A. (1993). Enhancement of daunorubicin accumulation, retention, and cytotoxicity by verapamil or cyclosporin A in blast cells from patients with previously untreated acute myeloid leukemia. *Blood* **82,** 1288–1299.
16. Noonan, K. E., Beck, C., Holzmayer, T. A., Chin, J. E., Wunder, J. S., Andrulis, I. L., Gazdar, A. F., Willman, C. L., Griffith, B., von Hoff, D. D. and Roninson, I. B. (1990) Quantitative analysis of *MDR*1 (multidrug resistance) gene expression in human tumors by polymerase chain reaction. *Proc. Natl. Acad. Sci. USA* **87,** 7160–7164.

17. Hegewisch-Becker, S., Faltz, C., and Hossfeld, D. K. (1996) Prolongation of medium exchange is associated with a decrease in function but not expression of the P-glycoprotein pump in leukaemic cells. *Eur. J. Haematol.* **56,** 12–22.
18. Young, I. T. (1977) Proof without prejudice: use of the Kolmogarov-Smirnov test for the analysis of histograms from flow systems and other sources. J: *Histochem. Cytochem.* **25,** 935–941.
19. Maslak, P., Hegewisch-Becker, S., Godfrey, L., and Andreeff, M. (1994) Flow cytometric determination of the multidrug-resistant phenotype in acute leukemia. *Cytometry* **17,** 84–93.

7

Measuring *MDR*-1 by Quantitative RT-PCR

Susan E. Bates, Zhirong Zhan, Joanna Regis, and Erick Gamelin

1. Introduction

Accurate determination of the expression of P-glycoprotein and its encoding mRNA, *MDR*-1, is key to determining the importance of this mechanism of drug resistance in the clinic. This understanding is critical to development of P-glycoprotein antagonists to block drug efflux and to overcome drug resistance. Reversal studies are best performed in diseases in which this mechanism represents the major component of drug resistance. The clearest approach to identifying these is to measure *MDR*-1 mRNA or P-glycoprotein in tumors at diagnosis, at the time of disease recurrence, and before and after treatment with P-glycoprotein reversal agents.

Multiple methods have been used to detect *MDR*-1 mRNA or P-glycoprotein *(1–3)*. RNA methods include Northern and slot blot measurement, RNA *in situ* hybridization, and the quantitative polymerase chain reaction (PCR), which is the topic of this chapter. Protein methods include immunoblotting, immunohistochemistry, and immunofluorescence. The RNA *in situ* hybridization and immunohistochemical methods have as a chief advantage the detection of *MDR*-1/P-glycoprotein expression in individual cells observed on a microscope slide. Although fewer cells are observed overall than in the other methods, the advantage of using microscopy is to exclude detection of expression in contaminating normal tissues. In contrast, the methods which measure expression in cell populations, including the PCR methods, lack the cell-based analysis. Yet, quantitative PCR offers a highly sensitive and specific approach to the detection of *MDR*-1 mRNA *(4–9)*. The problem of contaminating normal tissue can be dealt with by taking into account the basal level of expression in the normal tissue surrounding the tumor tissue. Thus, accurate results for *MDR*-1 mRNA quantitation can readily be obtained from metastatic sites in

From: *Methods in Molecular Medicine, Vol. 28: Cytotoxic Drug Resistance Mechanisms*
Edited by: R. Brown and U. Böger-Brown © Humana Press Inc., Totowa, NJ

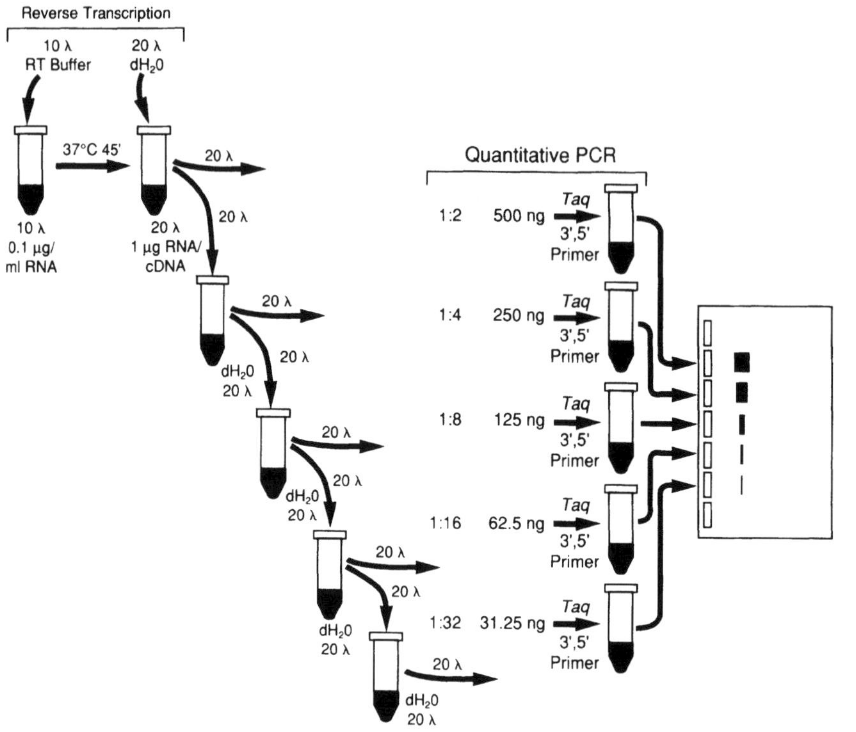

Fig. 1. Schematic diagram of quantitative PCR method. As shown in the schema, 1 µg total RNA is subjected to reverse transcription, and serially diluted in depH_2O for individual PCR reactions.

the lung, given the low level of expression in normal lung tissue. On the other hand, less confidence may be placed in *MDR*-1 mRNA values obtained from metastatic sites in the liver, given the high level of expression in normal liver. The fraction of contaminating normal cells should be assessed pathologically on every tumor sample biopsy.

Our approach for quantitating *MDR*-1 mRNA by PCR begins with reverse transcription of the mRNA to cDNA. Customarily, 1 µg total RNA is subjected to the reverse transcription reaction following gel electrophoresis that verifies the quality and quantity of the RNA measurements (*see* **Note 1**). The resulting cDNA is serially diluted and separate PCR reactions are performed on each of the serial dilutions (**Fig. 1**). This will allow determination of the exponential range of amplification. By convention, the quantity of cDNA in each serial dilution is referred to by either the dilution factor or the calculated "input RNA" for that dilution. When the PCR products are in the exponential range, the difference in the optical density of the PCR products from a two-fold dilution of the cDNA will be two-fold. The key to this method is that the amplification must be performed in the exponential range. In parallel and in separate reaction tubes, RNA from a standard cell line is amplified to provide a gauge for normalizing the results. We use total RNA from SW620 cells, which stably express a low level of *MDR*-1 mRNA. The exponential range is usually comparable to or below the level of PCR product amplified from the cDNA derived from 125 ng RNA isolated from the positive control, SW620 (*see* **Note 2**). In parallel tubes, serial dilutions are amplified for β_2-microglobulin, which provides a control for normalization of the RNA quantity (*see* **Note 3**). Because of the much higher level of expression of β_2-microglobulin, the dilutions are much greater in order to achieve the exponential range. Densitometry is performed on the ethidium-bromide stained gel containing PCR products separated by electrophoresis (*see* **Note 4**). Following densitometry, the signal in the sample of interest is normalized to the levels of expression of *MDR*-1 and β_2-microglobulin in SW620, which have been arbitrarily assigned values of 10 and 1, respectively. Subsequently, the *MDR*-1 level is divided by the β_2-microglobulin level to give the final result. Carefully performed, this method is reproducible to within two-fold.

Accurate quantitation with this PCR method relies upon several prerequisites. First, the quantity of RNA should be as accurately measured as possible. The quality of RNA is also important, as partially degraded RNA will not give good PCR results. The most accurate approach to confirming RNA quantity and quality is to run a denaturing RNA gel, including a comparable quantity of the control RNA for comparison. This gel can be stained with ethidium bromide and densitometry applied to quantitate differences in the RNA loading. This can be used as a second approach to normalizing the amount of input RNA, and provides a valuable way to verify the results of the normalization using β_2-microglobulin expression. Second, quantitative PCR begins with reverse transcription to transcribe the RNA to DNA, and this reaction must faithfully reflect the amount of mRNA in the sample. Third, the primers utilized and the conditions chosen for the PCR reaction should provide exponential amplification (*see* **Note 5**). A given primer set may not give exponential amplification due to differences in secondary structure in the PCR product which result in differences in amplification efficiency. Primers from regions in the gene which do not span an intron may give a PCR product with increased background due to amplification of contaminating genomic DNA. This problem can be eliminated by choosing primers which span an intron, resulting in either a product which is easily distinguished from the cDNA product, or a product which is too large to amplify. The only exception to this would be the detection of pseudogenes. While no pseudogenes have been described for *MDR*-1, they do exist for other genes and should be considered. If doubt exists, the PCR can be performed without the RT to determine their existence; or the

RNA sample can be treated with DNase to remove the pseudogene prior to reverse transcription.

A final and chief prerequisite for accurate quantitation is that it must be performed on reactions still in the exponential phase of amplification *(4,10,11)*. The plateau of PCR reaction is a well-described phenomenon, in which the efficiency of amplification decreases dramatically. For the method we utilize, quantitation in the plateau phase greatly underestimates gene expression. The cause of the PCR plateau is not well-understood, but has been attributed to insufficient primer concentrations *(12,13)*, insufficient *Taq* polymerase *(14)*, and competition between primers and products for reannealing and further amplification *(15)*. Whatever the cause, quantitation in the plateau phase is inaccurate. Early plateau can be induced by amplification of a second target in the same PCR tube (either an exogenous or an endogenous target included for quantitation in some PCR protocols), amplification of primer dimers, amplification of contaminants, or amplification of nonspecific background bands (*see* **Note 5**).

The three most frequently cited disadvantages to the protocol delineated here are: the lack of an internal control for the efficiency of the RT and PCR reactions; the requirement for the quantitation in the exponential phase of amplification; and the variability of expression of the control gene. The first argument suggests that the greatest variability in quantitative PCR arises from variable reaction efficiency from sample to sample. Our experience has been that the chief variability in performing quantitative PCR from clinical samples arises from difficulty in quantitating the amount of RNA generated from very tiny biopsy samples and needle aspirates. In this setting, careful measurement of the OD is often incorrect, and may not even be possible with small samples. As to the PCR efficiency, the simultaneous amplification of a control RNA sample derived from a large previously prepared RNA quantity (in our studies, RNA from SW620 is the control RNA), has allowed detection of problems with the RT or PCR reaction. When present, these problems affected all of the samples in an experiment and were recognized as reduced PCR product, relative to that normally obtained (*see* **Note 6**). The other two disadvantages are relative. The requirement for exponential amplification is indeed critical to the success of the method. However, exponential amplification with the *MDR*-1 primers is always obtained with 125 ng or less input cDNA/RNA from SW620. Thus, a test sample can be run at the same dilution to determine in which direction the serial dilutions need to go to perform the quantitation accurately (*see* **Note 2**). Finally, quantitation of a control gene to determine RNA loading is a necessity for any PCR quantitative method. We have found β_2-microglobulin most reliable, but this should be verified for each individual model system (*see* **Note 3**).

A number of other approaches to quantitative PCR have been described in recent reviews ***(10,11,15–17)***. As with any methodology, there are advantages and disadvantages to each approach. Some protocols incorporate a set of primers recognizing a housekeeping gene along with primers recognizing the target gene in the PCR reaction, which then serves as in our method, as a control for RNA loading, RT efficiency, and for PCR efficiency. The chief disadvantage of this approach is that amplification of the housekeeping gene mRNA, which is expressed at high levels, brings the PCR reaction to plateau much more quickly, suppressing amplification of the gene of interest, which is expressed at much lower levels. This results in a lower level of expression than would have been otherwise detected ***(4,18)***. Depending upon the level of gene expression in the sample, the competition has a greater or lesser effect, and provides inaccurate quantitation. Consequently, co-amplification should be avoided in quantitative protocols.

A commonly used approach, known as the competitive PCR method, exploits the competition and plateau features of PCR to quantitate the expression of the mRNA of interest ***(15,16)***. The reaction incorporates an RNA or DNA PCR template which is included with the sample and amplified along with the RNA of interest. The most frequently used alternate methods include the use of competitive RNA or DNA PCR templates that are different in size, contain a recognizable mutation detectable because of gel electrophoresis separation properties, or contain a restriction site to allow digestion following PCR. Typically, in these approaches, serial dilutions of a known concentration of the competitor RNA or DNA are added to tubes containing equal, but unknown quantities of the mRNA of interest. Subsequently, RT is performed, followed by PCR amplification. The differing PCR products are separated by gel electrophoresis, and the concentration in the unknown sample is obtained at the dilution where the product of the unknown sample is equal to the product of the competitor.

The chief advantage of the competitive PCR method is that the PCR reaction can proceed to plateau without affecting the equivalent concentration, where equal product and competitor ratios occur. While this is clearly a major advantage, several other elements of the competitive method are potential sources of error. A critical assumption of this method is that the amplification of the two PCR products will proceed with equal efficiency in the same PCR reaction tube. Comparable amplification efficiency of the two templates must be documented *a priori*, before using the competitive PCR in quantitation ***(19,20)***. Although one would not expect that a single base pair difference between two PCR products could yield a large difference in amplification efficiency, precisely such an observation has been reported ***(21)***. This potential disparity may be even greater when one considers that the templates used in these analyses often differ by more than one base pair. A second critical

Table 1
Primers Used for Quantitative PCR Analysis of *MDR*-1, *MRP*, and β_2-Microglobulin Expression *(4,5,22,23)*

3' *MRP*
5'ACCTCCTCATTCGCATCCACCTTGG3'
5'*MRP*
5'CGGAAACCATCCACGACCCTAATCC3'
5'*MDR*-1
5'GCCTGGCAGCTGGAAGACAAATACACAAAATT3'
3'*MDR*-1
5'CAGACAGCAGCTGACAGTCCAAGAACAGGACT3'
5'β_2-microglobulin
5'GTGGAGCATTCAGACTTGTCTTTCAGCA3'
3'β_2-microglobulin
5'TTCACTCAATCCAAATGCGGCATCTTC3'

assumption in the competitive PCR assay is that RNA O.D. measurements are accurate, since controls for RNA loading are not required in all assays. Although careful RNA quantitation may be planned prior to PCR, some samples, particularly small clinical samples, do not yield enough RNA to accurately quantitate by densitometry. In addition to potential errors introduced in measuring and aliquoting RNA before the reverse transcription, in competitive PCR there is also the potential error introduced in aliquoting the competitive template. Amplification of an endogenous or housekeeping gene can be performed to quantitate RNA loading, but requires establishment of a second reaction. A third variable in some competitive protocols is the use of DNA as the competitor template, which does not require reverse transcription prior to PCR, therefore omits a control for RT efficiency. The best control for the RT step is to perform RT on the competitor or control RNA, and on the sample RNA simultaneously. Regardless of the PCR approach chosen, the assay used must be carefully optimized and validated, with controls tailored to the types of questions being asked in the study.

Table 1 shows the primer pairs used successfully for *MDR*-1 and *MRP* detection by our laboratory and others *(4,7,22,23)*. We have observed that primers from other regions of *MDR*-1 do not always give the same intensity of signal, given identical loading and PCR conditions. This can be due to lower efficiency of amplification, or to competition from background giving nonspecific PCR products (*see* **Note 5**). These products are amplified along with the specific product, cause competition, and inaccuracy in quantitation. The primers listed in **Table 1** have repeatedly shown low background and exponential amplification.

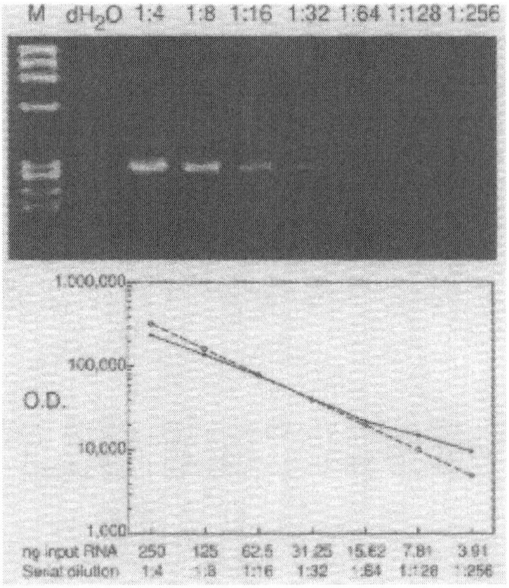

Fig. 2. Exponential range for *MDR*-1 amplification in a renal cell carcinoma line. Top panel: Ethidium-stained agarose gel demonstrating results of PCR amplification of *MDR*-1 mRNA in serially diluted cDNA. Bottom panel: Densitometric values are plotted on the y-axis, while the dilution and the calculated amount of input RNA in the

The results of the electrophoretic separation of PCR products are shown in **Figs. 2** and **3**. **Figure 2** shows the results of amplification of *MDR*-1 in cDNA derived from a renal cell carcinoma cell line. The ethidium-stained PCR products were evaluated by densitometry, and the results plotted on the graph. The ideal is shown as a dashed line, based on two-fold dilutions yielding two-fold differences in PCR product. **Figure 3** shows the results of *MDR*-1 and *MRP* quantitation for parental SW620 cells, a human colon carcinoma cell line used as a control for normalization; and for two drug resistant sublines, SW620 Ad 20 and Ad300 *(3)*. These sublines were selected in Adriamycin and cultured in 20 and 300 ng/mL Adriamycin, respectively. Results in the drug resistant sublines are normalized to the results for SW620, which is arbitrarily ascribed a value of 10. In the top panel, amplifications in the exponential range for *MDR*-1 are shown. For SW620 parental cells, densitometric results showing a 2.1-fold difference between the 125 ng sample and the 62.5 ng sample confirm the exponential range. For Ad20, the exponential phase was found by diluting the cDNA to 0.25 ng input RNA, and for Ad300, the exponential phase was found by diluting the cDNA to 0.06 The middle panel demonstrates the

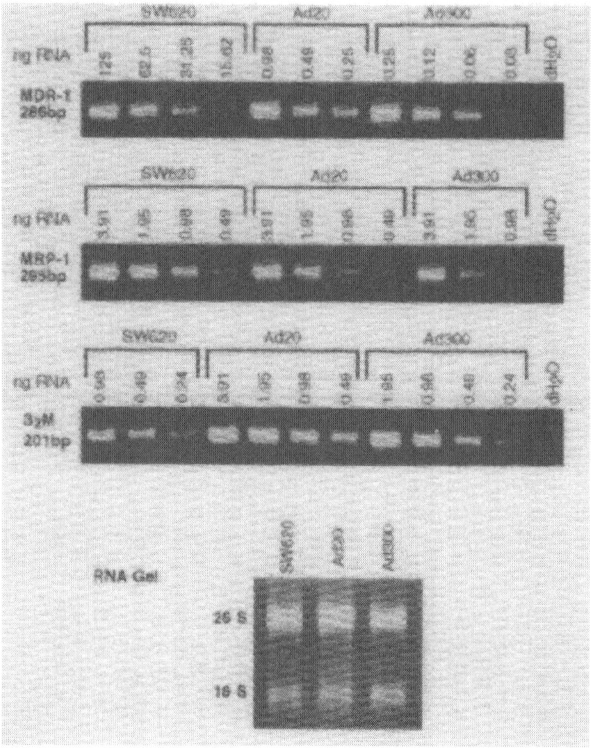

Fig. 3. Expression of *MDR*-1, *MRP*, and β_2-microglobulin mRNAs in drug resistant SW620 Ad20 and 300 cells. The three panels demonstrate the dilution series from which mRNA expression levels can be calculated. Dilution yields PCR products which are two-fold different when measured by densitometry from cDNA diluted to provide the exponential range. Serial dilutions in the exponential range for *MRP* and β_2-microglobulin are shown in the next two panels.

exponential range for *MRP* expression, which is comparable for the parental and the resistant sublines, since there is no *MRP* overexpression in these cells. The lowest PCR panel demonstrates the results for β_2-microglobulin, which is included as a control for RNA loading. Beneath the PCR figure, an ethidium-stained RNA gel demonstrates the intact, non-degraded, comparably loaded RNA used for the reverse transcription reaction. **Table 2** provides the calculated levels of mRNA present in the two sublines, relative to SW620. The expression level is normalized to the level of β_2-microglobulin and for comparison to the level of 28S ribosomal RNA measured by densitometry of the ethidium-stained RNA gel.

Table 2
Results of Quantitative PCR Assay Measuring *MDR*-1, *MRP*, and β_2-Microglobulin in SW620 Cells and Sublines

	MDR-1	*MRP*	β_2-M	28 S	*MDR*-1 / 28S	*MRP* / 28S	*MDR*-1 / β_2-M	MRP / β_2-M
SW620	10.0	10.0	1.0	1.0	10.0	10.0	10.0	10.0
Ad20	1263	6.4	0.79	1.12	1128	5.75	1599	8.15
Ad300	5147	4.5	0.76	0.92	5595	4.89	6733	5.92

2. Materials

2.1. Reverse Transcription

All reagents need to be RNase and DNase-free.

1. Sterile thin-walled microcentrifuge tubes for the reaction mixtures of appropriate size to be placed in the DNA thermal cycler.
2. 2'-Deoxyadenosine 5'-Triphosphate (dATP): 100 m*M* solution, pH 7.5 (Pharmacia Biotech, Piscataway, NJ)
3. 2'-Deoxycytidine 5'-Triphosphate (dCTP): 100 m*M* solution, pH 7.5 (Pharmacia).
4. 2'-Deoxyguanosine 5'-Triphosphate (dGTP): 100 m*M* solution, pH 7.5 (Pharmacia).
5. 2'-Deoxythymidine 5'-Triphosphate (dTTP): 100 m*M* solution, pH 7.5 (Pharmacia).
6. 5X First-strand buffer (Life Technologies, Gaithersburg, MD).
7. 3' oligonucleotide primer *MDR*-1 or *MRP* gene: 10 μ*M* (Life Technologies). While primers can be synthesized and purchased, the OD must always be checked and the concentration corrected prior to use in the RT and PCR reactions. Primers are diluted in DEPC-treated water (depH_20) and stored at –20°C.
8. 3' oligonucleotide primer β_2-microglobulin: 10 μ*M* (Life Technologies).
9. RNasin® RNase Inhibitor at 40 U/μL (Promega, Madison, WI).
10. 0.1 *M* Dithiothreitol (DTT) (Life Technologies).
11. Diethyl Pyrocarbonate (DEPC) (Sigma, St. Louis, MO).
12. Moloney Murine Leukemia Virus Reverse Transcriptase (M-MLV RT) at 200 U/μL (Life Technologies).
13. DNA Thermal Cycler (or water bath) at 37°C and at 95°C.
14. Autoclaved 0.1% DEPC-treated H_20 (depH_2O).
15. Autoclaved Eppendorf tubes and PCR tubes.

2.2. Quantitative PCR

All reagents RNase and DNase-free.

1. 1X PCR buffer: 50 m*M* KCl, 40 m*M* Tris-HCl, pH 8.3, 1.8 m*M* $MgCl_2$, and 0.1 mg/mL bovine serum albumin (BSA) and DEPC H_2O.
2. dATP: 100 m*M* solution, pH 7.5 (Pharmacia).
3. dCTP: 100 m*M* solution, pH 7.5 (Pharmacia).

4. dGTP: 100 m*M* solution, pH 7.5 (Pharmacia).
5. dTTP: 100 m*M* solution, pH 7.5 (Pharmacia).
6. 3'-oligonucleotide primer for *MDR*-1, *MRP*, or β_2-microglobulin gene: 10 μ*M* (Life Technologies). Primer concentrations should be verified prior to aliquoting and storing at –20°C.
7. 5'-oligonucleotide primer for *MDR*- 1, *MRP*, or β_2-microglobulin gene: 10 μ*M* (Life Technologies).
8. Ampli*Taq*® DNA Polymerase at 5 U/μL (Perkin Elmer, Foster City, CA).
9. AmpliWax™ PCR Gem 100 (Perkin Elmer).
10. Autoclaved dH_20, PCR tubes, and Eppendorf tubes.
11. Autoclaved 1 *M* KCl; 1 *M* Tris-HCl, pH 8.3; and 1 *M* $MgCl_2$ solutions. Store at 21°C.
12. DNA Thermal Cycler.
13. Multi-Block Heater.

2.3. Gel Electrophoresis and Analysis of PCR Products

1. Speed Vac.
2. Agarose Electrophoresis Grade (Life Technologies).
3. NuSieve® GTG® Agarose (FMC BioProducts, Rockland, ME).
4. 10X Tris/borate/EDTA, pH 8.3: DNase-free, RNase-free, and protease-free buffer.
5. An electrophoresis gel apparatus with combs.
6. An electrophoresis power supply.
7. Molecular base-pair marker.
8. DNA loading dye.
9. Ethidium bromide solution at 10 mg/mL.
10. Plastic container and shaker.
11. Densitometer.

3. Methods

3.1. Reverse Transcription

1. RNA can be isolated by a number of extraction methods. The Chomczynski method works well with tumor tissue samples because the multiple extraction steps in the protocol help eliminate the higher levels of protein found in tissue samples *(24)*. The RNA Stat-60 (Tel-Test, Inc., Friendswood, TX), kit works well with cell lines. The key is intact RNA accurately measured by spectrophotometry (*see* **Note 1**).
2. Typically, 1 μg of total cellular RNA is reverse transcribed; however, lower concentrations can be substituted when less RNA is available (*see* **Note 7**). All RNA should be diluted in 0.1% DEPC-treated water ($depH_2O$). For simplicity, RNA can be diluted to a concentration of 1 μg/10 μL.
3. Controls should be included in the reverse transcription reaction. Typically, $depH_2O$ is used as a negative control and is subjected to the RT reaction along with the RNAs of interest (*see* **Note 8**). RNA from the human colon carcinoma cell line SW620 is used as a positive *MDR*-1 control.

4. Prepare a 100 µL 20 m*M* stock of deoxynucleotide triphosphate (dNTP) mix by combining 20 µL aliquots of each of the four dNTPs, with 20 µL of depH_2O. This dNTP mixture is usually freshly prepared, although it can be stored at –20°C for a short period of time.
5. Prepare the reaction mixture as follows (10 µL needed for each RT reaction):

   4 µL of 5X First-strand buffer; 1 µL of dNTP 20 m*M* mix; 1 µL of 10 µ*M* 3' PCR primer (*MDR*-1 or *MRP*); 1 µL of 10 µ*M* 3' PCR primer (β_2-microglobulin); 0.5 µL of 40 U/µL RNasin®; 2 µL of DTT; 0.5 µL of 200 U/µL M-MLV reverse transcriptase; 10 µL total.

   Aliquot 10 µL of this reaction mixture into a microcentrifuge tube containing 1 µg of total cellular RNA in 10 µL dep$H_2$0. Heat at 37°C for 45 min, then at 95°C for 5 min to terminate the reverse transcription. The resulting cDNAs can be diluted for PCR. The cDNA not used in serial dilutions can be stored at –20°C for reuse if needed. If determination of other genes is anticipated, then the random primer protocol ought to be used to generate the cDNA (*see* **Note 9**).

3.2. Quantitative PCR

1. Prepare serial dilutions of the cDNA in dH_2O using appropriate sized sterile microcentrifuge tubes (**Fig. 1**). A good starting point for the *MDR*-1 gene is a 1:8 dilution; for the *MRP* gene, a 1:256 dilution; and for the β_2-microglobulin gene, a 1:2096 dilution (*see* **Note 2**).
2. After the dilutions are prepared, aliquot 20 µL into a sterile microcentrifuge tube. To this tube, add one AmpliWax™ PCR Gem, melt at 80°C for 5 min in a multiblock heater. On ice, allow the AmpliWax™ PCR Gem to solidify and to form a layer over the diluted cDNA; put aside until the PCR master mixture is made (*see* **Notes 10** and **11**).
3. Prepare 700 µL 1X PCR buffer as follows (70 µL needed per PCR reaction):

Aliquot		Stock	Final concentration
35 µL	KCl	1 *M*	50 m*M*
28 µL	Tris, pH 8.3	1 *M*	40 m*M*
1.26 µL	$MgCl_2$	1 *M*	1.8 m*M*
3.5 µL	BSA	20 mg/mL	0.1 mg/mL
632 µL	dH_2O		
700 µL			

   Prepare a master mixture for PCR as follows (82.3 µL needed per PCR reaction):

70 µL	1X PCR buffer
5 µL	10 µ*M* 5' primer
5 µL	10 µ*M* 3' primer
2 µL	10 m*M* dNTP mix (note change from concentration used for the RT)
0.3 µL	5 U/µL *Taq* polymerase
82.3 µL	

   Aliquot 82.3 µL master mix into the waxed, diluted cDNA layer.

The final reaction volume is 102.3 µL.

Place in a DNA thermal cycler.

4. Depending on the type of DNA thermal cycler used, the tubes may need to be placed in the thermal cycler in mineral oil to facilitate adequate and even heating of the tubes. In the DNA thermal cycler the reaction mixture is heated at 94°C for 7 min to denature the cDNA. Amplification is accomplished in sequential cycles of denaturing (at 94°C), annealing product and primers (at 55°C), and extension by the *Taq* polymerase (at 72°C) according to the following protocol: 20 cycles: 94°C, 75 s; 55°C, 75 s; and 72°C, 90 s; followed by: 10 cycles: 94°C, 75 s; 55°C, 75 s; and 72°C, 120 s; followed by: a final extension phase at 72°C for 10 min.

   In the standard protocol, samples are amplified a total of 30 cycles, this can be varied as needed (*see* **Notes 12** and **13**). The negative control, depH_2O, is allowed to amplify yet another 5–10 sequential cycles for a total number of 35–40 sequential cycles in order to detect contamination.

3.3. Gel Electrophoresis of PCR Products

1. Prepare a 2% NuSieve/1% agarose gel as follows; for 100 mL add: 1 g agarose, 2 g NuSeive, 10 mL of 10X TBE, and deionized water. (Add a little extra water to allow for vaporization owing to boiling.) Melt the agarose until boiling to ensure proper mixing. After the agarose is thoroughly mixed, allow to cool to 68°C, and pour into gel box using a graduated cylinder. Remove any bubbles that may form with a pasteur pipet. After the gel has polymerized, add 1X TBE to cover the gel, and remove the comb.
2. Prepare the PCR products: label an appropriate number of microcentrifuge tubes corresponding to the reactions and transfer an aliquot of at least 33 µL into the labeled microcentrifuge tube. Because this aliquot is a fraction of the original PCR reaction, this electrophoresis can be repeated with the remaining sample if there are problems.
3. Using a Speed Vac concentrator, reduce the volume of the aliquotted PCR product from 33 µL to 5–7 µL.
4. Add 1 µL of DNA loading dye; briefly, centrifuge in a microcentrifuge.
5. Load the marker as a standard reference in the first well followed by the PCR products.
6. Initially, electrophorese in 1X TBE buffer at 100 volts until the PCR product has migrated out of the wells and then turn down the voltage to 75 volts. Allow the dyes to migrate approximately three-quarters of the gel length. Do not discard the running buffer.
7. Place the gel in a container and cover with used running buffer to which 1.0 µg/mL ethidium bromide has been added.
8. Shake the gel for 10 min and then discard the diluted stain with the chemical waste. De-stain the gel with the remainder of the ethidium bromide-free running buffer for at least 20 min.

3.4. Analysis of PCR Products

1. Perform densitometry on the ethidium stained gels.
2. Analyze using the densitometric results to determine final *MDR*-1 or *MRP* expression level (*see* **Note 14**). The calculations are performed as follows:

$$\frac{\dfrac{\text{Sample OD}}{\text{Control OD}} \times \dfrac{\text{Sample Dilution Factor}}{\text{Control Dilution Factor}} \times 10 = MDR\text{-}1 \text{ level}}{\dfrac{\text{Sample OD}}{\text{Control OD}} \times \dfrac{\text{Sample Dilution Factor}}{\text{Control Dilution Factor}} \times 1 = B_2 \text{ level}} = MDR\text{-}1 / B_2 \text{ level}$$

or

$$\frac{\dfrac{\text{Sample OD}}{\text{Control OD}} \times \dfrac{\text{Control Input RNA/ cDNA}}{\text{Sample Input RNA/ cDNA}} \times 10 = MDR\text{-}1 \text{ level}}{\dfrac{\text{Sample OD}}{\text{Control OD}} \times \dfrac{\text{Control Input RNA/ cDNA}}{\text{Sample Input RNA/ cDNA}} \times 1 = B_2 \text{ level}} = MDR\text{-}1 / B_2 \text{ level}$$

The Sample Dilution Factor relates the dilution from the reverse transcription reaction, based on a 1 µg RNA sample (equivalent to a 1:1 dilution) used directly in the PCR reaction. For example, a 1:8 dilution contains 125 ng input RNA, and the Sample Dilution Factor used in the equation is 8. A 1:2048 dilution contains 0.49 ng input RNA, and the Sample Dilution Factor used in the equation is 2048. The expression of the control gene, β_2-microglobulin,varies between tissues and cell lines. In lymphoma samples, we found that overall, RNA expression was fourfold higher than in cell lines. This did not appear to be cell type specific, since RNA from 60 cell lines had comparable levels of β_2-microglobulin ***(25)***. We thus instituted a correction factor for tissues, dividing the β_2-microglobulin level by 4 (*see* **Note 15**).

4. Notes

1. Any RNA preparation method can be used that provides intact, undegraded RNA. Biopsy samples can be flash frozen, pulverized, and suspended in guanidinium thiocyanate prior to extraction by the Chomczynski method ***(24)***. Small, fresh samples may also be suspended in guanidinium thiocyanate. In order to shear the sample for improved extraction, the samples should be passed several times through a 22-g needle, attached to a plastic syringe. The extraction steps can be repeated several times in order to get a clean RNA preparation prior to precipitation.
2. It is best to make a large quantity of total RNA from the control cell line (SW620), to be included in every PCR reaction. Typically, the maximum concentrations which allow exponential amplification at 30 cycles for SW620 are: cDNA derived from 125 ng input RNA (a 1:8 dilution from the 1 µg RT reaction) for *MDR*-1 mRNA; cDNA derived from 3.91 ng RNA (a 1:256 dilution from the 1 µg RT reaction) for *MRP* mRNA; and cDNA derived from 0.49 ng RNA (a 1:2048 dilution from the 1 µg RT reaction) for β_2-microglobulin mRNA. For quantitation of each of these in unknown samples, an initial test PCR reaction is performed using an amount of RNA/cDNA equivalent to that used from SW620. Optimal dilutions of the test sample cDNA for a definitive

PCR are suggested by the results of the initial reaction. If a sample is undetectable at this level, then the subsequent PCR reaction can be carried out at a lower dilution or at an increased number of cycles.

3. There is no perfect control for normalization of RNA loading. Most accurate results are ensured when RNA can be carefully measured, and the comparable loading verified by running formaldehyde gels to assess the quantity and quality of the RNA. Housekeeping genes used with Northern analyses are equally applicable to quantitative PCR. β_2-microglobulin expression has proven an acceptable control for our studies, and the expression level was largely comparable in a panel of 60 cell lines derived from a variety of human cancers *(25)*. However, we have identified some drug resistant sublines which do not have β_2-microglobulin expression. In a study with lymphoma samples, comparison with β-actin, GPDH, and β_2-microglobulin using ethidium staining of ribosomal RNA as a gold standard suggested that the β_2-microglobulin was the best control *(5)*. The use of PCR amplified ribosomal RNA fragments has also been used as a control, equivalent to ethidium staining an RNA gel for determination of comparability of loading *(10)*. This could be a superior control, since reverse transcription of the ribosomal RNA would also provide a control for the RT reaction. Whatever the control gene chosen, it must be amplified in a separate tube, parallel to the *MDR*-1 or *MRP* reaction. Otherwise, the high level of expression of the control gene will result in early plateau and inaccurate quantitation due to competition of the PCR products from the control gene.
4. Just as in the amplification itself, there is also a range in which the densitometry of the ethidium-stained gels containing the PCR product will provide linear measurements. A gel can be run separately with known quantities of serially diluted PCR product to check the linear range of the densitometer. Very low and very high signals may not give accurate results. Most accurate measurements require subtraction of the background. In earlier studies, 10 μCi [^{32}P] dCTP were added to the PCR reaction, and autoradiography was performed. Densitometry of PCR products in an ethidium-stained gel has proven to be just as accurate as autoradiography, with some increase in sensitivity. Detection methods using chemiluminescence have been described, dramatically decreasing the PCR product analysis time *(9,26)*. These methods are quicker because separation of PCR products by gel electrophoresis is not required. However, certain problems, such as background bands, may not be detectable without gel separation.
5. Two-fold differences in PCR product from 2-fold serial dilutions have been documented for PCR reactions with the primer sets for *MDR*-1 and *MRP* shown in **Table 1**. PCR reactions which do not show two-fold differences from 2-fold serial dilutions may be affected by one of several problems, including those due to PCR reaction components (*see* **Note 6**) and those due to competition. Competition limits exponential amplification and accurate quantitation, and can be due to contaminating DNA found in the RNA sample, contaminating PCR products from previous PCR reactions, or amplification of non-specific PCR products. Some samples may have very high levels of *MDR*-1 mRNA, and therefore competition

from one of these sources would be less marked; however, quantitation will be compromised. RNA samples contaminated with significant quantities of DNA may need to be treated with DNase, and the RNA re-extracted, in order to provide accurate quantitation. Contamination of the PCR reaction with PCR products from prior reactions is a common problem (*see* **Note 8**). When extrapolating this method to other primer sets, it is important to determine whether a new primer set will give exponential amplification. Increased background can result from hybridization of the primers to non-specific regions in the cDNA. This background results in competition which prevents exponential amplification because the total reaction is in plateau at an earlier time point.

6. Unexpectedly low levels of PCR product in positive controls are seen periodically. On different occasions, we identified problems with *Taq* polymerase, primers, or RNA degradation. Primer concentrations may need to be remeasured, for verification that the amount being added is correct. Unknown differences in quantity of primer will result in problems with the PCR efficiency *(13)*. Degradation of primers or of RNA will result in high background and low PCR product.
7. In this approach, β_2-microglobulin is included as a control for RNA loading but also provides an endogenous control for the reverse transcription reaction and for the PCR reaction. It has been our anecdotal experience that very low concentrations of RNA do not give comparable RT reactions, and consequently, we make an effort to include 1 microgram of RNA in the RT reaction. If that is not available, the RT and PCR reactions are conducted as usual, with the understanding that significantly decreased input RNA may have a deleterious influence on the efficiency of the RT reaction. This was our anecdotal experience; a limited study reported similar findings *(27)*.
8. Contamination is a major problem in quantitative PCR methods. The most common type of contamination is with PCR product from previous reactions, which may be aerosolized during preparation for gel analysis. PCR product contamination can be found on the benchtop, on pipetmen, and on the thermal cycler itself. The use of dedicated sets of PCR pipetmen (one pre-PCR, and one post-PCR), and pipette tips with aerosol filters helps prevent this problem. We monitor for contamination by amplifying a water-alone sample for 10 cycles more than the PCR reaction being performed. When contamination is detected, new PCR buffers are generated and reactions are run again.
9. Random primers can be used in the RT reaction, rather than the specific downstream primer. Comparable results are obtained, and this method allows for long-term storage of the RT reaction and the serial dilutions for later PCR reactions. The following RT buffer is made:

   4 µL 5X first-strand buffer
   1 µL dNTP 20 m*M* mix
   2 µL 0.1 *M* DTT
   0.5 µL 40.0 U/µL RNAsin
   1.0 µL 500 µ*M* random primer
   1.5 µL 200 U/µL MMLV RT enzyme

10. Samples that have very low target mRNA concentrations often display increased background, particularly if amplification above 35 cycles is required. The initial formation of these products can occur at low initial (ambient) temperatures, and are reduced or eliminated by the "hot start" approach, in which wax beads are added, melted to form a solid layer above the cDNA, and then the PCR master mix added on top. The two solutions are mixed and the PCR reaction begins after the thermocycler heats to 94°C. Background is sometimes due to the formation of primer dimers, a double-stranded PCR product consisting of the two primers and their complementary sequences. Sometimes these primer dimers contain extra sequences between the primers ***(14)***. When primer dimers form, they can be a major problem as they are very efficiently amplified and compete with amplification of the target cDNA. This is not a major problem with the primer sets described in Table 1, but can be a problem with other primer sets. With persistent problems, the hot start approach could be modified to add the cDNA, the primers, and the *Taq* polymerase separately.
11. The RT reaction mixture, PCR buffer, and PCR reaction mixture are freshly prepared.
12. We have previously shown that exponential amplification can be demonstrated by either serial dilutions or serial cycles ***(4)***. Thus, an alternate approach is to use multiple aliquots of a standard dilution, e.g. equivalent to 31.25 ng RNA, and to remove a one PCR reaction each PCR cycle. This approach can be very accurate, because the serial dilutions which require great technical precision to perform correctly are not used, but consumes more RNA/cDNA. One investigator removed of a small aliquot from the PCR tube each cycle, dotting on nitrocellulose, and generating a dot blot of products from sequential cycles ***(28)***. Although considerably more efficient than starting with multiple reaction tubes for each cycle, this method, in our hands, has lead to significant problems with contamination due to spillage of PCR products as the tubes are opened and closed repeatedly.
13. In addition to using sequential cycles to avoid the process of serial dilution, the principle of sequential cycles can be very useful when low amounts of RNA are present. We have quantitated *MDR*-1 mRNA from 40 cycles in extreme cases. In that situation, SW620 is diluted to 0.12 ng input RNA since amplification 40 cycles should give a PCR product equivalent to 125 ng input RNA amplified 30 cycles. Since greater variability results from this approach, the better solution is larger biopsy samples.
14. The results are normalized to the level of expression found in the SW620 cells. This unselected human colon cancer cell line has served well as a positive control for *MDR*-1 expression, since levels are in the range found for clinical samples, and the expression level is stable over time in culture. The SW620 cell line has an *MDR*-1 level which is barely detectable by Northern analysis and is sensitized 1.2-fold to Adriamycin and 3 to 11-fold to vincristine by verapamil ***(3,29)***. Although the assigned level of 10 is arbitrary, previous studies incorporating ^{32}P-dCTP in the PCR reaction allowed us to calculate the level of *MDR*-1 mRNA at 2.3 mRNA molecules/ng of input total RNA ***(4)***.

15. During our studies with cell lines, the use of β_2-microglobulin as a control for RNA loading appeared quite reliable. However, when clinical samples derived from lymphomas were examined, it became evident that β_2-microglobulin expression was significantly higher than in the cell lines. Ethidium stained formaldehyde gels confirmed comparable loading of the RNA *(5)*, while the calculated PCR result for β_2-microglobulin in the lymphoma samples was typically 4-fold higher than the result for SW620. We concluded that a correction had to be made for RNA derived from clinical samples, dividing the β_2-microglobulin results by 4. For new cell types, the need for this correction can be validated by hybridizing an RNA gel containing 1 μg total RNA from the control cell line (SW620) and 1 μg total RNA from the tumors or tissues of interest.

References

1. van der Heyden, S., Gheuens, E., DeBruijn, E., Van Oosterom, V., and Maes, R. (1995) P-glycoprotein: Clinical significance and methods of analysis. *Crit. Rev. Clin. Lab. Sci.* **32,** 221–264.
2. Beck, W. T., Grogan, T. M., Willman, C. L., Cordon-Cardo, C., Parham, D. M., Kuttesch, J. F., Andreeff, M., Bates, S. E., Berard, C. W., Boyett, J. M., Brophy, N. A., Broxterman, H. J., Chan, H. S. L., Dalton, W. S., Dietel, M., Fojo, A. T., Gascoyne, R. D., Head, D., Houghton, P. J., Srivastava, D. K., Lehnert, M., Leith, C. P., Paietta, E., Pavelic, Z. P., Rimsza, L., Roninson, I. B., Sikic, B. I., Twentyman, P. R., Warnke, R., and Weinstein, R. (1996) Methods to detect P-glycoprotein-associated multidrug resistance in patients' tumors: consensus recommendations. *Cancer Res.* **56,** 3010–3020.
3. Herzog, C. E., Trepel, J. B., Mickley, L. A., Bates, S. E., and Fojo, A. T. (1992) Various methods of analysis of *mdr-1*/P-glycoprotein in human colon cancer cell lines. *J. Natl. Cancer Inst.* **84,** 711–716.
4. Murphy, L. D., Herzog, C. E., Rudick, J. B., Fojo, A. J., and Bates, S. E. (1990) Use of the polymerase chain reaction in the quantitation of mdr-1 gene expression. *Biochemistry* **29,** 10,351–10,356.
5. Kang, Y. K., Zhan, Z., Regis, J., Robey, R., Meadows, B., Dickstein, B., Lee, J. S., Otsuki, T., Stetler-Stevenson, M. A., Jaffe, E. S., Solomon, D., Wilson, W. H., Fojo, A., and Bates, S. E. (1995) Expression of *mdr*-1 in refractory lymphoma: quantitation by polymerase chain reaction and validation of the assay. *Blood* **86,** 1515–1524.
6. Lyttelton, M. P. A., Hart, S., Ganeshaguru, K., Hoffbrand, A. V., and Mehta, A. B. (1994) Quantitation of multidrug resistant MDR 1 transcript in acute myeloid leukemia by non-isotopic quantitative cDNA-polymerase chain reaction. *Br. J. Haematol.* **86,** 540–546.
7. Noonan, K. E., Beck, C., Holzmayer, T. A., Chin, J. E., Wunder, J. S., Andrulis, I. L., Gazdar, A. F., Willman, C. L., Griffith, B., Von Hoff, D. D., and Roninson, I. B. (1990) Quantitative analysis of *MDR1* (multidrug resistance) gene expression in human tumors by polymerase chain reaction. *Proc. Natl. Acad. Sci. USA* **87,** 7160–7164.

8. Clifford, S. C., Thomas, D. J., Neal, D. E., and Lunec, J. (1994) Increased *mdr*-1 gene transcript levels in high-grade carcinoma of the bladder determined by quantitative PCR-based assay. *Br. J. Cancer* **69,** 680–686.
9. Zhao, S., Consoli, U., Arceci, R., Pfeifer, J., Dalton, W. S., and Andreeff, M. (1997) Semi-automated PCR method for quantitating MDR-1 expression. *BioTechniques* **21,** 726–731.
10. Foley, K. P., Leonard, M. W., and Engel, J. D. (1993) Quantitation of RNA using the polymerase chain reaction. *Trends Genet.* **9,** 380–385.
11. Ferre, F. (1997) Quantitative or Semi-quantitative PCR: reality versus myth. *PCR Methods Appl.* **2,** 1–9.
12. Czerny, T. (1996) High primer concentration improves PCR amplification from random pools. *Nucleic Acids Res.* **24,** 985–986.
13. Sugimoto, T., Fujita, M., Taguchi, T., and Morita, T. (1993) Quantitative detection of DNA by coamplification of polymerase chain reaction: a wide detectable range controlled by the thermodynamic stability of primer template duplexes. *Nucleic Acids Res.* **21,** 557–583.
14. Erlich, H. A., Gelfand, D., and Sninsky, J. J. (1991) Recent advances in the polymerase chain reaction. *Science* **252,** 1643–1651.
15. Cross, N. C. P. (1995) Quantitative PCR techniques and applications. *Br. J. Haematol.* **89,** 693–697.
16. Zimmerman, K. and Mannhalter, J. W. (1996) Technical aspects of quantitative competitive PCR. *BioTechniques* **21,** 268–279.
17. Killeen, A. A. (1997) Quantification of nucleic acids. *Clin. Lab. Med.* **17,** 1–19.
18. Braga, V. M. M and Gendler, S. J. (1997) Co-amplification of two cDNAs in RT-PCR can alter the yield of both products. *BioTechniques* **17,** 228–230.
19. Raeymaekers, L. (1993) Quantitative PCR: theoretical considerations with practical implications. *Anal. Biochem.* **214,** 582–585.
20. Pannetier, C., Delassus, S., Darche, S., Saucier, C., and Kourilsky, P. (1993) Quantitative tiration of nucleic acids by enzymatic amplification reactions run to saturation. *Anal. Biochem.* **193,** 231–235.
21. Liu, Q., Thorland, E. C., and Sommer, S. S. (1997) Inhibition of PCR amplification by a point mutation downstream of a primer. *BioTechniques* **22,** 292.
22. Zhan, Z., Sandor, V. A., Gamelin, E., Regis, J., Dickstein, B., Wilson, W., Fojo, A. T., and Bates, S. E. (1997) Expression of the multidrug resistance-associated protein gene in refractory lymphoma: quantitation by a validated polymerase chain reaction assay. *Blood* **89,** 3795–3800.
23. Gussow, D., Rein, R., Ginjaar, I., Hochstenbach, F., Seeman, G., Kottman, A., and Ploegh, H. L. (1987) The human beta$_2$-microglobulin gene. Primary structure and definition of the transcriptional unit. *J. Immunol.* **139,** 3132–3138.
24. Chomczynski, P. and Sacchi, N. (1987) Single-step method of RNA isolation by acid guanidinium thiocyanate-phenol-chloroform extraction. *Anal. Biochem.* **162,** 156–159.
25. Alvarez, M., Paull, K., Monks, A., Hose, C., Lee, J. S., Weinstein, J., Grever, M. R., Bates, S. E., and Fojo, A. T. (1995) Generation of a drug resistance progile by

quantitation of mdr-1/P-glycoprotein in the cell lines of the NCI anticancer drug screen. *J. Clin. Invest.* **95,** 2205–2214.

26. Landgraf, A., Reckmann, B., and Pingoud, A. (1991) Quantitative analysis of polymerase chain reaction (PCR) products using primers labeled with biotin and a flourescent dye. *Anal. Biochem.* **193,** 231–235.
27. Williams, W. V., Rosenbaum, G., and Weiner, D. B. (1992) Effect of RNA concentration on cDNA synthesis for DNA amplification. *PCR Methods Appl.* **2,** 86.
28. Bishop, G. A., Rokahr, K. L., Lowes, M., McGuinness, P. H., Napoli, J., DeCruz, D. J., Wong, W-Y., and McCaughan, G. W. (1997) Quantitative reverse transcriptase-PCR amplification of cytokine mRNA in liver biopsy specimens using a non-competitive method. *Immunol. Cell Biol.* **75,** 142–147.
29. Lai, G.-M., Chen, Y.-N., Mickley, L. A., Fojo, A. T., and Bates, S. E. (1991) P-glycoprotein expression and schedule dependence of Adriamycin cytotoxicity in human colon carcinoma cell lines. *Int. J. Cancer* **49,** 696–703.

8

Microtiter Plate Technique for the Measurement of Glutathione in Fresh and Cryopreserved Lymphoblasts Using the Enzyme Recycling Method

Pamela R. Kearns and Andrew G. Hall

1. Introduction

Glutathione is an intracellular, nonprotein thiol that appears to play an important role in protection of the cell against cytotoxic drugs *(1)* and has been implicated in the control of cell cycling *(2,3)* and apoptosis *(4,5)*. It can exist in an oxidized (disulfide, [GSSG]) and a reduced (sulphydryl, [GSH]) form. In general, GSSG comprises less than 1% of the total intracellular glutathione. In circumstances of oxidative stress, GSH dimerizes to form glutathione disulfide (GSSG), making protons available to neutralize reactive oxygen species (*Reaction 1*). In vivo, reduction of GSSG is catalysed by glutathione reductase, efficiently regenerating high intracellular GSH levels (*Reaction 2*)

1. GSH + GSH ——> $GSSG^+ 2H^+$
2. GSSG + glutathione reductase + (NADPH) ——> 2 GSH

A number of methods are available for the measurement of intracellular glutathione. Owen and Belcher first described the enzyme recycling method in 1965 *(6)*. This was subsequently modified by Tietze in 1969 *(7)* and by Anderson in 1985 *(8)*. Vandeputte et al. 1994 *(9)* adapted the assay for use in microtiter plates. It provides a sensitive and specific assay for the measurement of total intracellular glutathione, i.e., both GSH and GSSG.

The enzyme recycling assay is particularly valuable in the study of stored cells because total reduced and oxidized glutathione is measured and therefore alterations in the intracellular ratio of reduced and oxidized glutathione that

From: *Methods in Molecular Medicine, Vol. 28: Cytotoxic Drug Resistance Mechanisms*
Edited by: R. Brown and U. Böger-Brown © Humana Press Inc., Totowa, NJ

may result from cryopreservation or thawing do not influence the results. Comparative studies using fresh cells have shown concordance between data achieved using this technique and other methods of glutathione measurement; for example, high-performance liquid chromatograph (HPLC) techniques measuring monobromobimane-GSH adducts ***(10,11)*** and flow cytometric techniques using a GSH-specific fluorescent dye ***(11)***.

In the assay described here cells are permeablized using a detergent-based lysis method. Care must be taken to inhibit the membrane-bound enzyme, γ glutamyl-transferase (γ-GT), which metabolizes glutathione released from the cell ***(12)***. This is achieved by the use of an acidified lysis buffer ***(8)***. The lysate is then assayed for total protein and glutathione content.

Inhibition of glutathione reductase has been noted in some cell lines, which can lead to falsely low measurement of glutathione ***(10)***. Therefore, for each sample, glutathione is measured in the sample itself, and following the addition of a known quantity of glutathione. The recovery of glutathione can then be calculated for each sample. Spiking the samples in this way also determines if there is any residual γ-GT activity.

In brief, the method involves the glutathione reductase-catalyzed reduction of GSSG by NADPH, followed by the reaction of GSH with Ellman's reagent, (5,5'-dithiobis-2-nitrobenzoic acid; DTNB). The chromophoric product, TNB, has an absorbance between 405–412 nm. The reaction can therefore be followed spectrophotometrically (*Reaction 3*).

3. $GSSG + NADPH + H^+ \longrightarrow 2GSH + NADP^+$
$2GSH + DTNB \longrightarrow GSSG + TNB$

The method will be described for lymphoblasts prepared from bone marrow or peripheral blood samples; however, it can be readily adapted to study cell lines.

2. Materials

2.1. Sample Preparation; Thawing Cryopreserved Cell Pellets

1. Phosphate buffered saline (PBS) (Dulbecco's PBS tablets, ICN).
2. Fetal calf serum (FCS, GIBCO Life Sciences, Gaithersburg, MD).
3. 100 U/mL Penicillin, 100 mg/mL streptomycin, and 0.125 mg/mL fungizone (PSF; all from GIBCO Life Sciences): Prepare and divide into 10-mL aliquots for storage at –20°C.
4. Tissue culture medium (RPMI-1640): Dutch modified solution without glutamine (Gibco Life Sciences) with 2% PSF and 1% FCS added.

2.2. Red Cell Lysis

1. Stock solution A: 8.29 mg NH_4Cl, 37 mg Na_2EDTA in 100 mL H_2O. Store at 4°C.
2. Stock solution B: 1.0 g $KHCO_3$ in 100 mL. Store both stock solutions at 4°C.

3. Final red cell lysis mixture A:B: H_2O = 1:1:8. Prepare immediately before use and store on ice.

2.3. Lymphoblast Lysis

Lymphoblast lysis buffer; Triton-X 100 (Sigma) 0.1% (v/v) in 10 m*M* HCl. Store at 4°C.

2.4. Enzyme Recycling Assay

1. Stock phosphate buffer: 143 m*M* (1.9 g/100 mL) sodium phosphate, 6.3 m*M* (234 mg/100 mL) ethylenediaminetetraacetic acid (EDTA), pH 7.0. Store at 4°C (*see* **Note 1**).
2. Glutathione reductase (type IV from Baker's yeast, Sigma) 2.4 IU/mL in phosphate buffer (stable for 4 wk at 4°C).
3. DTNB (Sigma): 100 m*M* of a 20-fold stock solution (3.93 mg/100 mL) should be prepared in stock phosphate buffer, aliquoted, and stored at –80°C. An aliquot of the stock DTNB is thawed and diluted to 5 m*M* using stock phosphate buffer. This should be prepared just prior to use.
4. βNADPH (Sigma): 40 m*M* of 20-fold stock solution (3.32 mg/100 mL) should be prepared in stock phosphate buffer, aliquoted, and stored at –80°C. An aliquot of the stock βNADPH is thawed and diluted to 2 mmol/L using stock phosphate buffer. This should be prepared just prior to use.
5. Reaction mixture: 18.25 mL phosphate buffer, 2.5 mL DTNB, 4.25 mL NADPH (prepare just prior to use). The final concentration of reagents per well is 0.345 m*M* DTNB, 0.24 m*M* NADPH, and 0.34 IU/mL glutathione reductase.
6. GSSG (Sigma): 100 μ*M* stock solution: Prepare a 0.1 *M* solution (0.328g GSSG/ 5 mL phosphate buffer) and dilute 1:1000 to 100 μ*M* with phosphate buffer.
7. GSSG standard curve: 100 μ*M* stock solutions: store 800 μL aliquots at –80°C. The standard curves are prepared as described in **Subheading 3.4.1.**
8. GSSG quality controls: The 100 μ*M* GSSG stock solution is used to prepare 4 and 12 μ*M* quality control samples which are stored at –80°C (*see* **Note 2**).

3. Methods

3.1. Thawing Cryopreserved Samples

1. The ampoule containing the cell pellet is removed from liquid nitrogen, placed immediately into a 37°C waterbath, and continuously agitated.
2. Immediately the pellet is thawed and the contents of the ampoule are transferred to a 50-mL tube.
3. Two mL of ice-cold FCS are added dropwise, followed by 18 mL of RPMI. The mixture is gently agitated throughout (*see* **Note 3**).
4. The cells are left to recover for 90 min at room temperature (*see* **Note 4**).

3.2. Red Cell Lysis

Erythrocytes have high GSH levels; therefore, it is important to ensure the samples are free of red cells prior to white cell lysis and glutathione analysis.

Table 1
Dilutions Used for Preparing the Standard Curve and Spiking Solutions

GSH equivalent (m*M*)	100 m*M* GSSG (mL)	[a]Buffer vol (mL)
0	0	1000
1	5	995
2	10	990
4	20	980
8	40	960
16	80	920
24	120	880
30	150	850

[a]Lysis buffer is used to prepare standards and phosphate buffer to prepare the 'spiking' solutions.

The red cells are lysed by osmotic shock in ice-cold ammonium chloride solution.

1. The cells are spun at 300g for 10 min and then resuspended in ice-cold red lysis buffer and incubated on ice for 4 min.
2. The white cells are then washed in 4 mL of ice-cold PBS and spun at 300*g* for 10 min.
3. White cells are then resuspended in 4 mL of ice-cold PBS (*see* **Note 5**).
4. A sample is taken for counting (the trypan blue exclusion technique can be used to identify the percentage of dead cells) (*see* **Note 6**).
5. The cells are respun at 4°C for 10 min and resuspended at a density of 1×10^7/mL in PBS.
6. A sample is taken for cytospin to evaluate the percentage of blasts.
7. Aliquots of 4×10^6 cells are sufficient for glutathione analysis.

3.3. Lymphoblast Lysis

1. The cells are pelleted by spinning at 300*g* at 4°C for 10 min.
2. The cell pellet is lysed by resuspension in 250 mL of ice-cold Triton-X 100 0.1% in 10 m*M* HCl and incubated on ice for 10 min.
3. The cells are centrifuged for 10 min, 300*g* at 4°C.
4. A 40-µL sample of the supernatant is removed for total protein analysis. The Bradford protein assay ***(14)*** is suitable, because it is compatible with the lysis buffer.

3.4. Glutathione Enzyme Recycling Assay

3.4.1. Preparation of Standard Curve

1. An 800-µL aliquot of the 100 µ*M* stock GSSG is thawed to prepare the standard curve.
2. Preparation of standards: The dilutions are prepared as shown in **Table 1**. The standards expressed in GSH equivalents are 0, 1, 2, 4, 8, 16, 24, and 30 µ*M* (*see* **Note 7**).

s 0	s 0	high qc	high qc	sample2	sample2						
s 0.5	s 0.5	high qc	high qc	sample2 +spike 2	sample2 +spike2						
s 1.0	s 1.0	low qc	low qc	sample2 +spike 4	sample2 +spike4						
s 2.0	s 2.0	low qc	lowqc								
s 4.0	s 4.0										
s 8.0	s 8.0	sample1	sample1								
s 12	s 12	sample1 +spike2	sample1+ spike2								
s 15	s 15	sample1 +spike4	sample1+ spike4								

Fig 1. Microtiter plate layout.

3.4.2. Preparation of Microtiter Plate

1. Standards, samples, and assay solutions should be kept on ice.
2. The assay is performed in a 96-well microtiter plate (Costar, flat-bottomed cell-culture cluster dish).
3. 20 µL of phosphate buffer or GSSG-spiked phosphate buffer is added to each well.
4. 20 µL of standard sample or quality-control sample are pipetted into the appropriate well (**Fig. 1**). The prepared plate is kept at 4°C while the reaction mixture is being prepared.
5. Prepare the reaction mixture and, using an eight-channel, pipet, add 200 µL to each well.
6. The plate is then incubated for 5 min at room temperature.
7. The plate is placed in the plate reader and the enzyme recycling reaction initiated by the addition of glutathione reductase, 40 µL to each well, again using a multi-channel pipet. Care should be taken to ensure that there are no bubbles in the wells.
8. The reaction is followed kinetically, measuring the absorbance at 405nm at 4-min intervals from time 0–16 min. The plate is shaken prior to each reading.
9. The linear range over time is determined for each GSH concentration in the standard curve (**Fig. 2**).
10. The linear range of the standard curve over the time period measured is also determined (**Fig. 3**).
11. The standard curve is a plot of GSH equivalent against absorbance at 405 nm at a given time point within the linear range of the reaction (**Fig. 4**).
12. GSH levels are derived from standard curves constructed for each plate (*see* **Note 8**).
13. For each sample, curves are derived with and without spiking with known amounts of GSH to evaluate the possibility of cytosolic glutathione reductase inhibitors and residual γ-GT activity.

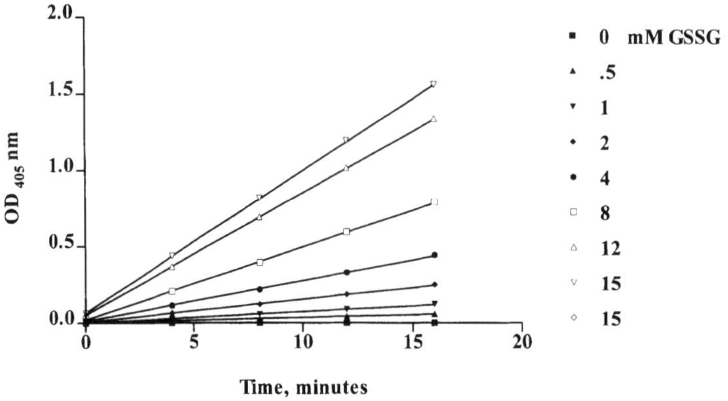

Fig. 2. Plot of rate of OD change with time. (Used to determine the linear range.)

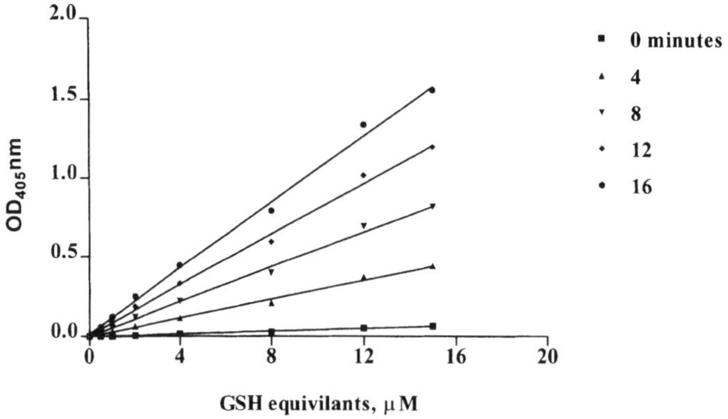

Fig. 3. Plot of OD change with concentration of GSSG. (Used to determine linear range for assay.)

4. Notes

1. The enzyme recycling assay is very sensitive to differences in the ionic strength of this buffer *(13)*. Therefore, sufficient stock buffer should be prepared for all experiments in a comparative series.
2. The quality control samples are used to control for intra-assay variability.
3. Optimal conditions for thawing cells may differ depending on the cell type.
4. A considerable improvement in cell recovery is achieved when the cells are allowed to rest at this stage.
5. Maintaining the cells at 4°C prevents transmembrane loss of glutathione.
6. Dead cells, as defined by Trypan blue exclusion, have been found not to contribute to the glutathione measurement.

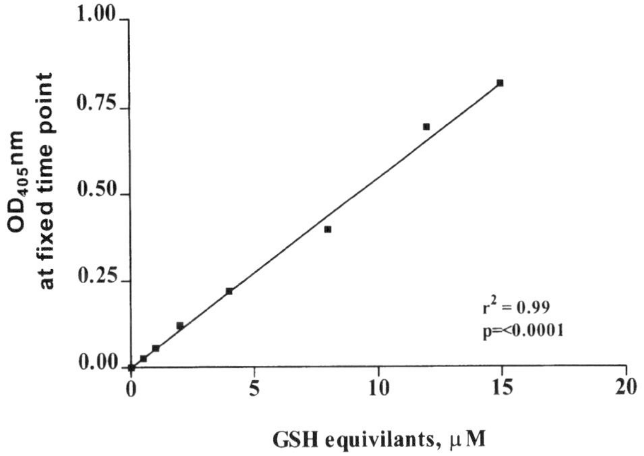

Fig. 4. Sample standard curve. (Plot of OD at fixed time point vs GSH concentration.)

7. Each mmol of GSSG produces the equivalent of 2 mmols of GSH. Because the assay measures total glutathione, i.e., both GSSG and GSH, the results are best expressed in terms of GSH equivalents.
8. The assay can be considered reliable if the quality-control values lay within the accepted coefficient of variability.

References

1. Obrien, M. L. and Tew, K. D. (1996) Glutathione and related enzymes in multidrug resistance . *Eur. J. Cancer* **32A,** 967–978.
2. Kavanagh, T. J., Grossmann, A., Jaecks, E. P., Jinneman, J. C., Eaton, D. L., Martin, G. M., and Rabinovitch, P. S. (1990) Proliferative capacity of human peripheral blood lymphocytes sorted on the basis of glutathione content. *J. Cell. Physiol.* **145,** 472–480.
3. Iwata, S., Hori, T., Sato, N., Ueda-Taniguchi, Y., Yamabe, T., Nakamura, H., Masutani, H., and Yodoi, J. (1994) Thiol-mediated redox regulation of lymphocyte proliferation: possible involvement of adult T cell leukemia-derived factor and glutathione in transferrin receptor expression. *J. Immunol.* **152,** 5633–5642.
4. Watson, R. W. G., Rotstein, O. D., Nathens, A. B., Dackiw, A. P. B., and Marshall, J. C. (1996) Thiol mediated redox regulation of neutrophil apoptosis. *Surgery* **120,** 150–158.
5. Chiba, T., Takahashi, S., Sato, N., Ishii, S., and Kikuchi, K. (1996) Fas mediated apoptosis is modulated by intracellular glutathione in human T cells. *Eur. J. Immunol.* **26,** 1164–1169.
6. Owens, C. W. I. and Belcher, R. V. (1965) A colorimetric micro-method for the determination of glutathione. *Biochem. J.* **94,** 705–711.
7. Tietze, F. (1969) Enzymatic method for quantitative determination of nanogram amounts of total and oxidized glutathione. *Anal. Biochem.* **27,** 502–522.

8. Anderson, M. E. (1985) Determination of glutathione and glutathione disulfide in biological samples. *Methods Enzymol.* **113,** 548–555.
9. Vandeputte, C., Guizon, I., Genestie-Denis, I., Vannier, B., and Lorenzon, G. (1994) A microtiter plate assay for total glutathione and glutathione disulfide contents in cultured/isolated cells: performance study of a new miniaturized protocol. *Cell Biol. Toxicol.* **10,** 415–521
10. Eady, J. J., Orta, T., Dennis, M. F., Stratford, M. R., and Peacock, J. H. (1995) Glutathione determination by the Tietze enzymatic recycling assay and its relationship to cellular radiation response. *Br. J. Cancer* **72,** 1089–1095
11. Beaver, J. P and Waring, P. (1995) A decrease in intracellular glutathione concentration precedes the onset of apoptosis in murine thymocytes. *Eur. J. Cell Biol.* **68,** 47–54.
12. Khalaf, M. R. and Hayhoe, F. G. J. (1987) Cytochemistry of gamma-glutamyltransferase in haemic cells and malignancies. *Histochem. J.* **19,** 385–395.
13. Eyer, P. and Podhradsky, D. (1986) Evaluation of the micromethod for determination of glutathione using enzymatic cycling and Ellman's reagent. *Anal. Biochem.* **153,** 57–66.
14. Bradford, M. (1976) A rapid a sensitive method for the quantitation of microgram quantities of protein using the principle of protein-dye binding. *Anal. Biochem.* **72,** 248–254.

9

Measurement of Reduced Glutathione Using High-Pressure Liquid Chromatography

Linda A. Hogarth, Celia M. A. Rabello, and Andrew G. Hall

1. Introduction

As outlined in Chapter 8, glutathione in the intact cell is maintained predominantly in its reduced form by the cytosolic enzyme, glutathione reductase. Cell lysis can lead to rapid oxidation to the oxidized form, GSSG, and degradation by γ-glutamyl transpeptidase. In order to obtain a true measurement of the amount of reduced glutathione (GSH) in living cells we have utilized the method of Cotgreave and Moldeus *(1)* in which GSH is derivatized using monobromobimane (MBBr), which can freely cross the cell membrane (**Fig. 1**). The GSH–MBBr adduct is then extracted and the amount formed measured by high-performance liquid chromatography (HPLC) with fluorescence detection.

2. Materials

2.1. Preparation of Glutathione Standards, Quality Controls, and Samples

1. 30 m*M* DL-dithiothreitol (DTT): 45 mg dissolved in 10 mL of distilled deionized water on the day of assay (Sigma)
2. 1 *M* hydrochloric acid (HCl): 1 *M* stock solution (Fisons)
3. 8 m*M* MBBr: 54.25 mg (Calbiochem-Novabiochem Corporation) dissolved in a minimum volume of acetonitrile. In a separate tube, 158 μL of N-ethylmorpholine (Sigma) is mixed with 23.5 mL of deionized water and added to the previously dissolved MBBr. The pH is adjusted to 8.0 by the addition of 1 *M* HCl and the final volume made up to 25 mL with distilled deionized water. The final reagent may be divided into 500 μL aliquots and stored at –80°C (*see* **Note 1**).

From: *Methods in Molecular Medicine, Vol. 28: Cytotoxic Drug Resistance Mechanisms*
Edited by: R. Brown and U. Böger-Brown © Humana Press Inc., Totowa, NJ

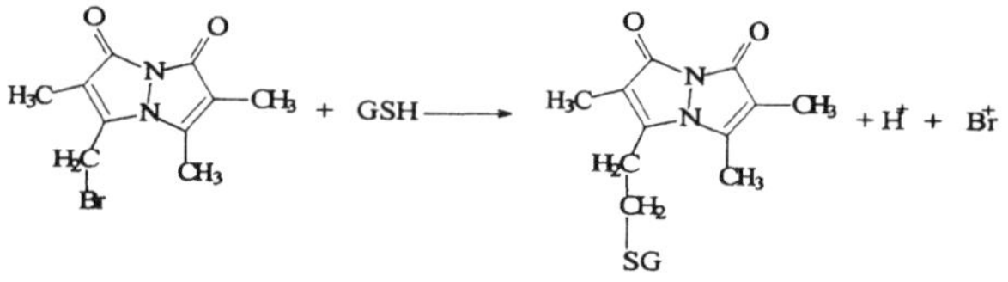

Fig. 1. Reaction of monobromobimane with glutathione.

Table 1
Preparation of GSH Standards

	105 μ*M* GSH (mL)	PBS (mL)	Final GSH concentration (μ*M*)[a]
A	1.0	0.0	100
B	0.8	0.2	80
C	0.6	0.4	60
D	0.4	0.6	40
E	0.2	0.8	20
F	0.1	0.9	10
G	0.05	0.95	5
H	0.025	0.975	2.5

[a]After addition of DTT.

4. GSH stock solution: 32.26 mg (Sigma) dissolved in 25 mL of phosphate buffered saline (PBS; Dulbecco's; ICN Biomedicals). Prepare fresh on day of assay.
5. Trichloroacetic acid (TCA): 100% solution (Sigma) (*see* **Note 2**).

2.2. Reagents for HPLC

1. Deionized, distilled water (purchase high-performance liquid chromatography [HPLC] grade from Fisons if necessary). Pass through a 0.2-μm polytetrafluoroethylene (PTFE) filter (Whatman) prior to use.
2. Acetonitrile (Fisons, HPLC-grade). Pass through a 0.2 μm PTFE filter (Whatman) prior to use.
3. Glacial acetic acid (Fisons, HPLC grade). Mix with HPLC-grade water to give a 2.5% (v/v) solution. Pass through a 0.2-μm PTFE filter (Whatman) prior to use.

3. Methods

3.1. Preparation of GSH Standards

1. Make up 250 μL of GSH stock solution to 10 mL with PBS in a volumetric flask giving a final concentration of 105 μ*M*.
2. Dilute in PBS as shown in **Table 1**.
3. Add 50 μL of 30 m*M* DTT to 1 mL of each standard solution

4. Incubate for 30 min at room temperature to reduce any oxidized glutathione.
5. Mix 150 µL of each concentration with 150 µL of the MBBr stock solution.
6. Incubate at room temperature in the dark for 5 min.
7. Add 15 µL of TCA (100%).
8. Centrifuge at 13,000*g* in a microfuge for 10 min, to remove particulate matter.

3.2. Preparation of Quality Control (QC) Samples

1. Prepare 50 mL of 5 and 80 µ*M* GSH and store as 1-mL aliquots at –80°C. One high and one low concentration QC should be analyzed at the beginning, middle, and end of batch of samples.
2. On the day of analysis, defrost one aliquot of each and incubate with DTT and MBBr, as previously described.
3. Centrifuge at 13,000*g* in a microfuge for 10 min, to remove particulate matter.

3.3. Sample Preparation

1. Wash cells twice in PBS to remove GSH in medium or plasma.
2. Resuspend washed cells in 250 µL of PBS at a concentration of 2×10^6/mL (*see* **Note 3**).
3. Mix with 250 µL of the stock MBBr solution.
4. Incubate for 5 min in the dark at room temperature.
5. Add 25 µL of 100% TCA and keep at 4°C for 30 min to insure complete protein precipitation.
6. Centrifuge at 13,000*g* for 5 min using a microfuge and remove supernatant for analysis. Samples may be stored at –80°C prior to HPLC.

3.4. Quantitation of MBBr-GSH Adducts by HPLC

1. Separation of fluorescent compounds is achieved using reverse phase gradient HPLC (RP-HPLC) using a 4.6 × 150 mm Spherisorb ODS 5 µm column (Jones Chromatography) kept at 19°C (*see* **Note 4**).
2. Peaks are detected using a fluorescent detector set with an excitation wavelength of 384 nm and an emission wavelength of 480 nm.
3. The sample volume injected is 25 µL.
4. Acetonitrile (100%), acetic acid (2.5%), and water are used as the mobile phase, with a flow rate of 1 mL/min. A linear gradient from 10% acetonitrile, 0.25% acetic acid to 75% acetonitrile, 0.25% acetic acid is used for elution (*see* **Table 2**). The total analysis time, including flushing and equilibration of the column, is 26 min.
4. The concentration in the unknowns is calculated from a standard curve, prepared using integrated peak areas.

4. Notes

1. Because MBBr is light-sensitive, all steps should be performed in the dark.
2. Purchase as solution to reduce risk of handling.

Table 2
Gradient Used to Separate MBBr-GSH Adducts

Time	Flow rate (mL/min)	Water (%)	Acetonitrile (%)	Acetic acid[a] (%)
0	1	80	10	10
5	1	80	10	10
13	1	15	75	10
17	1	15	75	10
19	1	80	10	10

[a]2.5% solution.

3. This concentration of cells is appropriate for lymphoblasts. Dilution experiments should be performed for larger cells to establish the optimum cell concentration to use.
4. Flush and store the column in 80% water and 20% acetonitrile.

Reference

1. Cotgreave, I. A. and Moldeus, P. (1986) Methodologies for the application of monobromobimane to the simultaneous analysis of soluble and protein thiol components of biological systems. *J. Biochem. Biophys. Methods* **13,** 231–249.

10

Topoisomerase I and II Activity Assays

**Philippe Pourquier, Glenda Kohlhagen,
Li-Ming Ueng, and Yves Pommier**

1. Introduction

DNA topoisomerases I and II (top1 and top2, respectively) are ubiquitous enzymes that play an essential role in transcription, replication, chromosome segregation, and DNA repair. The basic enzymatic reaction of topoisomerases, namely reversible DNA nicking, is a transesterification reaction where a DNA phosphodiester bond is transferred to a specific enzyme tyrosine residue. Eukaryotic top1 and top2 exhibit major differences concerning their mechanism of action. Top1 acts as a monomer and forms a covalent bond with the 3'-terminus of a DNA single-strand break *(1–3)* whereas top2 acts as an homodimer and forms a covalent bond with the 5'-terminus of the DNA double-strand break with a four base-pairs overhang (**Fig. 1**) *(1–4)*. No energy cofactor is required for top1 activity, whereas top2 hydrolyzes adenosine triphosphate (ATP) during its catalytic cycle.

Both top1 and top2 can remove supercoils by making transient nicks in DNA and allowing the passage of another single- or double-stranded DNA molecule through the nick. However, only top2 is able to catenate or decatenate closed duplex DNA.

Both topoisomerases have been shown to be important targets for numerous classes of anticancer agents (see refs. *4–7* for reviews). Top2 inhibitors have been separated into two main categories: topoisomerase poisons such as anthracyclines (doxorubicin), epipodophyllotoxins (etoposide [VP-16] and teniposide [VM-26]), and aminoacridines (*m*-AMSA), which trap the cleavage step. The second category is the topoisomerases suppressors, such as ICRF 187 or 193, which do not stabilize the cleavage complexes but rather inhibit the catalytic activity of the enzyme *(4)*. The main top1 poisons to date belong

From: *Methods in Molecular Medicine, Vol. 28: Cytotoxic Drug Resistance Mechanisms*
Edited by: R. Brown and U. Böger-Brown © Humana Press Inc., Totowa, NJ

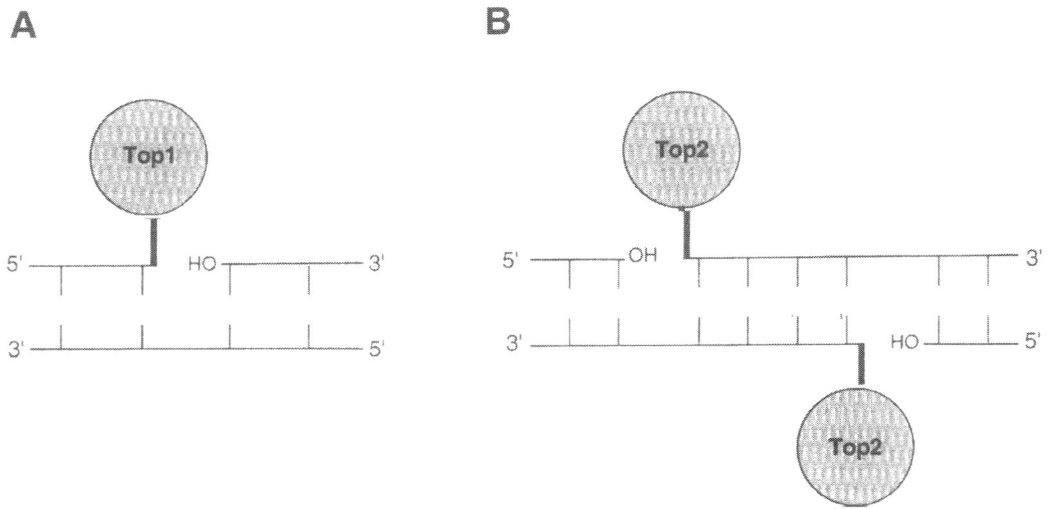

Fig. 1. Top1- and top2-cleavage complexes. **(A)** Top1 acts as a monomer, makes a single-strand break and covalently binds to the 3'-end of the break, leaving a 5'-hydroxyl end. **(B)** Top2 acts as a dimer, and generally makes a double-strand break. Each strand is cleaved by one monomer, with a 4-base overhang. Each monomer covalently binds to the 5'-end of the break and leaves a 3'-hydroxyl end.

to the camptothecins family *(5)*. Topoisomerase poisons can be used to map topoisomerase cleavage sites because they enhance top1 or top2 cleavage. However, they show specific base preferences depending on the class of the compound *(4,5)*

Here, we describe simple and commonly used in vitro assays (**Table 1**) to measure mammalian top1 and top2 activities and the response of topoisomerases to drugs.

2. Materials

Both top1 and top2 cleavage assays can be performed using two different substrates: either short duplex oligonucleotides containing a unique top1 or top2 cleavage site, or DNA fragments from genes, DNA viruses, or plasmids.

2.1. Oligonucleotide Assay for Top1-Mediated Cleavage

1. Oligonucleotides: One duplex oligonucleotide is derived from Tetrahymena rDNA hexadecameric sequence *(8)* where the A was changed to a G at the +1 position relative to the top1 cleavage site (indicated by the caret) to enhance camptothecin sensitivity *(9)*:
   5' - GATCTAAAAGACTT^GGAAAAATTTTTAAAAAAGCTC - 3' (scissile strand)
   3' - CTAGATTTTCTGAA-CCTTTTTAAAAATTTTTTCGAG - 5' (nonscissile strand)
   Another oligonucleotide is derived from a strong cleavage site in simian virus 40 DNA *(9)*:
   5' - CAAAGTCAGGTTGAT^GAGCATATTTTACTC - 3' (scissile strand)
   3' - GTTTCAGTCCAACTA-CTCGTATAAAATGAG - 5' (non scissile strand)
   Oligonucleotides are high-performance liquid chromatography (HPLC)-purified and resuspended in distilled water at 10 picomoles/μL and stored at 4°C (*see* **Note 1**).
2. Terminal deoxynucleotidyl transferase (Gibco BRL, Grand Island, NY).
3. Labeling buffer (5X: 500 m*M* potassium cacodylate, pH 7.2, 1 m*M* DTT). Store at –20°C.
4. [α^{32}P]-cordycepin (New England Nuclear, Boston, MA; specific activity: 5000 μCi/μL). Store at –20°C.
5. G25 Sephadex spin columns.
6. Annealing buffer (10X): 100 m*M* Tris-HCl, pH 7.8, 1 *M* NaCl, 10 m*M* Na_2 ethylenediaminetetracetic acid (EDTA). Store at –20°C.
7. Catenation buffer (10X): 100 m*M* Tris-HCl, pH 7.5, 500 m*M* KCl, 50 m*M* $MgCl_2$, 1 m*M* Na_2EDTA, 150 μg/mL bovine serum albumin (BSA). Store at –20°C.
8. 10X dithiothreitol (DTT): 2 m*M* stock solution. Store at –20°C.
9. Purified top1.
10. 10 m*M* camptothecin (CPT) stock solution in dimethylsulfoxide (DMSO). Aliquots can be stored at –20°C, but making fresh solution is recommended.

Table 1
Topoisomerase Reactions and Assays Described in this Chapter[a]

Substrate Gel	Supercoiled unlabeled DNA Agarose	^{32}P End-labeled DNA fragments Agarose	kDNA Agarose	^{32}P End-labeled DNA (Gene fragments or oligonucleotides) Denaturing Acrylamide
Top2	DNA relaxation Cleavage complexes: SSB: nicks[b]	Cleavage complexes: DSB	Decatenation	Cleavage complexes: SSB + DSB (5'-end-labeled DNA)
Top1	Cleavage complexes: SSB: nicks[b] DSB: form III linear	Cleavage complexes: SSB[c]	N/A	Cleavage complexes: SSB (3'-end-labeled DNA)

[a]This table provides a simple guide to choose the suitable technique for the different top1 or top2 activities measurements (cleavage, relaxation, decatenation).

[b]Addition of chloroquine or ethidium bromide in the running buffer resolves nicked DNA vs relaxed DNA **(21)**.

[c]In this case, the agarose gel loading buffer needs to be denaturing, and electrophoresis needs to be started quickly after loading to avoid renaturation **(12)**.

DSB, DNA double-strand break; SSB, DNA single-strand break; N/A, not applicable.

11. Sodiumdodecylsulfate (SDS): 5% (w/v) stock solution in distilled water.
12. Beta scintillation counter.
13. DNA sequencing gels and loading buffer (*see* **Subheading 2.7.**).

2.2. Long DNA Fragment Assay for Top1-Mediated Cleavage

1. Various fragments can be used: for instance, SV40 DNA, pBR322 plasmid, pBluescript SK(–) phagemid, c-*myc* proto-oncogene fragments or human top1 cDNA *(10–12)*.
2. Restriction enzymes from commercial sources (*see* also **Note 2**).
3. Dialysis membrane for electroelution.
4. [α^{32}P]-dCTP (New England Nuclear: specific activity: 3000 Ci/mmol). Stored at 4°C.
5. 0.5 m*M* of dATP, dTTP, and dGTP Mix.
6. Labeling buffer (10X): 500 m*M* Tris, pH 8.0, 100 m*M* $MgCl_2$, 500 m*M* NaCl.
7. Klenow fragment of DNA polymerase I.
8. Phenol (1X TBE saturated).
9. Chloroform/isoamyl alcohol (25:1).
10. TE buffer (1X): 10 m*M* Tris-HCl, pH 7.5, 1 m*M* Na_2EDTA.
11. Sodium acetate 3 *M*, pH 5.2.
12. 100% and 70% ethanol, stored at –20°C.
13. Catenation buffer (10X): 100 m*M* Tris-HCl pH 7.5, 500 m*M* KCl, 50 m*M* $MgCl_2$, 1 m*M* Na_2EDTA, 150 µg/mL BSA. Store at –20°C.
14. 10X DTT: 2 m*M* stock solution. Store at –20°C.
15. Purified top1.
16. 10 m*M* CPT stock solution in DMSO. Aliquots can be stored at –20°C, but making fresh solution is recommended.
17. SDS: 5% (w/v) stock solution in distilled water.
18. Alkaline precipitation solution: 0.6 *M* sodium acetate, 100 µg/mL tRNA (final concentrations).
19. Beta scintillation counter.
20. DNA sequencing gels and loading buffer (*see* **Subheading 2.7.**).

2.3. Oligonucleotide Assay for Top2-Mediated Cleavage

1. Oligonucleotides: Three oligonucleotides for top2 cleavage have been described:
   a. One oligonucleotide is derived from the SV40 DNA (from position 4235 to 4270) and contains a top2 site in the absence of drug (indicated by the carets). This oligonucleotide contains 3 additional sites in the presence of idarubicin, and few additional sites in the presence of *m*-AMSA and VM-26 *(13)*:
      5' - GTATGTTATGATT^ATAA-CTGTTATGCCTACTTATAA - 3'
      3' - CATACAATACTAA-TATT^GACAATACGGATGAATATT - 5'
   b. Another oligonucleotide is derived from the T4rIIB gene that contains a strong and unique *m*-AMSA-induced cleavage site (indicated by the carets) *(14)*:
      5' - GATCCAAGCTAAAGTT^ATAT-AACTTTATTCAAGGTCGA - 3'
      3' - CTAGGTTCGATTTCAA-TATA^TTGAAATAAGTTCCAGCT - 5'

c. The third oligonucleotide is a pBR322 fragment (from position 87–126) and contains a unique top2 cleavage site (indicated by the carets). However, cleavage at this site is only enhanced three-fold by high concentrations of etoposide (200 µ*M*) ***(15)***:
   5' - TGAAATCTAACAATG^CGCT-CATCGTCATCCTCGGCACCGT - 3'
   3' - ACTTTAGATTGTTAC-GCGA^GTAGCAGTAGGAGCCGTGGCA - 5'
2. T4 polynucleotide kinase (Gibco BRL).
3. Forward reaction buffer (5X): 350 m*M* Tris-HCl, pH 7.6, 500 m*M* KCl, 5 m*M* 2-mercaptoethanol, 50 m*M* $MgCl_2$. Store at –20°C.
4. [γ^{32}P]-ATP (New England Nuclear: specific activity: 6000 Ci/mmol).
5. Na_2EDTA: 0.5 *M* stock solution.
6. Annealing buffer (10X): 100 m*M* Tris-HCl, pH 7.8, 100 m*M* NaCl, 10 m*M* Na_2EDTA.
7. Catenation buffer (10X): 100 m*M* Tris-HCl, pH 7.5, 500 m*M* KCl, 50 m*M* $MgCl_2$, 1 m*M* Na_2EDTA, 150 µg/mL BSA. Store at –20°C.
8. 10X DTT: 2 m*M* stock solution. Store at –20°C.
9. ATP: 10 m*M* stock solution. Store at –20°C.
10. Purified top2.
11. 10 m*M* VM-26 stock solution in DMSO. Store at –20°C. Aliquots can be stored at –20°C, but making fresh solution is recommended.
12. SDS: 5% (w/v) stock solution in distilled water.
13. Proteinase K (Gibco BRL): 5 mg/mL stock solution in distilled water. Store at –20°C.
14. Beta scintillation counter.
15. DNA sequencing gels and loading buffer (*see* **Subheading 2.7.**).

2.4. Long DNA Fragment Assay for Top2-Mediated Cleavage

1. SV40 DNA, pBluescript SK(-) phagemid, pBR322 plasmid and c-*myc* proto-oncogene can be used in this assay ***(9,10,16–18)***.
2. Restriction enzymes from commercial source.
3. Shrimp alkaline phosphatase (SAP) (United States Biochemical, Cleveland, OH). This enzyme is preferred to calf intestinal phosphatase (CIP) because it is heat-labile in its 10X reaction buffer: 200 m*M* Tris-HCl, pH 8.0, 100 m*M* $MgCl_2$.
4. T4 polynucleotide kinase (Gibco BRL).
5. Forward reaction buffer (5X): 350 m*M* Tris-HCl, pH 7.6, 500 m*M* KCl, 5 m*M* 2-mercaptoethanol, 50 m*M* MgCl2. Store at –20°C.
6. [γ^{32}P]-ATP (New England Nuclear): specific activity: 6000 Ci/mmol.
7. G50 Sephadex spin columns.
8. Catenation buffer (10X): 100 m*M* Tris-HCl, pH 7.5, 500 m*M* KCl, 50 m*M* $MgCl_2$, 1 m*M* Na_2EDTA, 150 µg/mL BSA. Store at –20°C.
9. 10X DTT: 2 m*M* stock solution. Store at –20°C.
10. ATP: 10 m*M* stock solution. Store at –20°C.
11. Purified top2.
12. 10 m*M* VM-26 stock solution in DMSO (store at –20°C).

13. SDS: 5% (w/v) stock solution in distilled water.
14. Proteinase K (Gibco BRL): 5 mg/mL stock solution in distilled water. Store at –20°C.
15. Alkaline precipitation solution (for 10 mL solution): 2 mL 3 *M* sodium acetate, 100 µg/mL tRNA solution, distilled water up to 10 mL. Store at –20°C.
16. Beta scintillation counter.
17. DNA sequencing gels and loading buffer (*see* **Subheading 2.7.**).

2.5. Top1 and Top2 Relaxation and Cleavage Assays

1. Supercoiled native SV40 DNA, form I (Gibco BRL) or pBR322 plasmid DNA.
2. Catenation buffer (10X): 100 m*M* Tris-HCl, pH 7.5, 500 m*M* KCl, 50 m*M* $MgCl_2$, 1 m*M* Na_2EDTA, 150 µg/mL BSA; store at –20°C.
3. 10X DTT: 2 m*M* stock solution. Store at –20°C.
4. ATP: 10 m*M* stock solution (for top2 assays only). Store at –20°C.
5. Purified top1 or top2.
6. SDS: 5% (w/v) stock solution in distilled water.
7. Proteinase K (Gibco BRL): 5 mg/mL stock solution in distilled water. Store at –20°C.
8. Agarose gel and agarose loading buffers (*see* **Subheading 2.8.**).

2.6. Decatenation Assays

1. Kinetoplast DNA (kDNA) (TopoGEN Inc., Columbus, OH).
2. Markers: linear kDNA (*Xho*I cut) and decatenated kDNA.
3. Decatenation buffer (10X): 100 m*M* Tris-HCl, pH 7.4, 1 *M* KCl, 50 m*M* $MgCl_2$, 10 m*M* ATP, 1 m*M* Na_2EDTA, 150 µg/mL BSA. Store at –20°C.
4. ATP: 10 m*M* stock solution. Store at –20°C.
5. Purified top2.
6. SDS: 5% (w/v) stock solution in distilled water.
7. Proteinase K (Gibco BRL): 5 mg/mL stock solution in distilled water. Store at –20°C.
8. Standard agarose gel (1% in TBE 1X) and standard agarose loading buffer (*see* **Subheading 2.8.**).

2.7. Sequencing Gels

1. Sequencing loading buffer: 80% formamide, 10 m*M* NaOH, 1 m*M* Na_2EDTA, 0.1% xylene cyanol, 0.1% bromophenol blue.
2. Acrylamide solution (50%): dissolve 100 g acrylamide into 100 mL of distilled water, and add up to 200 mL.
3. N, N' methylenebisacrylamide (bisacrylamide) 2% solution.
4. TBE (10X): 108 g Tris base, 55 g boric acid, 4 mL 0.5 *M* Na_2EDTA, pH 8.0; add up to 1 L with distilled water.
5. Ammonium persulfate: 10% (w/v) solution (make fresh).
6. N,N,N',N',tetramethylenediamine (TEMED).
7. Sequencing gel electrophoresis apparatus.
8. PhosphorImager system or X-ray films and developer.

2.8. Agarose Gels

1. Standard agarose loading buffer (10X): 20% Ficol 400, 0.1 *M* Na_2EDTA, pH 8.0, 1% SDS, 0.25% bromophenol blue.
2. Denaturing agarose loading buffer (10X): 0.45 *M* NaOH, 30 m*M* Na_2EDTA, 15% sucrose, 0.25 mg/mL bromocresol green (12).
3. Agarose (molecular-biology grade).
4. TBE (10X): 108 g Tris base, 55 g boric acid, 4 mL 0.5 *M* Na_2EDTA, pH 8.0; add up to 1 L with distilled water.
5. Ethidium bromide: 10 mg/mL stock solution.
6. $MgSO_4$: 1 *M* stock solution for destaining.
7. Molecular-weight markers: usually the 1 kb ladder and/or the λDNA/*Hin*dIII.
8. Sequencing gel electrophoresis apparatus.
9. Ultraviolet (UV) transilluminator system.

3. Methods

3.1. Oligonucleotides Labeling

3.1.1. 3'-End Labeling

1. Standard 40 μL reaction: mix 1 μL scissile strand oligonucleotide (approximately 10 picomoles) with 20 μL purified distilled water, 8 μL 5X labeling buffer, 10 μL [α^{32}P]-cordycepin and 1 μL terminal deoxynucleotidyl transferase (TdT) (15 units).
2. Incubate for 1 h at 37°C.
3. Prepare the G25 Sephadex spin column by removing the buffer by two centrifugations at 1000*g* for 5 min. Then, load the reaction mixture on top of the column and spin for 5 min at 1000*g*. The unincorporated [α^{32}P]-cordycepin remains in the column. Make sure to load the sample in the middle of the top of the column.
4. Check the labeling efficiency by counting 1 μL of the flow-through. The counts should be over 100,000 dpm/μL (*see* **Note 4**).
5. An additional purification step can be performed (for both labeled and unlabeled oligonucleotide) by loading single-stranded DNA on a denaturing polyacrylamide gel and electroeluting the corresponding band ***(19)***, or using commercially available gel extraction protocols (*see* **Note 5**).

3.1.2. 5'-End Labeling

1. Standard 20 μL reaction: mix 1 μL of one oligonucleotide (approximately 10 picomoles) with 8.5 μL purified distilled water, 4 μL 5X forward reaction buffer, 6 μL [γ^{32}P]-ATP, 0.5 μL T4 DNA polynucleotide kinase (5 units).
2. Incubate for 1 h at 37°C.
3. Stop the reaction by adding 1 μL of 0.5 *M* Na_2EDTA, and heat the reaction tube at 70°C for 10 min.
4. Purification of the oligonucleotide is performed with a G25 Sephadex spin column as described in **Subheading 3.1.1, steps 3–5**.

3.1.3. Annealing Reactions

1. The labeled oligonucleotide (flow-through) is mixed with the same amount of unlabeled complementary strand (1 µL or approximately 10 picomoles) and a final concentration of 1X annealing buffer (adjust the volume with distilled water).
2. Heat the mixture at 95°C for 5 min on a dry heating block.
3. Switch off the block and let the mixture cool down to room temperature.

3.2. pBluescript SK(-) Fragments Labeling

pBluescript SK(-) is taken as an example. Principles are similar with other DNA fragments.

3.2.1. 3'-End Labeling (Fill-in Reaction)

1. 2 µg of pBluescript SK(-) phagemid is digested for 1 h at 37°C with 10 units of *Pvu*II and *Hin*dIII in a final volume of 50 µL.
2. Add 5 µL 10X standard agarose loading buffer and load the sample on a 1% agarose gel.
3. The *Pvu*II-*Hin*dIII-digested pBluescript SK(-) 161 bp fragment is electrophoresed overnight in a 1% agarose gel (*see* **Subheading 3.4.2.**).
4. After ethidium bromide staining, the 161 bp band is excised from the gel and electroeluted ***(19)*** before ethanol precipitation. Any commercially available agarose gel extraction protocol can be used at this stage.
5. Approximately 200 ng of *Pvu*II-*Hin*dIII fragment is labeled with 2 units (1 µL) Klenow fragment from DNA polymerase I, 4 µL [α^{32}P]-dCTP, and 0.05 m*M* dNTP Mix in 1X Klenow buffer. Final reaction volume is 30 µL.
6. Incubate the reaction mixture at room temperature for 15 min.
7. Add an equal volume (30 µL) of phenol:chloroform/isoamyl alcohol (v:v). Vortex for 10 s and microcentrifuge to separate phases (usually 30 s).
8. Transfer the top (aqueous) layer to a new tube, and re-extract the first tube with 30 µL of 1X TE buffer.
9. Pool the aqueous phases and extract with 1 volume of chloroform/isoamyl alcohol (24/1).
10. Transfer the upper phase to a new tube and ethanol precipitate: add 1 volume of alkaline precipitation solution and 2.5 volumes of cold 100% ethanol (mix gently) and incubate for at least 20 min at –20°C.
11. Centrifuge at 12,000*g* for 30 min at 4°C, remove the supernatant, add 500 µL cold ethanol 70% to wash the pellet and centrifuge at 12,000*g* for another 30 min at 4°C.
12. Remove the supernatant, lay the tube near a 70°C heat block to dry, check the labeling by counting the dry tube, and resuspend the DNA in distilled water.

3.2.2. 5'-End Labeling

1. 2 µg of pBluescript SK(-) phagemid is digested for 1 h at 37°C with 10 units of PstI in a final volume of 50 µL.

2. Add to the former 50 μL reaction mixture 6 μL of 10X SAP buffer and 1 μL (1 unit) of SAP. Add distilled water up to 60 μL and incubate for 1 h at 37°C.
3. Heat-inactivate the phosphatase for 30 min at 65°C.
4. Take a 4 μL aliquot (approximately 130 ng) of the aforementioned solution and add 2 μL 10X kinase buffer, 10 μL [γ^{32}P]-ATP, and 1 μL (10 U) of T4 polynucleotide kinase. Add distilled water up to 20 μL and incubate for 1 h at 37°C.
5. Heat-inactivate for 15 min at 70°C.
6. Add 1 μL (10 U) of *Hin*dIII to the aforementioned solution and incubate for another hour at 37°C. This step will generate two 5'- end-labeled fragments of 22 and 2936 bp. Only the 2936 bp fragment is used to sequence topoisomerase cleavage sites.
7. Remove the excess of unincorporated [γ^{32}P]-ATP through a G50 Sephadex spin column as described in **Subheading 3.1.1. step 3**. This step should also remove the 22 bp fragment.
8. Count 1 μL of the flow through to check the labeling efficiency.

3.3. Topoisomerase Reactions

3.3.1. Top1 Cleavage Reactions

1. For a typical 10 μL reaction: use approximately 50,000 dpm from the 3'-labeled DNA, 1 μL 10X catenation buffer, 1 μL 10X DTT, 1 μL DMSO and approximately 1 μL the enzyme solution. Add distilled water up to 10 μL (*see* also **Note 6**).
2. Run controls in the absence and presence of purified top1.
3. If reactions are performed in order to test new top1 inhibitors, run a reaction with 1 μL of a 100 μ*M* solution of CPT (10 μ*M* final concentration) as a positive control.
4. Incubate reactions at room temperature for 30 min and stop reactions by adding 1 μL of SDS 5%.
5. For oligonucleotides experiments, add 3–4 volumes of sequencing loading buffer. Only a fraction of the samples (generally 5 μL) is loaded on the gel. **Figure 2A** shows a typical gel is shown for top1 cleavage in the Tetrahymena oligonucleotide.
6. An extra purification step is needed when long DNA fragments are used: after **step 4**, add 1 volume of alkaline precipitation solution and 2.5 volumes of cold 100% ethanol (mix gently) and incubate for at least 20 min at –20°C (*see* **Note 7**).
7. Repeat **steps 11** and **12** from **Subheading 3.2.1.** and resuspend the DNA directly in sequencing loading buffer instead of distilled water. Heat the samples 1 min at 95°C before loading. A representative gel for top1 cleavage in pBluescript SK(–) fragment is shown in **Fig. 2B**.
8. Top1-mediated cleavage complexes (single-strand breaks) can also be detected using agarose gels ***(12)***. In that case, approximately 0.5 volumes of agarose denaturing buffer is added directly to the samples after reactions are stopped by 0.5% SDS. A fraction of the sample is quickly loaded in a standard 1% agarose gel.

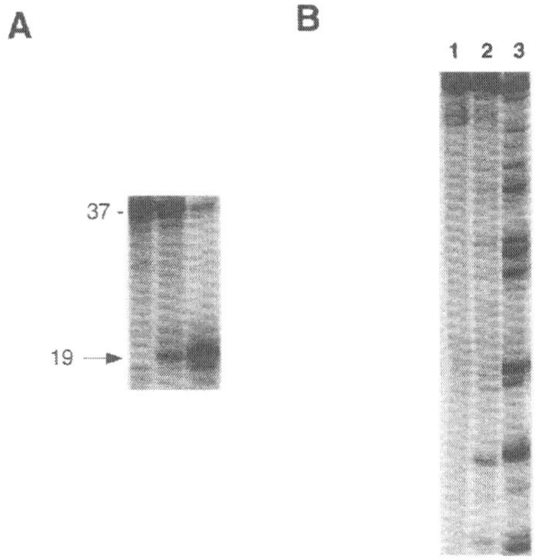

Fig. 2. **(A)** Purified top1-mediated cleavage in the 3'-labeled Tetrahymena oligonucleotide. Lane 1, DNA alone; lane 2: + top1; lane 3: + top1 + 10 µ*M* CPT. The unique cleavage product is indicated by the arrow. **(B)** Purified top1-mediated cleavage in the *Pvu*II–*Hin*dIII fragment of the pBluescript SK(–) phagemid. Lanes are the same as in Panel A. The gel shows the multiple CPT-enhanced cleavage of top1 sites (compare lane 2 to lane 3).

3.3.2. Top2 Cleavage Reactions

Reactions are performed in the same conditions except that the DNA is 5'-end labeled and that the reactions are modified as follows for a typical 10 µL reaction:

1. Add 1 µL 10 m*M* ATP stock solution to reactions (1 m*M* final concentration).
2. After stopping the reaction with SDS, a digestion with proteinase K is recommended for samples run in nondenaturing agarose gels: usually, add 1 µL 5 mg/mL Proteinase K solution and incubate for 1 h at 50°C.
3. If reactions are performed in order to test new top2 poisons, run a reaction with 1 µL of a 100 µ*M* solution of VM-26 (10 µ*M* final concentration) as a positive control (*see* **Note 3**).

3.3.3. Relaxation Assays with Native Supercoiled DNA (Top1 or Top2 Reactions)

1. For a typical 10 µL reaction: 0.3–0.4 µg SV40 DNA is mixed with 1 µL 10X catenation buffer, 1 µL 10X DTT, 1 µL 10 m*M* ATP, 1 µL DMSO (control for drugs diluted in DMSO), generally 1 µL topoisomerase or cellular extract, and distilled water up to 10 µL.
2. If reactions are performed in order to test new topoisomerases inhibitors, run a reaction with 1 µL of a 100 µ*M* solution of the appropriate positive control drug (either CPT or VM-26; 10 µ*M* final concentration).

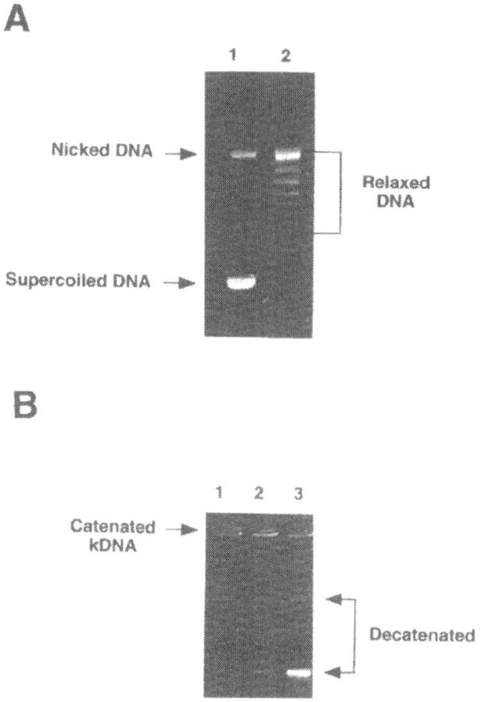

Fig. 3. **(A)** Relaxation of SV40 DNA by purified top1. Lane 1, DNA alone. The majority of the DNA is in its supercoiled form, but a fraction of the DNA is nicked. Lane 2: SV40 + top1. Relaxed DNA appears as multiple bands corresponding to the different changes in linking numbers between the supercoiled and the nicked DNA. **(B)** Decatenation of kDNA by top2. Lane 1, DNA alone; lane 2 and 3: kDNA + top2 for 15 min and 30 min incubation, respectively. Decatenation is measured by the disappearance of the band in the well and appearance of lower bands (indicated by arrows).

3. Incubate the reaction mixture for 30 min at 37°C or 30°C.
4. Stop reactions with 1 µL SDS 5% (0.5% final concentration).
5. Add 1 µL of 5 mg/mL proteinase K and incubate the reaction mixture for 15 min at 50°C.
6. Add 1.2 µL of 10X loading buffer for agarose gel electrophoresis.
7. A representative gel for top1-induced relaxation assay is shown in **Fig. 3A** (top2-induced relaxation gives the same type of pattern).

3.3.4. Decatenation Assays (Top2 Reactions)

1. To 0.3 µg of kDNA, add 2 µL 10X decatenation buffer, 1 µL DMSO, generally 1 µL of top2 or cellular extracts, and distilled water up to 20 µL.
2. If reactions are performed to assay new top2 inhibitors, run a control reaction with 1 µL of a 100 µ*M* VM-26 solution as a positive control.

3. Incubate for 30 min at 37°C or 30°C.
4. Stop the reaction with 2.5 µL of SDS 5% (0.5% final concentration).
5. Add 2 µL 5 mg/mL proteinase K and incubate the reaction mixture for 15 min at 50°C.
6. Add 2.5 µL 10X loading buffer for agarose gel electrophoresis.
7. A representative gel is shown in **Fig. 3B**.

3.4. Gels

3.4.1. Polyacrylamide Gels

1. Glass plates (42 × 33 cm) are separated by 0.4-mm plastic spacers. The edges and the bottom of the plates are sealed with clamps (*see* **Note 8**).
2. Standard 16% polyacrylamide gels (preparation for 100 mL): Mix 42 g of urea in 32 mL of 50% acrylamide, 8 mL of 2% bisacrylamide, and 10 mL of 10X TBE (*see* **Note 9**). Microwave the acrylamide solution (avoid boiling) and wait until complete solubilization. Add distilled water up to 100 mL.
3. Cool down the solution to room temperature while stirring and filter with a 0.2-µm Millipore membrane.
4. To the 100 mL solution, add 45 µL TEMED, and 800 µL freshly prepared 10% ammonium persulfate.
5. Pour the mixture between the glass plates at an angle of approximately 45°. When the level of acrylamide reaches the top, slowly lay down the plates horizontally and insert the 32-tooth comb (0.4-mm thick). Polymerization takes at least 30 min.
6. After polymerization, remove slowly the comb and flush the wells with 1X TBE (running buffer) using a Pasteur pipet or a large syringe. Pre-run the gel until the temperature reaches 50°C (indicated by the temperature sensor).
7. Load 5 µL of the samples and run the gel at 120 W until the bromophenol blue reaches the 3/4 of the plates for the oligonucleotides assays, or until the bromophenol blue reaches the bottom of the gel for the pBluescript SK(–) fragment assays. If necessary, decrease electric power in order not to exceed 50°C during the electrophoresis (to avoid cracking of the glass plates).
8. At the end of electrophoresis, the plates are carefully separated (the gel should remain stuck to the nonsiliconized plate). The gel is transferred to a 3MM Whatman paper, covered with a plastic wrap and dried at 80°C for at least 1 h.
9. Gels are exposed for autoradiography or in a PhosphorImager cassette.

3.4.2. Agarose Gels

1. 1% (w/v) standard agarose gel solutions:
   Large gels (22 × 25 cm): 3 g agarose in 300 mL of 1X TBE buffer.
   Medium gels (11.5 × 14.2 cm): 1 g agarose in 100 mL of 1X TBE buffer.
2. Microwave agarose solution until complete dissolution (the solution should boil). Let the solution cool down while stirring. Pour the gel when the temperature is around 40–50°C. Insert the comb.
3. When polymerized, add enough 1X TBE buffer to cover the gel and load samples.
4. Different markers can be used depending on the reaction:

For pBluescript SK(–) fragments purification: 1 Kb ladder.
For relaxation: linear and supercoiled samples.
For decatenation reactions: linear kDNA and decatenated kDNA markers.
For detection of cleavable complexes: ^{32}P-end-labeled 1Kb ladder or the *Hin*dIII or *Eco*RI digested DNA fragment used in the assay.

5. Electrophorese overnight at 80–100 volts for large gels or 40–60 V for medium gels in 1X TBE buffer (the bromophenol blue should be near the end of the gel).
6. Agarose gels are stained in TBE 1X containing 0.5 mg/mL ethidium bromide for 30–45 min and destained with a 1 m*M* $MgSO_4$ solution for an additional 30 min.
7. DNA visualization is made with an UV transilluminator (*see* **Notes 10** and **11**).

4. Notes

1. Oligonucleotide working solutions can be stored at 4°C. However, each oligonucleotide should be aliquoted, vacuum-dried and stored at –20°C.
2. Usually restriction enzymes are supplied with the adequate 10X reaction buffer. Enzyme concentration and reaction buffer composition may vary from one source to another, and volumes need to be adjusted accordingly.
3. In the top2 reactions, VM-26 is used as a positive control. However, depending on the oligonucleotide or the DNA fragment used, other top2 inhibitors (etoposide [VP-16], or *m*-AMSA) can be used. It is preferable not to use doxorubicin as a positive control because of its strong DNA intercalating property, which suppresses top2 cleavage above 1 μ*M*.
4. The radiolabeled fragments (long pieces or oligonucleotides) have to be used within a reasonable time because of radiolysis (usually within a week if stored at 4°C), to avoid any laddering.
5. In some cases, two (or more) bands migrating slower than the predicted size can be detected in the control DNA after 3'-end labeling with [α^{32}P]-cordycepin. This could be owing to the presence of normal [α^{32}P]-ATP in the cordycepin vial. Generally, a new [α^{32}P]-cordycepin batch must be used.
6. 5'-end labeling is also possible for top1-mediated cleavage reactions. Then, proteinase K digestion is necessary before analysis of the cleavage products. Otherwise, the covalent topoisomerase-DNA complexes will remain in the wells. 5'-end labeling is not recommended, however, because proteinase K leaves the top1 catalytic tyrosine attached to the DNA and sometimes a small peptide.
7. Usually, for long fragments, a purine sequencing is performed according to Maxam Gilbert chemical sequencing protocol ***(20)***. Briefly, 25 μL formamide is added to 5 μL labeled DNA and incubated at room temperature for 5 min. DNA is precipitated with an equal volume of alkaline precipitation solution (30 μL) and 2.5 volumes of 100% ethanol. After 20 min incubation on ice, the tube is centrifuged 30 min at 12,000*g* at 4°C, rinsed with 70% ethanol and dried. 100 μL of freshly diluted piperidine (1:10 in distilled water) is added, heated at 90°C for 30 min, and the sample vacuum-dried. The pellet is washed with 20 μL of distilled water and vacuum-dried again. The DNA is resuspended in the denaturing loading buffer and heated at 95°C for 2 min before loading.

8. One plate is "siliconized" by washing with 2 mL nonstick plate-coating Acrylease solution (Stratagene, La Jolla, CA). After complete drying, the plate is buffed until clear. New plates have to be washed with 5 *M* NaOH and rinsed with distilled water before use. Before each electrophoresis, the plates are first washed with a glass-cleaning solution and then with methanol.
9. Higher percentage of acrylamide (20 or 25%) can be used when topoisomerase-mediated cleavage leads to small fragments. In that case, 0.5X instead of 1X TBE can be used for the acrylamide gel and for the running buffer.
10. Separation between relaxed and nicked DNA is possible using agarose gels containing 2 μg/mL chloroquine ***(21)***.
11. Some drugs at high concentration can retard the migration of DNA in agarose gels. Such a problem can be solved by adding 0.1% SDS in the gel. However, after electrophoresis, the gel has to be rinsed extensively in water to remove the SDS before adding the ethidium bromide staining solution.

References

1. Wang, J. C. (1996) DNA topoisomerases. *Annu. Rev. Biochem.* **65,** 635–692.
2. Champoux, J. (1990) Mechanistic aspects of type-I topoisomerases, in *DNA Topology and Its Biological Effects* (Wang, J. C. and Cozarelli, N. R., eds.), Cold Spring Harbor Laboratory Press, Cold Spring Harbor, NY, pp. 217–242.
3. Gupta, M., Fujimori, A., and Pommier, Y. (1995) Eukaryotic DNA topoisomerases I. *Biochim. Biophys. Acta* **1262,** 1–14.
4. Pommier, Y. (1997) DNA topoisomerase II inhibitors, in *Cancer Therapeutics: Experimental and Clinical Agents* (Teicher, B. A., ed.), Humana Press, Totowa, NJ, pp. 153–174.
5. Pommier, Y. (1996) Eukaryotic DNA topoisomerase I: genome gatekeeper and its intruders, camptothecins. *Semin. Oncol.* **23,** 3–10.
6. Chen, A. Y. and Liu, L. F. (1994) DNA Topoisomerases: essential enzymes and lethal targets. *Annu. Rev. Pharmacol. Toxicol.* **94,** 194–218.
7. Osheroff, N., Corbett, A. H., Elsea, S. H., and Westergaard, M. (1994) Defining functional drug-interaction domains on topoisomerase II by exploiting mechanistic differences between drug classes. *Cancer Chemother. Pharmacol.* **34,** 19–25.
8. Bonven, B. J., Gocke, E., and Westergaard, O. (1985) A high affinity topoisomerase I binding sequence is clustered at DNAase I hypersensitive sites in Tetrahymena R-chromatin. *Cell* **41,** 541–551.
9. Jaxel, C., Capranico, G., Kerrigan, D., Kohn, K. W., and Pommier, Y. (1991) Effect of local DNA sequence on topoisomerase I cleavage in the presence or absence of camptothecin. *J. Biol. Chem.* **266,** 20418–20423.
10. Leteurtre, F., Fujimori, A., Tanizawa, A., Chhabra, A., Mazumder, A., Kohlhagen, G., Nakano, H., and Pommier, Y. (1994) Saintopin, a dual inhibitor of DNA topoisomerases I and II, as a probe for drug-enzyme interactions. *J. Biol. Chem.* **269,** 28,702–28,707.
11. Sorensen, B. S., Jensen, P. B., Sehested, M., Jensen, P. S., Kjeldsen, E., Nielsen, O. F., and Alsner, J. (1994) Antagonistic effect of aclarubicin on camptothecin induced cytotoxicity: role of topoisomerase I. *Biochem. Pharmacol.* **47,** 2105–2110.

12. Hsiang, Y. H., Hertzberg, R., Hecht, S., and Liu, L. F. (1985) Camptothecin induces protein-linked DNA breaks via mammalian DNA topoisomerase I. *J. Biol. Chem.* **260,** 14,873–14,878.
13. Bigioni, M., Zunino, F., Tinelli, S., Austin, C. A., Willmore, E., and Capranico, G. (1996) Position-specific effects of base mismatch on mammalian topoisomerase II DNA cleaving activity. *Biochemistry* **35,** 153–159.
14. Freudenreich, C. H. and Kreuzer, K. N. (1994) Localization of an aminoacridine antitumor agent in a type II topoisomerase-DNA complex. *Proc. Natl. Acad. Sci. USA* **91,** 11,007–11,011.
15. Kingma, P. S. and Osheroff, N. (1997) Apurinic sites are position-specific topoisomerase II poisons. *J. Biol. Chem.* **272,** 1148–1155.
16. Burden, D. A., Kingma, P. S., Froelich-Ammon, S. J., Bjornsti, M.-A., Patchan, M. W., Thompson, R. B., and Osheroff, N. (1996) Topoisomerase II–etoposide interaction direct the formation of drug-induced enzyme-DNA cleavage complexes. *J. Biol. Chem.* **271,** 29,238–29,244.
17. Pommier, Y., Orr, A., Kohn, K. W., and Riou, J. F. (1992) Differential effects of amsacrine and epipodophyllotoxins on topoisomerase II cleavage in the human c-*myc* proto-oncogene. *Cancer Res.* **52,** 3125–3130.
18. Nelson, E. M., Tewey, K. M., and Liu, L. F. (1984) Mechanism of antitumor drug action: poisoning of mammalian DNA topoisomerase II on DNA by 4'-(9-acridinylamino)-methanesulfon-*m*-anisidide. *Proc. Natl. Acad. Sci. USA* **81,** 1361–1365.
19. Sambrook, J., Fritsch, E. F., and Maniatis, T. (1989) *Molecular Cloning; A Laboratory Manual, 2nd ed.,* Cold Spring Harbor Laboratory Press, Cold Spring Harbor, NY.
20. Maxam, A. and Gilbert, W. (1980) Sequencing end-labeled DNA with base-specific chemical cleavages. *Methods Enzymol.* **65,** 499–560.
21. Jaxel, C., Kohn, K. W., Wani, M. C., Wall, M. E., and Pommier, Y. (1989) Structure-activity study of the actions of camptothecin derivatives on mammalian topoisomerase I: evidence for a specific receptor site and a relation to antitumor activity. *Cancer Res.* **49,** 1465–1469.

11

5-Fluorouracil Metabolizing Enzymes

Howard L. McLeod, Lesley H. Milne, and Stephen J. Johnston

1. Introduction

The uracil analog 5-fluorouracil (5-FU) is used as part of combination therapy for the treatment of breast, head/neck, and gastrointestinal malignancies, and has single-agent activity in colorectal cancer. 5-FU itself is inactive and requires intracellular conversion to form cytotoxic nucleotides *(1)*. Several cellular targets for fluoropyrimidines have been well-characterized, including inhibition of thymidylate synthase (TS) by fluorodeoxyuridine monophosphate (FdUMP) and false base incorporation into RNA or DNA. Most investigations into cellular resistance factors regulating 5-FU activity have focused on alterations in (TS) levels and reduced folate pools, the required cofactor for binding dUMP to thymidylate synthase *(1)*. However, the majority of an administered 5-FU dose undergoes metabolism to inactive species through a three-enzyme process, which is initiated and rate-limited by dihydropyrimidine dehydrogenase (DPD; EC 1.3.1.2). Following a bolus injection of 5-FU, 80% is degraded via DPD after 24 h after administration *(2)*. Studies of ^{19}F nuclear magnetic resonance (NMR) spectroscopy in mice bearing colon tumors found catabolites made up 51% of labeled drug in the tumor, compared with 26% for the anabolic products *(3)*.

DPD activity is found in most tissues, with the highest content in liver and peripheral mononuclear cells. Peripheral mononuclear cells are used as an easily accessible surrogate tissue for assessing in vivo DPD activity, and a high degree of variation in activity is observed in the general population (up to 20-fold) *(2)*. Although 5-FU is usually well-tolerated, patients with low or undetectable DPD activity have been described who exhibit severe, even life-threatening, toxicity such as pancytopenia, mucositis, and neurological toxicity *(4)*.

Several methods for measuring DPD activity have been described, including thin-layer chromatography (TLC), high-pressure ligand chromatography

From: *Methods in Molecular Medicine, Vol. 28: Cytotoxic Drug Resistance Mechanisms*
Edited by: R. Brown and U. Böger-Brown © Humana Press Inc., Totowa, NJ

(HPLC), and ultraviolet (UV) spectroscopy methods for measuring the ability of the enzymes to affect test substrates *(5)*. These methods have used several different substrates, including radiolabeled uracil, thymine, or 5-FU. Until recently, the assays used have been cumbersome, preventing efficient, high-throughput analysis of enzyme activity in biological tissues in a reproducible manner. In this chapter, we describe a method for measuring ex vivo DPD activity using ^{14}C-labeled 5-FU as the preferred substrate. This assay is useful in peripheral mononuclear cells, solid tissues, and cell lines, and has been applied to mouse, rat, monkey, dog, cow, pig, and human tissues *(6,7)*.

Another relatively under-investigated pathway of 5-FU metabolism is conversion of 5-FU to 5-fluoro-2'deoxyuridine (FDUR) by thymidine phosphorylase (TP; E.C. 2.4.2.4) *(1)*. FDUR is the first step in one pathway for the metabolic activation of 5-FU to deoxyribonucleotides. Studies into its regulation of 5-FU activity were first stimulated by the findings that interferon induces TP expression at doses that modulated 5-FU activity *(8)*. Further experiments have indicated that the enzyme has angiogenic and endothelial cell chemotactic activities, and that its expression may have prognostic significance in colorectal and breast cancer *(9,10)*. Levels of TP expression vary up to 15-fold in different human tissues. Studies in colorectal, stomach, and ovarian cancers have demonstrated that TP activity is consistently higher in tumor tissue when compared to adjacent normal tissues (up to 10-fold) *(11)*.

Until recently, there were two methods for analysis of TP activity; spectrophotometry and TLC, both of which were based on the conversion of thymidine to thymine. The spectrophotometric assay is based on the difference in molar-extinction coefficients between thymidine and thymine at alkaline pH. A fixed time-point at 90 min *(12)* or 16 h *(13)* has been used.

The second method uses the conversion of [^{14}C]-thymidine to [^{14}C]-thymine or vice versa as separated by TLC. Unlike the spectrophotometric assay, data on linearity with time and protein concentration is available for the TLC assay *(14)*. The main disadvantage of this particular method is the limitation of the number of samples that can be analyzed at one time owing to the capacity of the available chromatography equipment.

Milne et al. recently described a new assay for the measurement of TP activity in cell lines and tissues, which is sensitive, automated, and allows the processing of multiple assays simultaneously *(15)*. This method exploits the ability of TP to convert 5-FU to 5-FDUR in the presence of deoxyribose-1-phosphate (dR-1-P).

2. Materials

2.1. DPD

2.1.1. Peripheral Blood Cell Preparation

1. Ficoll-hypaque 1.077 g/mL (e.g., lymphoprep, histopaque, and so forth).
2. Phosphate buffered saline (PBS), pH 7.4.

3. 35 m*M* sodium phosphate buffer, pH 7.4
   $NaH_2PO_4 \cdot 2H_2O$ 2.73 g in 500 mL
   Na_2HPO_4 2.48 g in 500 mL
   Combine ~400 mL Na_2HPO_4 with ~100 mL NaH_2PO_4 and adjust to pH 7.4 by addition of Na_2HPO_4, if pH too high, or NaH_2PO_4, if pH too low. For final buffer, combine 10 mL glycerol (e.g., Sigma, Poole, UK, cat. no. G7893) with 90 mL $NaPO_4$ buffer.

2.1.2. HPLC

1. 25 m*M* $MgCl_2$.
2. 100 m*M* β-mercaptoethanol.
3. 10 m*M* benzamidine.
4. 10 m*M* aminoethylisothiouronium bromide (AEITU Br; Sigma).
5. 2.5 *M* sucrose.
6. 50 m*M* ethylenediaminetetraacetic acid (EDTA).
7. Nicotinamide adenine dinucleotide phosphate (NADPH).
8. [^{14}C]-5-FU (Amersham 54 mCi/mmol, Amersham, Arlington Heights, IL).
9. Ethanol.
10. 37°C shaking water bath.
11. 7.5-mL borsilicote glass culture tubes (Corning Glassworks, Corning, NY).
12. HPLC system (isocratic pump; UV detector helpful, but not required).
13. On-line HPLC radioactivity monitor (e.g., Berthold LB506C, Berthold, Leeds, UK).
14. Columns (in sequence): Hypersil ODS 25 × 0.46 cm, 5 μm packing; and Spherisorb ODS 25 × 0.46 cm, 5 μm packing.
15. 35 m*M* potassium phosphate buffer, pH 7.4. Combine 400 mL 35 m*M* K_2HPO_4 with 100 mL 35 m*M* KH_2PO_4 and pH to 7.4 by addition of K_2HPO_4, if pH is too low, or KH_2PO_4, if pH is too high.
16. Buffer A: (make 10 mL/5 samples): 8.9 mL of 35 m*M* phosphate buffer, pH 7.4, 1.0 mL 25 m*M* $MgCl_2$, and 100 μL of 100 m*M* β-mercaptoethanol.
17. Homogenization buffer (make 50 mL/10 samples): 4.9 mL of 35 m*M* phosphate buffer, pH 7.4, 1.0 mL of 25 m*M* $MgCl_2$, 1.0 mL of 10 m*M* benzamidine, 1.0 mL of 10 m*M* AEITU Br, 1.0 mL of 2.5 *M* sucrose, 1.0 mL of 50 m*M* EDTA, and 100 μL of 100 m*M* β-mercaptoethanol.
18. HPLC mobile phase. Place 3.4 g tetrabutylammonium hydrogen sulfate + 0.648 g K_2HPO_4, and 0.408 g KH_2PO_4 into a 2-L container and add 1.5 L of H_20; bring pH to 8.0 with NaOH. Make up to 2 L to give 0.005 *M* tetrabutylammonium hydrogen sulfate, 0.0015 *M* potassium phosphate buffer.

2.2. Thymidine Phosphorylase

2.2.1. Preparation of Cell Pellets

1. Trypsin (Gibco, BRL, Paisley, UK).
2. Phosphate-buffered saline (PBS) containing diaminoethanetetra-acetic acid disodium salt and 1 m*M* EDTA.
3. Liquid nitrogen or dry ice.

2.2.2. Preparation of Cell Extracts

1. 50 m*M* Tris-HCl, 1 m*M* EDTA, pH 7.4, (BDH Laboratory Supplies, Poole, UK).
2. Bio-Rad protein dye (Bio-Rad Laboratories GmbH, Hertfordshire, UK).
3. Bovine serum albumin (BSA), (Sigma).

2.2.3. Enzyme Assay

1. dR-1-P (Fluka Chemicals, Dorset, UK).
2. 5-FU, Iodouracil (5-IU), 5-Fluorodeoxyuridine (5-FDUR), (Sigma).
3. 50 m*M* Tris-HCl and 1 m*M* EDTA, pH 7.4, (BDH).
4. 37°C water bath.
5. 1.5 mL, screw-cap Eppendorf tubes.
6. Isopropanol (Fisons, Loughborough, UK).

2.2.4. Solid-Phase Extraction

1. Glass centrifuge tubes.
2. Vortex evaporator.
3. Potassium dihydrogen orthophosphate (KH_2PO_4), 0.1 *M*, pH 5.5, (BDH).
4. 1.5-mL, screw-cap Eppendorf tubes.
5. Isolute NH_2 (aminopropyl) cartridges, (International Sorbent Technology Ltd., Mid Glamorgan, UK).
6. Acetone (Fisons).
7. Methanol (Fisons).

2.2.5. HPLC

1. Tetrabutylammonium phosphate, pH 5.5, (10^{-4}M) (Sigma).
2. 0.02 *M* KH_2PO_4, pH 5.5, adjust pH with 2 *M* KOH.
3. Two Spherisorb (ODS-1) HPLC columns (150 × 4.6 mm and 250 × 4.6 mm) (Jones Chromatography, Mid-Glamorgan, UK).
4. ^{18}C guard columns.
5. HPLC system, including photodiode array detector.

3. Methods

3.1. DPD

3.1.1. Peripheral Blood Cell Preparation

1. Warm required amount of ficoll-hypaque for 15 min. Then add 15 mL to each 50 mL conical centrifuge tube.
2. Withdraw blood from the heparinized patient blood sample (*see* **Note 1**) and gently place onto the top of the ficoll-hypaque. Spin the tubes at 500*g* for 25 min at 25°C (room temperature).
3. Remove and discard the upper layer (plasma) with a Pasteur pipet to within 0.5 cm of the opaque interface (which contains mononuclear cells). Carefully transfer the opaque interface with a Pasteur pipet into a clean 50-mL conical centrifuge

tube (*see* **Note 2**). Dilute the cells with an equal volume of cold (4°C) PBS and spin at 200*g* for 10 min at 4°C.

4. Pour off the PBS from the pellet and gently resuspend pellet. Add 30 mL of cold (4°C) PBS and spin at 200*g* for 10 min at 4°C.
5. Repeat **step 4** (total of three washes)
6. Pour off excess PBS and resuspend cells in 1 mL sodium phosphate-glycerol buffer. Transfer to labeled Eppendorf tube. Pellet cells (10-s pulse) and store at –20°C, leaving the supernatant on top of the pellet.

3.1.2. Cytosol Preparation: Solid Tissue

1. Homogenize <1 g of tissue in 4 mL homogenization buffer.
2. Remove cell debris by centrifugation at 100,000*g* for 60 min at 4°C.
3. Store cytosols on ice until required (*see* **Note 3**).

3.1.3. Cytosol Preparation: Cell Pellets (Peripheral Blood Cells, Tumor Lines)

1. Thaw cells on ice and discard supernatant.
2. Resuspend cells in 300 µL buffer A by passing up and down a pipet tip.
3. Freeze/thaw the suspension on dry ice (or –80°C freezer) three times.
4. Remove cell debris by centrifugation in a desktop centrifuge at maximum speed for 20 min at 4°C.
5. Store on ice until required (*see* **Note 3**).

3.1.4. Ex vivo DPD Metabolism of ^{14}C-5-FU

1. While samples are spinning, weigh out NADPH and dissolve in buffer A to final concentration of 1.0835 mg/mL (*see* **Note 4**).
2. For each tube prepare a reaction mixture containing 125 µ*M* NADPH, 125 µ*M* ^{14}C-5-FU in buffer A. (42.5 µL buffer A, 20 µL ^{14}C-5-FU, 12.5 µL NADPH/reaction) (*see* **Note 5**).
3. A negative control with no NADPH added is carried out for each sample. (55 µL buffer A, 20 µL ^{14}C-5-FU, a single control is carried out for each sample).
4. Aliquot 75 µL of the reaction or control mix to 7.5 mL borosilicote-glass culture tubes and add 50 µL cytosol (*see* **Note 6**).
5. Cover tubes with parafilm to prevent loss of sample owing to evaporation and incubate in a 37°C water bath. Liver cytosol = 45 min incubation; other tissues and cell pellets = 90 min incubation (*see* **Note 7**).
6. Stop the reaction by the addition of 125 µL cold ethanol (4°C), cover with parafilm, and store at –20°C for 30 min.

3.1.5. Measuring Cytosolic Protein Concentration

To compare activity between samples, all are normalized for total cytosolic protein. We carry this out using the BioRad protein assay (a commercial preparation of the Bradford assay), and a standard curve from BSA protein standard

(BioRad) (*see* **Note 8**). The protein concentrations are then determined by spectrophotometry at wavelength 595 nm in 1-mL cuvets.

3.1.6. Separation of Metabolites by HPLC

DPD activity is determined by the amount of metabolite(s) produced per unit of time. The metabolites are quantified by HPLC with on-line radioactivity detection. The retention time of the metabolites of 5-FU is approximately 7 min, whereas the parent is retained for approximately 15 min.

1. Prepare mobile phase and degas with helium before running through column for 30 min prior to loading of the first sample. This allows the columns to equilibrate.
2. Centrifuge samples at 2000*g* for 10 min at 4°C to remove precipitated protein.
3. Inject 100 µL of the supernatant. Run at ambient temperature (22°C) at a flow rate of 1 mL/min for 22 min/sample

3.1.7. Determining DPD Activity in the Samples

In most tissue samples, three metabolite peaks are apparent, whereas only a single metabolite is produced in peripheral blood cells (*see* **Note 9**). For systems using the Berthold LB506C detector (*see* **Note 10**), the software allows quantitation of the counts contained in each peak. Alternatively, fraction collection and scintillation counting can be applied. From the counts per peak for metabolites (*see* **Note 11**), the activity of an individual sample can be calculated using the equation:

$$\begin{aligned} &\text{counts (cpm)} \times 1\ \text{dpm}/0.1302\ \text{cpm}^{b} \times 4.5 \times 10^{-7}\ \mu\text{Ci}/1\ \text{dpm} \\ &\times 0.0188679\ \mu\text{mol}/1\ \mu\text{Ci} \times 1000\ \text{nmol}/1\ \mu\text{mol} \times 2.5^{a} \end{aligned} \tag{1}$$

([a]*see* **Note 12**, [b]*see* **Note 13**).

This yields nmols produced divided by incubation time and amount of protein (in mg) to yield the final units of nmol/min/mg protein.

3.2. Thymidine Phosphorylase

3.2.1. Preparation of Cell Pellets

1. Grow cells to 70% confluence in 75-cm² tissue culture flasks.
2. Dissociate cells from culture flasks by first removing the medium, then adding 2.5 mL of PBS containing EDTA (1 m*M*) and trypsin (0.25%).
3. Deactivate trypsin by adding 8.5 mL of 10% serum containing medium. Transfer to a 10-mL universal container.
4. Pellet the cells by centrifugation at 4°C.
5. Wash the cell pellet three times in 10 mL of ice-cold PBS, centrifuging between each wash.
6. Resuspend the final washed pellet in 1 mL of PBS and transfer to a 1.5-mL Eppendorf tube. Centrifuge to pellet the cells.

7. Remove supernatant and snap-freeze the pellet by placing in liquid nitrogen or dry-ice; store at –70°C until required. (The enzyme should be stable for up to 3 mo.)

3.2.2. Preparation of Cell Extracts from Pellets

1. Thaw the cell pellet on ice and re-suspend in an appropriate volume, (e.g., 200 µL) of 50 m*M* Tris-HCl buffer containing 1 m*M* EDTA, pH 7.4 (*see* **Note 14**).
2. Sonicate the suspension on ice for three 5-s cycles at maximal output with intervals of 10 s.
3. Prepare a 10,000*g* supernatant (30 min, 4°C).
4. Transfer the supernatant to a clean Eppendorf tube.
5. Determine the protein concentration of the extract (*see* **Note 15**).

3.2.3. Preparation of Cell Extracts from Tissue Samples

1. Homogenize tissues in 3 times v/w of 0.05 *M* Tris/HCl, 0.25 *M* sucrose, pH 7.5.
2. Prepare cytosolic fractions by centrifugation at 100,000*g* for 1 h at 4°C.
3. Aliquot supernatant and store at –70°C.
4. Determine protein concentration.

3.2.4. Enzyme Assay

1. Set up a reaction mixture containing final concentrations of 2.5 m*M* dR-1-P; 2 mg/mL cell extract or 0.25 mg/mL tissue cytosol; 50 m*M* Tris-HCl, and 1 m*M* EDTA, pH 7.4 (*see* **Note 16**).
2. Place labeled sampling tubes containing 200 µL of isopropanol and 50 µL of internal standard (5-Iu 50 mg/mL) on ice.
3. Pre-incubate the reaction mixture in the 37°C water bath for 5 min (*see* **Note 17**).
4. Start the reaction by the addition of the substrate, 5-FU (final concentration 0.5 m*M*).
5. Mix and remove 50 µL and add to sampling tubes on ice and vortex for 5 s.
6. Remove further 50 µL samples at 15-min intervals up to 1 h for cell-line analysis. For tissue analysis, remove samples at 7-min intervals up to 28 min.

3.2.5. Solid-Phase Extraction

1. Centrifuge the samples (in isopropanol) at 550*g* for 15 min at 4°C.
2. Transfer the supernatants to glass centrifuge tubes and evaporate to dryness.
3. Reconstitute the residues in 100 µL of 0.1 *M* KH_2PO_4, pH 5.5, and vortex mix twice for 10 s to ensure that all the material is in suspension.
4. Add 400 µL of ice-cold acetone and vortex mix for 10 s.
5. Transfer the samples from glass tubes to clean Eppendorf centrifuge tubes.
6. Centrifuge at 550*g* for 5 min at 4°C.
7. Condition isolute NH_2 (aminopropyl) cartridges with 1 mL of acetone.
8. Load the supernatants onto the cartridges and collect the eluent (*see* **Note 18**).
9. Wash the columns with 2 mL of methanol, collecting the eluent in the same glass centrifuge tube as in **step 6**.

10. Evaporate eluates to dryness.
11. Re-constitute the final residue in 200 μL of mobile-phase ready for analysis by HPLC (*see* **Note 19**).

3.2.6. HPLC

1. Make up mobile phase: 0.02 *M* KH_2PO_4 and $10^{-4}M$ tetrabutylammonium phosphate, pH 5.5 with 2 *M* KOH (*see* **Note 20**).
2. Equilibrate the columns with 500 mL of HPLC mobile phase; flow-rate of mobile-phase is 1 mL/min.
3. Set-up the UV detector to monitor at 270 nm.
4. Ensure a run-time of 30 min.
5. Inject 150 μL of each 200 μL sample (*see* **Notes 21** and **22**).
6. Wash column (*see* Notes **Subheading 4.2.**, **Notes 23** and **24**).

4. Notes

4.1. DPD

1. To obtain an adequate number of peripheral mononuclear cells, use a minimum of 20 mL of whole blood.
2. Remove the cell layer with as little ficoll-hypaque as possible.
3. Proceed with incubation steps within 2 h of completing preparations.
4. Prepare fresh NADPH each day and protect from light.
5. All reactions are carried out in triplicate, and it is best to allow for 5 extra tubes when calculating the amount of cocktail mix to be prepared.
6. The assay is linear from 5–150 μg cytosolic protein. Alter the volume accordingly to achieve 50–100 μg protein.
7. Liver samples are linear for 60 min and other tissues for 120 min.
8. Run a standard curve with every protein assay. Also, most assays lose linearity at 20–25 μg protein, so dilute accordingly.
9. Peripheral mononuclear cells do not have dihydropyrimidinase, the second step in conversion of 5-FU to fluoro-β-alanine. Three peaks are not always seen, depending on the HPLC column and conditions.
10. We use the dry cell for ^{14}C detection, and thereby avoid the cost and mess of scintillation fluid.
11. Use the sum of all catabolites.
12. Multiplication by 2.5 gives the total counts for the whole sample, because only 100 μL out of 250 μL was injected onto the columns.
13. 0.1302 = efficiency of the detector. This was calculated from: E = counts × flow rate/dpm × volume. This factor will be different for each individual system.

4.2. Thymidine Phosphorylase

14. Cell pellets from a 70% confluent 75-cm^2 flask should be resuspended in 200 μL of buffer. Pellets larger than this should be divided into two, otherwise, the protein concentration will be too high and clarity of the supernatant will be reduced.

15. The Bio-Rad protein assay (based on the method described by Bradford in 1976) is sufficient for this purpose. This stage in the assay determines the amount of enzyme present in the incubation; therefore it is important to be consistent.
16. Make up 10X concentrations of co-factor and substrate and dilute 1:10 into the incubation mixture, (normally a total volume of 350 μL is sufficient, allowing 100 μL extra for mistakes in sampling).
17. Keep caps on the Eppendorf tubes while incubating to avoid evaporation. Ensure buffer, dR-1-P, and cell lysate are mixed thoroughly before pre-incubation and addition of the substrate, by pulsing in a microcentrifuge for a few seconds, followed by vortex mixing and pulsing again.
18. Try to keep samples from each cell line/tissue together. Results should be less variable if samples for each cell line/tissue are processed through the solid-phase extraction method simultaneously, usually 2 cell lines, 12 samples at one time, depending on the capacity of the extraction apparatus.
19. If you possess an auto-sampler, then it is best to process samples during the day and run overnight on HPLC. If HPLC difficulties arise, it is possible to store the samples in the final dry state at 4°C, with a covering of Parafilm or equivalent for up to 3 d.
20. It is possible to make up a 10X concentrate of mobile-phase, (excluding methanol) for storage. Make it up using ultrapure water if possible, filter and store at 4°C. Then as required, dilute 1:10 in ultra-pure water and add methanol; there is no need to filter again, just degas.
21. Always inject standards at the beginning of a run to ensure that the column has equilibrated with the mobile-phase. (This will also check that you have made up the mobile-phase correctly.)
22. Run three unextracted internal standards (50 μL and 150 μL of mobile-phase; inject 150 μL) at the start of each run. The mean peak area can then be used to correct the peak areas in the unknown samples.
23. You will find that the ^{18}C-guard column will become clogged after approximately 50 samples; therefore, it is best to replace it at this stage to avoid shoulders on peaks or splitting.
24. After running approximately 100 samples on HPLC, wash the column overnight with water, (1 mL/min), followed by 30% methanol for a few hours, then water again for a few hours prior to re-equilibration. This may seem laborious, but will ensure that samples are not wasted, especially when you are absent during an overnight run.

References

1. Pinedo, H. M. and Peters, G. J. (1988) Fluorouracil: biochemistry and pharmacology. *J. Clin. Oncol.* **6,** 1653–1664.
2. McMurrough, J. and McLeod, H. L. (1996) Analysis of the dihydropyrimidine dehydrogenase polymorphism in a British population. *Br. J. Clin. Pharmacol.* **41,** 425–427.
3. Kamm, Y. J. L., Rietjens, I. M. C., Vervoort, J., Heerschap, A., Rosenbusch, G., Hofs, H. P., and Wagener, D. J. T. (1994). Effect of modulators on 5-fluorouracil

metabolite patterns in murine colon carcinoma determined by in vitro ^{19}F nuclear magnetic resonance spectroscopy. *Cancer Res.* **54,** 4321–4326.

4. Wei, X., McLeod, H. L., McMurrough, J., Gonzalez, F. J., and Fernandez-Salguero, P. (1996) Molecular basis for the human dihydropyrimidine dehydrogenase deficiency and 5-FU toxicity. *J. Clin. Invest.* **98,** 610–615.
5. Gonzalez, F. J. and Fernandez-Salguero, P. (1995) Diagnostic analysis, clinical importance and molecular basis of dihydropyrimidine dehydrogenase deficiency. *Trends Pharmacol. Sci.* **16,** 325–327.
6. McLeod, H. L., Sludden, J., Murray, G. I., Keenan, R. A., Davidson, A. I., Park, K., Koruth, M., and Cassidy, J. (1998) Characterisation of dihydropyrimidine dehydrogenase in human colorectal tumors. *Br. J. Cancer* **77,** 461–465.
7. Sludden, J., Hardy, S. C., VandenBranden, M. R., Wrighton, S. A., and McLeod, H. L. (1998) Liver dihydropyrimidine dehydrogenase activity in human, cynomolgus monkey, rhesus monkey, dog, rat, and mouse. *Pharmacology* **56,** 276–280.
8. Makower, D., Wadler, S., Haynes, H., and Schwartz, E. L. (1997) Interferon induces thymidine phosphorylase/platelet-derived endothelial cell growth factor expression in vivo. *Clin. Cancer Res.* **3,** 923–929.
9. Folkman, J., (1996) What is the role of thymidine phosphorylase in tumor angiogenesis? *J. Nat. Cancer Inst.* **88,** 1091–1092.
10. Takebayashi, Y., Akiyama, S., Akiba, S., Yamada, K., Miyadera, K., Sumizawa, T., Yamada, Y., Murata, F., and Aikou, T. (1996) Clinicopathological and prognostic significance of an angiogenic factor, thymidine phosphorylase, in human colorectal carcinoma. *J. Nat. Cancer Inst.* **88,** 1110–1117
11. Peters, G. J., Vangroeningen, C. J., Laurensse, E. J., and Pinedo, H. M. (1991) A comparison of 5-fluorouracil metabolism in human colorectal cancer and colon mucosa. *Cancer* **68,** 1903–1909.
12. Friedkin, M. and Roberts, D. (1954) The enzymatic synthesis of nucleosides. I. Thymidine phosphorylase in mammalian tissue. *J. Biol. Chem.* **297,** 245–256.
13. Patterson, A. V., Zhang, H., Moghaddam, A., Bicknell, R., Talbot, D. C., Stratford, I. J., and Harris, A. L. (1995) Increased sensitivity to the prodrug 5'-deoxy-5-fluorouridine and modulation of 5-fluoro-2'-deoxyuridine sensitivity in MCF-7 cells transfected with thymidine phosphorylase. *Br. J. Cancer* **72,** 669–675.
14. Gan, T. E., Hallam, L., Pilkington, G. R., and Vanderweyden, M. B. (1981) A rapid and simple radiometric assay for thymidine phosphorylase of human peripheral blood cells. *Clin. Chim. Acta* **116,** 231–236.
15. Milne, L. H., Blackie, R. G., Twelves, C., and McLeod, H. L. A sensitive and automated assay for thymidine phosphorylase activity (submitted).

12

Measuring DNA Adducts by Immunoassay (ELISA)

Michael J. Tilby

1. Introduction

A large proportion of anti-cancer drugs act by causing chemical modifications to DNA, often involving the addition of part of the drug molecule to DNA to form DNA adducts. As discussed in Chapter 1, resistance mechanisms can act to diminish the extent of drug-target access or to alter the responses of cells to a given level of target modification. Measurement of the extent of drug-DNA interaction permits direct analysis of the contribution of the former type of mechanisms. Measurement of drug-DNA adduct levels can also be important for experiments focused on cellular responses because, first, it may be necessary to prove that observed differences in response are not owing to variation in drug-DNA access. Second, such measurements can be used to measure directly the rate of DNA repair processes, and hence, the influence on these processes of other variables, such as expression of specific genes. Finally, a knowledge of the DNA adducts levels formed in patients during therapy permits direct assessment of the clinical relevance of the levels of DNA modification employed in in vitro experiments. This could be important because the nature and significance of the various types of cellular responses will be dependent on the level of drug-target interaction initiating those responses.

Measurement of clinically relevant levels of DNA modification faces technical problems because these levels of modification are very low—a few adducts per million DNA bases. A number of established techniques have achieved the necessary sensitivity and specificity of detection needed by taking advantage of large changes in DNA molecular weight associated with single cross-linkage or strand-scission events per large molecule (e.g., centrifugational and membrane-elution techniques). However, there are a number of circumstances where such methods are not appropriate or are applicable with

From: *Methods in Molecular Medicine, Vol. 28: Cytotoxic Drug Resistance Mechanisms*
Edited by: R. Brown and U. Böger-Brown © Humana Press Inc., Totowa, NJ

difficulty. Of the other sensitive techniques currently available, immunological detection of drug-modified sites on DNA has a number of useful features. Immunological assays:

1. are not dependent upon radioactive labeling of DNA or drug,
2. can give an absolute determination of adduct level,
3. are relatively straightforward,
4. can be sufficiently sensitive and specific to detect clinical levels of adducts, and
5. can be extended to the analysis of individual cells (*see* Chapter 13).

Antibodies that recognize drug-induced DNA modifications can be raised by immunization with either drug-modified polymeric DNA or drug-modified mononucleoside/tide (covalently conjugated to a carrier protein). The latter approach is likely to provide antibodies with a specificity optimal for detection of DNA adducts in, for example, HPLC fractions from hydrolyzed DNA samples. However, they are less likely to be useful for techniques dependent on analysis of polymeric DNA, such as cytological staining or immunoaffinity fractionation of DNA fragments. Immunization with polymeric DNA is likely to yield antibodies optimal for these techniques although less likely to be suitable for application to HPLC analysis. It also has the potential to result in antibodies that recognize an aspect of DNA-conformation, rather than a specific base modification. Finally, it benefits from potentially simpler procedures for the preparation of the immunogen because it is not necessary to chemically synthesize, purify, and conjugate specific drug-nucleoside adducts.

Antisera or monoclonal antibodies (MAbs) have been described that recognize DNA adducts formed by many carcinogens. With regard to anticancer drugs, antibodies have been described that recognize DNA modifications formed by methylating agents *(1)*, cisplatin *(2)*, and melphalan *(3)*.

1.1. Principle of the Assay

The present protocol concerns antibodies raised against drug-modified polymeric DNA, and, although it attempts to be of general use, it is illustrated by including specific details relevant to the use of a rat MAb that recognizes cisplatin-induced DNA modifications *(2)*.

This is a competitive enzyme-linked immunosorbent assay (ELISA) involving competition between a constant amount of antigen bound to the wells of a 96-well plate and a variable quantity and/or quality of antigen in solution. These compete for an invariant small quantity of antibody in solution. The amount of antibody that binds to the immobilized antigen is measured and expressed as a percentage of the amount that binds in the absence of competing dissolved antigen. In this situation, the amount of immobilized antigen is not known (probably a few ng per well); however, this is of no consequence because the essential feature is that the amount bound is uniform from well to well. This type of assay has two features that are essential for many of its applications. First, accurately known amounts of soluble competing antigens can be included in the assay well with no dependency on their ability to bind to the plastic surface. Second, the quantity of competing antigen is not limited to what can be adsorbed to plastic, which means that small amounts of adducts in many micrograms of DNA can be determined (*see* ref. ***4*** for a general treatise on enzyme immunoassays).

To maximize assay sensitivity, the smallest possible amount of antibody should be included in each assay well. This amount, which must be determined empirically for each antibody, depends on the sensitivity of the enzyme detection method, the affinity constant of the antibody/antigen interaction and the background signal generated as the result of nonspecific binding of immunological reagents to the assay wells. An extremely sensitive and robust detection method, detailed in **Subheading 3.2.**, involves the enzyme β-galactosidase and a substrate, 4-methylumbelliferyl β-D-galactoside, which becomes enzymatically hydrolyzed to yield 4-methylumbelliferone. This product can be detected with great sensitivity (about 50 pmol/assay well) through its strong fluorescence. Under ideal circumstances, the system is capable of detecting a few amol of antibody bound to each well *(5)*.

Unfortunately, the sensitivity of detection of the competing antigen generally appears to be less than that of the immobilized antigen. Using this assay system, we have achieved sensitivities (50% inhibition) of 30 and 2 fmol/assay well for melphalan *(3)* and cisplatin *(2)* adducts on DNA, respectively. The properties of the antibodies being used are clearly a major factor in determining the sensitivity that can be achieved in an assay.

2. Materials

All the following solutions contain sodium azide (0.02% w/v) as an antimicrobial agent. SAFETY NOTE: Sodium azide is toxic.

1. Plate coating buffer: 1 *M* NaCl, 50 m*M* sodium phosphate, pH 7.0
2. Phosphate buffered saline (PBS): The simple recipe: 140 m*M* NaCl, 10 m*M* sodium phosphate, pH 7.0 is sufficient, but Dulbecco's PBS (available as tablets) can also be used.
3. PBSTw: PBS containing Tween-20 detergent at 0.1% v/v.
4. Stop buffer: 0.1 *M* glycine adjusted to pH 10.3 with NaOH solution.
5. Multiway pipets (50–250 µL and (ideally) 5–100 µL ranges).
6. 96-well plates: Ordinary flat and V-bottomed microtitration plates for diluting and mixing solutions and flat-bottomed immunosorbent assay plates for coating with DNA. The latter should be the high binding type. (We have found those supplied by Greiner or Dynatech to be satisfactory.)

7. Solution A: PBS containing Tween 20 (0.2% v/v) and BSA (1% w/v). Phenol red (10 μg/mL) is included to improve visibility of solutions in wells of the microtiter plates.
8. Solution B: Solution A containing primary antibody at double the desired final concentration (*see* **Note 1**).
9. Biotinylated second antibody. We routinely use affinity purified $F(ab')_2$ sheep anti-rat (from Sigma). This is supplied as a solution that we routinely dilute ×2,500 into PBSTw containing 1% w/v BSA.
10. Streptavidin-β-galactosidase conjugate. We routinely use the product from Boehringer Mannheim (Mannheim, Germany). It is supplied as a powder which is reconstituted with water and then, to avoid repeated freeze-thawing, this is stored in aliquots at –20°C. These are stable for many months and, once thawed, each aliquot is stable at 4°C for up to about 4 wk. Before use, aliquots of this stock solution are diluted ×10,000 into PBSTw containing 1% w/v BSA.
11. Substrate solution: Dissolve 4-methylumbelliferyl β-D galactoside (0.2 mg/mL) in PBS by gentle warming. Filter through filter paper and then add 1 *M* $MgCl_2$ solution to give a final concentration of 10 m*M*.
12. Incubator at 37°C. (This does not need to be humidified).
13. Fluorescence plate reader capable of reading fluorescence with excitation and emission wavelengths of 380 and 450 nm, respectively.

3. Methods

3.1. Coating Assay Plates

The method described supersedes a previously described method (*see* **Note 2**).

1. Place into each internal well (*see* **Note 3**) of the ELISA plates, 50 μL of a solution of highly modified DNA in plate coating buffer (50 ng DNA/mL; *see* **Note 4**). Tap the plate gently from different directions to ensure that the solution completely covers the bottom of each well.
2. Place the plates in an airtight box (to prevent dessication) in a 37°C incubator over-night (*see* **Note 5**).
3. Next morning, empty the wells and remove most of the liquid by 'banging' the inverted plates on paper towels. Then add to each coated well, 150 μL of PBS containing 1% BSA.
4. Leave the plates, with lids on, on the bench for at least 60 min, to allow the BSA to block sites of nonspecific binding.
5. Before use, wash the plates twice with PBSTw, it is important to remove all unbound DNA.

3.2. Competitive Assay

Each assay plate must include, in addition to wells containing various concentrations of soluble competing antigen, wells with no competitor and wells with no primary antibody. These indicate the maximum and minimum signals, respectively, to be expected. It is important to determine the maximum signal accurately. Therefore we routinely use columns 5 and 11 for zero competitor with one well in each of these columns containing no primary antibody. This layout minimizes the effects of any systematic variation across the plate in level of antigen coating

1. Minimum volumes of 260 µL of appropriate starting dilutions (*see* **Note 6**) of the competing antigens are placed in a screw-capped 1.5 mL polypropylene tube and heated at 100°C for 5 min to denature the DNA, thereby maximizing immunoreactivity of the cisplatin-DNA adducts (*see* **Note 7**).
2. Serially dilute the competing antigens in 96-well plates. For accurate assays, the two-fold dilution steps described here are appropriate. Larger steps could be used for preliminary tests. Place 120 µL of PBS in columns 3–11 of a flat-bottomed 96-well microtiter plate, using a multi-way pipettor. Place the initial dilutions of the competing antigens in the wells of column 2. Serially dilute 120 µL across the plate using the multiway pipettor, but do not dilute into columns 5 and 11, as these correspond to the wells without competitor.
3. For each row of serial dilutions, transfer 55 µL volumes to two rows of wells of a V-welled plate that has had the wells D5 and D11 ringed with a marker pen to identify them as wells for no primary antibody.
4. Next, add to each well 55 µL of solution A or B (i.e., without or with primary antibody). Because the accuracy of the assay depends on the accuracy of pipeting, some care is advisable, especially as solutions A and B contain protein and detergent, which cause them to wet the inside of pipet tips (*see* **Note 8**). The use of phenol red in these solutions makes it easy to see which wells have had the antibody solution added.
5. The plates containing the mixtures of antibody and competing antigen are mixed for a few seconds on a plate shaker before adding the lids and incubating for 30 min (*see* **Note 9**).
6. From each of the V-wells, transfer 50 µL, in a row-by-row fashion, to wells of duplicate DNA-coated assay plates. Thus, four assay wells, two on each assay plate, are used for each dilution of competing antigen. These plates are incubated for 1 h.
7. Next, wash the plates 5 times with PBSTw.
8. Add biotinylated second antibody solution (50 µL/well) and incubate the plates for 30 min.
9. Wash the plates 3 times with PBSTw.
10. Add streptavidin-enzyme conjugate solution (50 µL/well) and incubate the plates for 30 min.
11. Wash the plates extensively with PBSTw (5–7 times).
12. Add substrate solution (50 µL per well) and incubate the plates for the appropriate period, which will be dependent upon the particular assay (*see* **Note 10**).
13. Read the plates directly in the fluorescence plate reader (*see* **Note 11**).

3.3. Analysis of Data

1. For simple analysis, express the mean fluorescence intensity (F) for each dilution of competing antigen as a percentage of the mean reading for those wells without competing antigen (i.e., maximum reading):

$$F = ([S - BG]/[MAX - BG]) \times 100\% \quad (1)$$

where BG, mean value for wells without primary antibody; MAX, mean value for wells with no competing antigen; S, mean value for sample wells containing a given concentration of competing antigen.

2. Plot these values against concentration of competing antigen to generate a sigmoid curve from which the concentration necessary to give 50% inhibition of signal can be read as a measure of immunoreactivity of a particular antigen, or as an indication of assay sensitivity. Having plotted such a curve for a standard antigen it is possible to read off single values to determine the antigen concentration in unknown samples. However, we find it preferable to generate, for each unknown sample, data from a dilution series that can be fitted to a curve to determine the dilution required to give 50% inhibition. Not only is this more accurate, but also the shape of the curve can show up spurious results and reveal information about the quality of the antigen.
3. The analysis is best performed using curve fitting software, where all the individual readings contribute to the statistical analysis. The simplest fitting procedure uses the log-logit equation, but this is not very satisfactory for full sigmoid curves and more accurate fits are obtained using the logistic equation:

$$F = (M \times C^S)/(C^S + K^S) \quad (2)$$

Where F, assay signal at a given value of C; C, the concentration of competing antigen; M, fitted maximum fluorescence value; K, fitted competitor concentration for which F = M/2; S, fitted slope value.

4. The adduct level in the sample DNA is calculated from the determined concentration of the sample DNA (SA g DNA/assay well) and the determined concentration of adducts in the standard (STD moles adduct per assay well) that give 50% inhibition of assay signal.

adduct level in sample DNA = STD/SA moles adduct/g DNA

4. Notes

1. The final dilution at which the primary antibody is used must be determined for each antibody. It should be as high a dilution as possible, consistent with giving an assay signal that, in the absence of competing antigen, is at least 10 times the background signal observed in the wells from which primary antibody was omitted. For our MAbs that recognize DNA adducts caused by melphalan and cisplatin, we use unpurified hybridoma culture supernatants that are diluted 2,000 and 120,000 times, respectively.
2. The method described here supersedes a previously described method *(3)* that involved UV cross-linkage of DNA to BSA. The earlier method gave high back-

ground signals with the biotin-streptavidin reagents that are now in use and was more time consuming.

3. The outer wells of the 96-well immunoassay plates are often found to give poor reproducibility. These are not used, but water or buffer solution is placed in them to help maintain the uniformity of conditions of the inner wells.
4. For this assay, we use highly purified calf-thymus DNA (from Merck) that has been reacted with cisplatin to attain an adduct level of 20 µmole Pt adduct/g DNA.
5. Despite the instability of N7 alkylguanine in DNA alkylated by drugs such as melphalan, the overnight incubation at 37°C is optimal. We have found that overnight incubation at 4°C resulted in a high degree of inter-well variation in binding level.
6. The starting concentration is chosen (initially determined empirically) such that the immunoassay signals of the serial dilutions span a wide range of values—encompassing 50% of the maximum signal.
7. This heating step may not be appropriate for thermolabile DNA modifications such as N7-alkylpurine adducts. Partial hydrolysis of DNA has been found to be a useful alternative method to maximize immunoreactivity of such adducts ***(6)***.
8. The most convenient way to overcome this problem is to use an electronically controlled multiway pipettor such that, for example, 230 µL can be drawn up and then 4 × 55 µL dispensed, leaving 10 µL in the tips. A manual pipettor should be used in the reverse pipetting mode.
9. In the incubator, the plates should be arranged singly on the shelves. Stacking the plates will result in nonuniform warming within and between plates.
10. The β-galactosidase enzyme is very robust. It can be incubated overnight to generate a high fluorescence intensity. The reaction should not be permitted to proceed beyond the point where the substrate becomes significantly depleted so that the relationship between signal and incubation time is nonlinear. This situation would affect the relationship between antibody binding and signal.
11. The reaction can be terminated and the fluorescence intensity increased four-fold by the addition of 150 µL of stop buffer to each well. The plates should then be read right away because the fluorescence intensity of 4-methylumbelliferone is dependent on the pH of the solution and, being alkaline, the pH of the stopped wells will tend to fall as atmospheric CO_2 is absorbed. We do not find it necessary to use stop buffer routinely. Also, the plates (without stop buffer) can be sealed with proprietary self-adhesive sealing sheets and stored at –20°C prior to thawing and subsequent fluorescence measurement.
12. We use our own curve-fitting software based on program listings and explanations of curve-fitting procedures provided by Barlow *(7)*. However, current proprietary software packages for analysis of data generated by 96-well plate readers should permit this type of analysis.

References

1. Lee, S. M., Margison, G. P., Thatcher, N., O'Connor P. J., and Cooper, D. P. (1994) Formation and loss of O^6-methyldeoxyguanosine in human leucocyte

DNA following sequential DTIC and fotemustine chemotherapy. *Br. J. Cancer* **69,** 853–857.
2. Tilby, M. J., Johnson, C., Knox, R. J., Cordell, J., Roberts, J. J., and Dean, C. J. (1991) Sensitive detection of DNA modifications induced by cisplatin and carboplatin *in vitro* and *in vivo* using a monoclonal antibody. *Cancer Res.* **51,** 123–129.
3. Tilby, M. J., Styles, J. M., and Dean, C. J. (1987) Immunological detection of DNA damage caused by melphalan using monoclonal antibodies. *Cancer Res.* **47,** 1542–1546.
4. Maggio, E. T. (ed.) (1980) *Enzyme Immunoassay.* CRC Press, Boca Raton, FL.
5. Ishikawa, E. and Kato, K. (1978) Ultrasensitive enzyme immunoassay. *Scand. J. Immunol.* **8(Suppl.7),** 43.
6. Tilby, M. J., Newell, D. R., Viner, C., Selby, P. J., and Dean, C. J. (1993) Application of a sensitive immunoassay to the study of DNA adducts formed in peripheral blood mononuclear cells of patients undergoing high-dose melphalan therapy. *Eur. J. Cancer* **29A:** 681–686.
7. Barlow, R. B. (1983) *Biodata Handling with Microcomputers.* Elsevier, Amsterdam.

13

Measuring Drug-DNA Adducts in Individual Cells

Adrian J. Frank

1. Introduction

Many anticancer drugs and environmental carcinogens exert cytotoxic and or mutagenic effects through the direct reaction with DNA via in the formation of drug-DNA adducts or stabilized protein-DNA complexes *(1,2)*. The ability to determine the extent with which drugs, such as alkylating agents and platinum based drugs, interact with their cellular targets in tumor cells will permit further studies into cytotoxic and biological effects of these drugs. The use of antisera or antibodies directed against specific adducts has facilitated the development of immunologically based assays, such as ELISA methods, to determine the extent of drug-DNA interaction in cells. These techniques however, rely on the measurement of adducts on DNA isolated from millions of cells (described by Tilby in Chapter 12 and refs. ***3*** and ***4***).

The use of these assays is limited for studies on adduct formation and repair in clinically obtained biopsies because

1. In vivo adduct levels usually fall below the level of assay sensitivity.
2. Sample size is small.
3. Tumors exhibit intra-cell heterogeneity.

Immunocytological assays have been developed which permit the detection and quantification of drug/carcinogen-DNA adducts in individual cells. Staining techniques, based on standard immunocytochemistry, generally involve the fixation of cells to microscope slides through use of organic solvents (e.g., Methanol, acetone), application of antisera/antibodies followed by detection via secondary antibody conjugated with immunoperoxidase *(5)*. Assays of these sort have been used for qualitative or semi-quantitative analysis of DNA modifications resulting from exposure to cisplatin *(6)*, methylating agents and environmental car-

From: *Methods in Molecular Medicine, Vol. 28: Cytotoxic Drug Resistance Mechanisms*
Edited by: R. Brown and U. Böger-Brown © Humana Press Inc., Totowa, NJ

cinogens *(7)* in individual cells. Detection of DNA modification through the use of immunofluorescence staining of conventionally fixed cells followed by quantification of fluorescence has also been applied to alkylating agents *(8)*.

We have developed an immunofluorescence staining method for the detection and quantification of adducts formed between the bifunctional alkylating drug melphalan, and DNA in individual cells *(9)*. The method described here does not use classical fixing techniques prior to immunostaining and therefore avoids co-precipitation of proteins and DNA which may affect both the access of specific antibodies to the DNA adducts and DNA conformation. Instead, cells are embedded in agarose spread on microscope slides and lysed to remove most of the cellular material which is washed from the agarose leaving the DNA easily accessible to immunological staining reagents. A fluorescence microscope is used to detect fluorescence relating to both DNA content (blue Hoechst-DNA fluorescence) and DNA adduct (green FITC-adduct immunofluorescence). Through the use of a sensitive digital camera system followed by image analysis it is possible to quantify the fluorescence intensity from individual cells.

The basic immunostaining method is described here together with details of the camera system and image analysis used. Although specific systems have been suggested here, there are good alternatives which can be used. The principles underlying the use of the basic image analysis procedure has also been described together with a detailed protocol which was developed using a particular image analysis software package.

2. Materials

2.1. General

Many of the following solutions contain sodium azide (0.02% w/v) as an antimicrobial agent. **Take care, this is toxic.**

1. Dulbecco's phosphate-buffered saline (PBS): 10 m*M* Na and K phosphates, 140 m*M* NaCl, 2.7 m*M* KCl and 0.02% w/v azide. pH 7.4.
2. PBSTw: PBS containing 0.1% v/v Tween 20 detergent.
3. 1 m*M* stock solution of fluorescein in PBS, dilute to an appropriate concentration (e.g. 3 μ*M*) in PBS for use in shade correction procedures.
4. 1 m*M* stock of 4-methylumbeliferone (4-Me) in ethanol, dilute to an appropriate concentration (e.g., 200 μ*M*) in PBS for use in shade correction procedures.
5. Microscope slide with a 20 μ*M* deep observation chamber for use in correction procedures.

2.2. Agarose Embedding Procedure

1. Clean microscope slides (Menzel-Glaser from Weston Lab Services, Aldershot, UK) (*see* **Note 1**).

2. Glass staining tanks and racks.
3. Low melting-point agarose (LMP), (Seaprep, FMC, Rockland) 0.5% w/v in water and 2% w/v in PBS.
4. Lysis solution: 1% *v/v* sarkosyl NL30 detergent, 80 m*M* potassium phosphate, 10 m*M* EDTA pH 6.8.
5. 10% w/v Glycerol in PBS.

2.3. Immunostaining Procedure

1. Alkali: 0.1 *M* NaOH in water.
2. Antibody diluting solution: PBSTw containing 1% w/v bovine serum albumin (BSA).
3. Primary antibody directed against specific DNA adduct or complex (in this example MP5/73 rat monoclonal antibody *[3]* was used).
4. FITC-conjugated second antibody: IgG $F(ab)_2$ species specific preparation from Serotec (Oxford, UK).
5. Hoechst dye 33258: Can be prepared as a 1 m*M* stock in water, frozen (–80°C) until required, then thawed and diluted to 10 µ*M* in PBS.
6. Glass cover slips (22 × 50 mm No. 1 thickness).

2.4. Fluorescence Microscopy

1. Epifluorescence microscope with a 75W Xenon arc lamp fitted to a highly stabilized power supply (*see* **Notes 2** and **3**).
2. Multicavity interference band-pass filter sets (Omega Optical, Inc., Brattleboro, VT). Wavelengths (center of pass band ± half band width): Hoechst fluorescence (filter set XF06) ex. = 365 ± 12.5 nm, em. = 450 ± 32.5 nm; FITC immunofluorescence, (filter set XF22) ex. = 485 ± 11 nm, em. = 530 ± 15 nm (*see* **Note 4**).
3. Fluorescence images can be captured using sensitive detection system (such as a cooled slow-scan charge coupled device (CCD) camera [Astrocam Ltd., Cambridge, UK]) (*see* **Note 5**).

2.5. Quantification of Fluorescence

Analyze and quantify fluorescence using an image analysis package (such as Visilog version 4.1.3 (C) software by Noesis, France) which will permit adequate image processing functions (*see* **Note 6**).

3. Methods

3.1. Agarose Embedding Procedure

1. Boil the 0.5% and 2% LMP agarose for 5 min until molten and maintain in a 37°C waterbath until required.
2. Pre-coat microscope slides by adding 100 µL of 0.5% LMP agarose on to one end of each slide. Using another slide, spread the agarose thinly over each slide and dry at 37°C for approximately 2 h to form an adherent coating.

3. Following exposure of either cultured cells or cells derived from clinical material, with drug under study, wash with PBS (4°C) by centrifugation and resuspend in approximately 2 mL of PBS. Keep cell suspensions on ice until required.
4. Warm each cell suspension to 37°C and immediately mix an aliquot with a equal volume of molten 2% LMP agarose. Add approx. 100 µL of mixture on to one end of a pre-coated slide and spread thinly and evenly over the slide. Place slide onto a refrigerated surface to solidify the agarose and minimize evaporation of water.
5. Using the glass staining racks and tanks place slides into the lysis solution for approximately 15 min (*see* **Note 7**).
6. Wash slides thoroughly by immersion in each of three changes of PBS (5 min each).
7. Slides can be used immediately or frozen and stored until required for the immunostaining procedure. To freeze, carefully place 2 slides back to back into a 50 mL tube containing glycerol (10% w/v in PBS) and store at –20°C.
8. To thaw out the slides prior to immunostaining place frozen tubes into a 37°C incubator until fully thawed out. Carefully take slides out of the glycerol so as not to disturb the agarose and place into a glass staining rack. Wash slides thoroughly in 3 changes of PBS (**steps 7** and **8** are optional if immunostaining procedure can not be carried out on the same day as the embedding method).

3.2. Immunostaining Procedure

The immunostaining procedure described below can be applied, in principle, to the quantification of any stabilized drug/protein - DNA adduct or complex where antibodies are available for that adduct or complex. The protocol provided below describes the detection and measurement of the adducts formed between the bifunctional alkylating drug melphalan and DNA, where monoclonal antibodies have been elicited against the adducts *(3)*.

1. Treat slides for 5 min (in the dark) with 0.1 *M* NaOH to denature the DNA prior to immunostaining (*see* **Note 8**).
2. Wash slides in each of three changes of PBS (5 min each).
3. Incubate slides with primary antibody, elicited against the stabilized DNA adduct or complex, for 1 h at room temperature. (In this example MP5/73 rat monoclonal antibody diluted x100 in PBSTw containing 1% BSA was used).
4. Wash slides in each of three changes of PBSTw (5 min each).
5. Incubate slides with FITC-conjugated secondary antibody diluted x100 in PBSTw containing 1% BSA for 1 h at room temperature in the dark.
6. Wash slides in each of two changes of PBSTw (20 min each) and 1 overnight wash with PBS (4°C in the dark).
7. Stain slides with a solution of Hoechst dye for 5 min, remove excess and carefully place coverslip onto slide. Seal edges with clear nail varnish (or equivalent) to minimize evaporation of water.

3.3. Fluorescence Microscopy

Capture images of the blue Hoechst-DNA fluorescence and green FITC-adduct immunofluorescence separately using a sensitive digital camera (*see* **Note 5**).

1. Locate and focus onto a particular field of view using only the blue Hoechst-DNA fluorescence (preferably using reduced incident excitation light intensity) for a short period of time (*see* **Note 9**).
2. Take a short exposure of the blue DNA fluorescent objects (between 5–10 s) using the camera. Shut off the incident light immediately following the exposure.
3. Change to the filter set specific for the green FITC fluorescence and take a 20–40-s exposure, under reduced incident light, of the corresponding adduct immunofluorescence. (Illuminate the field of view with excitation light only during the exposure period).
4. Aim to capture at least 10 fields of view (5 from each duplicate slide per particular drug treatment), depending on the specimen this is between 50–150 fluorescent DNA objects.
5. Take images which can be used to perform the appropriate shade correction procedure. Fill the microscope slide, containing the 20 μM observation chamber, with either the 3 μM fluorescein solution or the 200 μM 4-methylumbeliferone solution. Find the correct focal plane by focusing on any particles in the solutions and then find a field without particles. Take, for example, a 10 second image of each fluorochrome using the appropriate filter set (*see* **Note 10**).
6. Take images which can be used to perform the appropriate background correction procedures. Fill another microscope slide, containing a 20 μM observation chamber, with PBS. Focus in the same way as **step 5** and take images of the PBS in 4 separate fields of view, one for each exposure time used in **steps 2**, **3**, and **5**. (For example 1 × 5–10 s exposure with blue filter set, 1 × 20–40 s exposure with green filter to correct sample images, 1 × 10 s exposure with blue filter set and 1 × 10 s exposure with green filter set to correct shade correction images). A list of initial starting images needed for application of the image analysis procedures in given as **Note 11**.

3.4. Quantification of Fluorescence

The Visilog image analysis software was used in the development of the analysis protocol described below, however the basic principles of the image processing steps should be applicable for use with any good software program.

Before quantification of fluorescence intensity from individual cells can be carried out using image analysis software, it may be necessary to perform correction procedures on each fluorescent object. Outlined below is a brief protocol for performing such corrections. (*See* **Note 11** for a list of the images needed before application of all corrections).

$$S_C = I_{S2} \times \frac{CMEAN}{I_{C2}}$$

where

S_C	=	Pixel in the final **CORRECTED SAMPLE IMAGE Sc short**
I_{S2}	=	Intensity of a pixel at a point in the background corrected **SAMPLE IMAGE S2 long**
CMEAN	=	Mean intensity of all pixels in the **SHADE CORRECTION IMAGE C2**
I_{C2}	=	Intensity of a pixel at the same position in the **SHADE CORRECTION IMAGE C2**

Fig. 1. Formula used to correct each pixel in the sample images. Words in **BOLD CAPITAL LETTERS** refer to image names.

3.4.1. Background and Shade Correction Procedures

Background and shade correction are basic procedures which should be applied to all sample images prior to quantification of fluorescence intensity to ensure that accurate measurements can made.

Background correction corrects images for stray light entering the optics and background dark current associated with the camera system. Shade correction of each image compensates for variations in intensity of illumination from the light source and non-uniformity in transmission of light through the optics.

Before any shade correction is carried out, the background correction process needs to be applied to all images including those which will be used to perform the shade correction on the sample images.

To apply a shade correction procedure to each sample image it is necessary to multiply the value of each pixel in the sample image by a factor which is calculated from the appropriate shade correction image (formula in **Fig. 1**).

Correction of each image was carried out on a pixel to pixel basis as shown in **Figs. 2A** and **B** (image analysis terms and image names are highlighted in **BOLD CAPITALS**). Each step below gives a basic description of the stages involved in the application of correction procedures. (This is followed by the exact image analysis commands used in Visilog to achieve the correction stages).

1. Using the image analysis software, perform an **ARITHMETIC SUBTRACTION** to subtract the appropriate (10 s) PBS image from the blue 4-MU shade correction image (**SHADE CORRECTION IMAGE C**, in **Fig. 2A**) on a pixel to pixel basis to form a new shade correction image (**SHADE CORRECTION IMAGE C2,** stage 1 in **Fig. 2A**). (Visilog software → Process → Point ops. → Arithmetic → subtract).

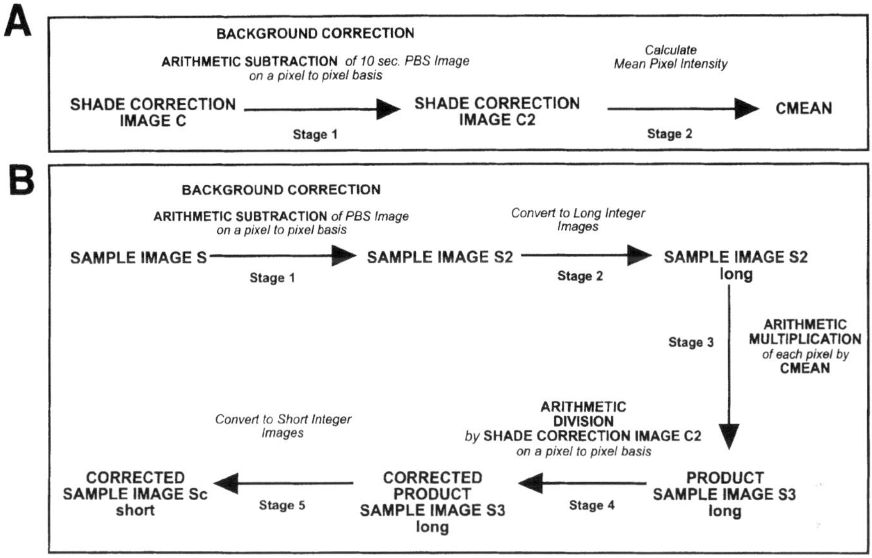

Fig. 2. Flow diagram showing the application of the background and shade correction processes to the sample images. **(A)** shows the background correction of the images used for shade correction. **(B)** shows the application of the shade correction process to sample images.

2. Use the software to calculate the mean pixel intensity of **SHADE CORRECTION IMAGE C2** (stage 2, **CMEAN** in Fig. 2A). (Visilog software → Analyze → Statistics → extrema).
3. Repeat **steps 1** and **2** using the fluorescein shade correction image and the appropriate (10 s) PBS image.
4. Before the shade correction procedure can be applied to sample images, the background correction procedure must be carried out on each sample image. Use the image analysis software to perform an **ARITHMETIC SUBTRACTION** to subtract the appropriate (5–10 s) PBS image from a Hoechst-DNA fluorescence image (**SAMPLE IMAGE S,** in **Fig. 2B**) on a pixel to pixel basis, to form a new sample image (**SAMPLE IMAGE S2**, stage 1 in **Fig. 2B**). (Visilog software → Process → Point ops. → Arithmetic → subtract).
5. Each sample image is stored as a 16-bit short integer image. To permit multiplication or division of two 16-bit images (as in **step 6**) all sample images must be converted to long integers, i.e., 32-bit images (**SAMPLE IMAGE S2 long**, stage 2 in **Fig. 2B**). (Visilog software → File → Convert → Arithmatic format changed to long integer).
6. Apply the shade correction procedure to each **SAMPLE IMAGE S2 long.** Perform an **ARITHMETIC MULTIPLICATION** by multiplying the image by **CMEAN** (stage 3 in **Fig. 2B**), to form a new **PRODUCT SAMPLE IMAGE S3 long**. (Visilog software → Process → Point ops. → Arithmetic → multiply).

7. Perform an **ARITHMETIC DIVISION** to divide the whole **PRODUCT SAMPLE IMAGE S3 long** by the **SHADE CORRECTION IMAGE C2** to produce a new image (**CORRECTED PRODUCT SAMPLE IMAGE S3 long**, stage 4 in **Fig. 2B**). (Visilog software → Process → Point ops. → Arithmetic → divide).
8. Convert **CORRECTED PRODUCT SAMPLE IMAGE S3 long** back into a short integer image to produce the final corrected Hoechst-DNA fluorescence image (**CORRECTED SAMPLE IMAGE Sc short**, stage 5 in **Fig. 2B**). (Visilog software → File → Convert → Arithmatic format changed to short integer).
9. Repeat **steps 4–8** using the appropriate 20–40 s PBS image for the background correction procedure and the **SHADE CORRECTION IMAGE C2** and **CMEAN** corresponding to the green fluorescein shade correction image to correct all FITC-adduct immunofluorescence sample images.

3.4.2. Quantification of Fluorescence Using Image Analysis

The next stage in the quantification of fluorescence is the application of image analysis processes which create new images that define the areas occupied by DNA from each cell. These images can then be refined and unwanted areas not associated with the DNA objects can be removed. The final image is used as an mask which can overlay the sample image, therefore, fluorescence measurements are made of areas corresponding to DNA or adduct fluorescence only (**Fig. 3**).

The principles of the image processing are given below, using Visilog software new images are produced after each process (image analysis terms and image names are highlighted in **BOLD CAPITALS**). *(This is followed by the exact image analysis commands used in Visilog to achieve the processing stages.)*

1. Using each sample Hoechst-DNA fluorescence image (**CORRECTED SAMPLE IMAGE Sc short**), create a new image (**BINARY IMAGE**) which contains objects or groups of pixels that correspond to the areas occupied by DNA from each cell. Creation of the **BINARY IMAGE** is the only subjective part of the analysis. This is carried out by setting **UPPER** and **LOWER THRESHOLD INTENSITIES** using the software. Set the **UPPER THRESHOLD** to the maximum measurable intensity (i.e., a 16 bit number = 64,000). Set the **LOWER THRESHOLD** as low as is consistent with the demarcation of the distinct DNA objects. The **BINARY IMAGE** denotes pixels with intensities that fall within the defined threshold limits as 1 (i.e., DNA and some background fluorescent objects) and those outside the limits as 0 (i.e., background). All subsequent processing is carried out on this **BINARY IMAGE**. (Visilog software → Process → Point ops → Segmentation → threshold).
2. Use the image analysis software to perform an **EROSION** of all objects in the **BINARY IMAGE**. This refining process removes pixels from the periphery of each object shown in the binary image. Using this process, areas defined in the

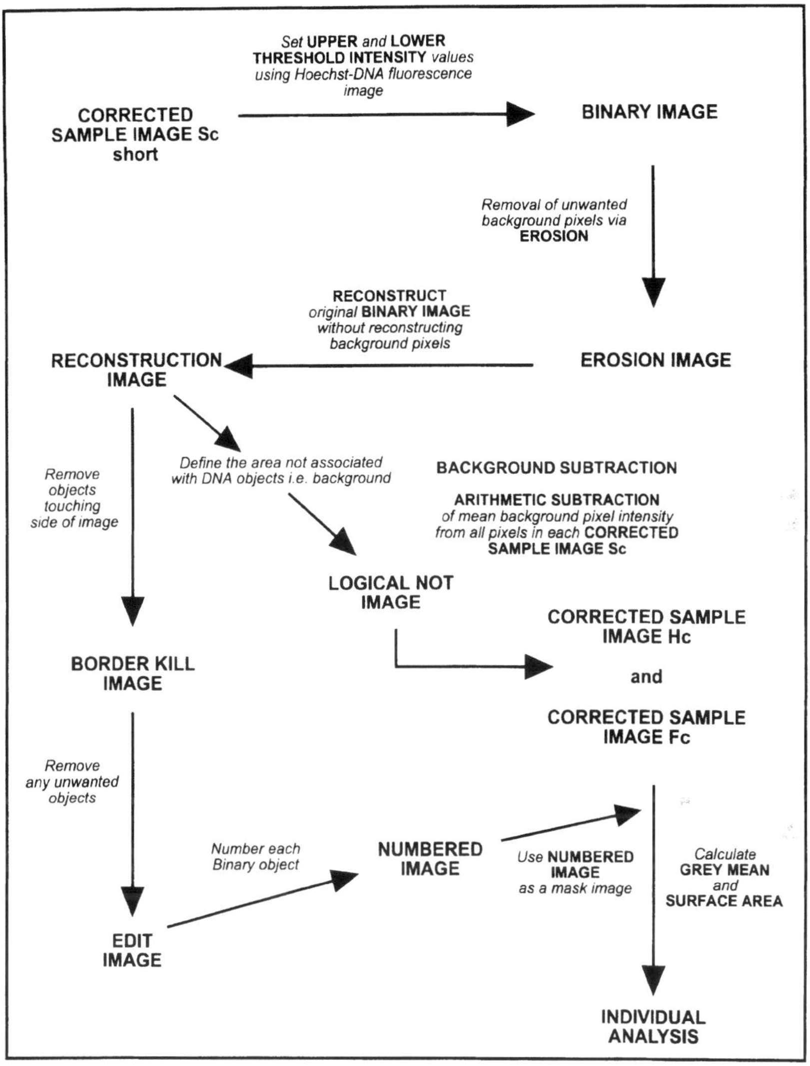

Fig. 3. Flow diagram of the image analysis procedure used to quantify the DNA and adduct fluorescence intensity from individual cells.

binary image which are not associated with DNA objects (i.e., background particles) can be removed. A new binary image is created (**EROSION IMAGE**). (Visilog software → Process → Morphology → Basic Operator → erode [perform approx. 4 erosions]).

3. The above process also removes pixels from the periphery of all objects in the binary image which do correspond to areas of DNA, therefore perform a

RECONSTRUCTION process to create a new binary image (**RECONSTRUCTION IMAGE**) in which the areas in the original **BINARY IMAGE,** corresponding to DNA, are reconstructed. Areas of pixels associated with the background are not reconstructed. (Visilog software → Process → Morphology → Conditional Op. → reconstruct).

4. The next stage in the image processing involves the application of a **BACKGROUND SUBTRACTION** procedure to all sample images to compensate for any local variations in the background level of fluorescence, due to the agarose or sample preparation, across the field of view. Using the **RECONSTRUCTION IMAGE,** create a new binary image (**LOGICAL NOT IMAGE**) in which all pixels that do not correspond to DNA objects, i.e., background, are defined. Use this new image as a mask to determine the mean intensity of all background pixels in each Hoechst-DNA fluorescence sample image (**CORRECTED SAMPLE IMAGE Sc short).** Perform an **ARITHMETIC SUBTRACTION** procedure to subtract the mean background pixel intensity from all pixels in that image (a new image is produced, **CORRECTED SAMPLE IMAGE Hc**). Repeat step 4 to determine mean intensity of all background pixels in each FITC-adduct immunofluorescence sample image and perform an **ARITHMETIC SUBTRACTION** to subtract the mean background pixel intensity from all pixels in that sample image (a new image is produced, **CORRECTED SAMPLE IMAGE Fc**). (Visilog software → Tools → AOI → addaoi → set AOI on → Process → Point ops. → Logical → not → Tools → AOI → addmask → Analyze → Statistics → extrema → Tools → AOI → set AOI off → Process → Point ops. → Arithmetic → subtract → Tools → AOI → set AOI on → Tools → AOI → addmask → Analyze → Statistics → extrema → Tools → AOI → set AOI off → Process → Point ops. → Arithmetic → subtract).
5. Remove from the **RECONSTRUCTION IMAGE,** objects which touch or overlap the boundary of the image using a **BORDER KILL** procedure, this produces a new binary image **BORDER KILL IMAGE**. (Visilog software → Process → Morphology → Classical Algo. → border_kill).
6. At this point the **BORDER KILL IMAGE** can be edited further, to remove any binary objects which overlap or correspond to large fluorescent objects in the agarose which are not areas of DNA. This produces a new image, **EDIT IMAGE**. (Visilog software → Tools → Graphics → toolbox → graphic area = image data → attributes = foreground = 0).
7. Finally, create a new image (**NUMBERED IMAGE**) in which each object area in the **EDIT IMAGE** is sequentially numbered. (Visilog software → Analyze → Measures → number).
8. Use the **NUMBERED IMAGE** as a mask which can be applied to each **CORRECTED SAMPLE IMAGE Hc** and **CORRECTED SAMPLE IMAGE Fc** to calculate various parameters associated with each DNA object such as average intensity (**GREY MEAN**) and total number of pixels occupied by each DNA object (**SURFACE AREA**). (Visilog software → Analyze → Individual → surface and GreyMean).

9. Because the spreadsheet functions in Visilog are basic, it is easier to export the data to another spreadsheet program, such as Microsoft EXCEL for calculation of the integrated fluorescence intensity for DNA and adduct fluorescence of each individual DNA object (**GREY MEAN** × **SURFACE AREA**). (Visilog software → Analyze → Individual → analysis → Display → to EXCEL).

4. Notes

1. This type of microscope slide was chosen because it was found that the agarose would not consistently spread over or stick to most of the other makes and type of slide.
2. An epifluorescence microscope such as the BH2-RFCA (Olympus, UK) fitted with objectives designed and suitable for transmission of fluorescence and UV light (e.g., ×10 DPlan Apo 10 UV, numerical aperture = 0.4) should be used.
3. Xenon arc lamp was chosen over the standard mercury option because Xenon lamps are a more stable light source than mercury. The stability was further maximized by connecting the lamp to a high stabilized power source. Xenon lamps emit excitation light over a broad spectral range (250–1000nm) where as mercury lamps emit discrete principal lines ***(10)***.
4. Multicavity Interference Optical filter sets consist of an excitation filter to selectively transmit a portion of the incident light, a dichroic mirror that reflects the selected light towards the sample and an emission filter to transmit light of a specific wavelength to the camera system. The choice of filter sets was made so that there was maximal excitation but no spectral overlap of excitation and emission signal between the two fluorochromes chosen.
5. To be able to detect the weak fluorescence, sensitive and accurate digital cameras or imaging systems must be used. The example given here was of a cooled slow scan charged coupled device camera (CCD) which contains a silicon based chip made up of three quarters of a million light-detecting pixels. The advantages of using a cooled CCD over a conventional CCD or video camera are firstly, that the dark current or background noise generated by the camera at all times is greatly reduced, thereby increasing the signal to noise ratio. Secondly, conventional CCD cameras can usually only read light intensities in each pixel to an accuracy of 8 bits, where the grey scale intensity of each pixel is on a scale of 0–255. The cooled slow scan CCD camera used, digitizes the light intensities of each pixel to a 16 bit number (i.e., a scale of 0–64,000). This means that the photometric accuracy is excellent and the dynamic range high, i.e., bright and dim pixel intensities can be measured accurately in the same exposure.
6. Visilog can be used to perform most of the image processing functions that may be needed. The main advantage is that it can handle and manipulate 16 bit numbers so that information provided by the camera is not lost. The version used here was adapted by Astrocam to incorporate manipulation, programming and execution of the CCD camera system.
7. The lysis solution and period of lysis described here provided optimal conditions for the detection of melphalan-DNA adducts. Optimization of conditions would have to be carried out for the detection of other complexes or adduct systems.

8. The 5 minutes alkali denaturation step was necessary to permit optimal access of the antibodies to the adduct epitopes on DNA. This step may not be required for detection of other complexes or adducts.
9. Accuracy in quantification of fluorescence intensity is optimized by increasing the length of exposure to the light source which results in an increase in number of photons detected by the camera. However exposure to light source will cause photobleaching of the fluorochromes. To ensure minimal photobleaching of the FITC immunofluorescence, the fluorochrome should only be exposed to incident light during the exposure times chosen therefore the time between exposure of incident light and taking the image should be minimal. To limit the amount of bleaching and permit longer exposure times images could taken under reduced levels of incident light, achieved by the use of a neutral density filter. This reduces the incident light to 25%.
10. Pure solutions of 4-methylumbelliferone and fluorescein are used for the shade correction process to provide a field of view with uniform fluorescence. Any non-uniformities present in the acquired images of these fields of view are owing to experimental variations. These variations such as non-uniformity in illumination of specimen or transmission of light will also be present in all sample images. To prevent further variations being added to the sample image following the shade correction process, the pixel intensity values in the shade correction images need to be high. Therefore appropriate exposure times such as 10 seconds are needed.
11. List of the starting images and the names assigned in **Figs. 1–3**, which are required before the application of appropriate image analysis correction and processing procedures:

10 s Images of 4-MU and fluorescein	= **SHADE CORRECTION IMAGE C**
10 s Images of PBS (with appropriate filters)	= **PBS IMAGE**
DNA and adduct fluorescence images	= **SAMPLE IMAGE S**
Images of PBS (same exposure conditions as samples	= **PBS IMAGE**

References

1. Lawley, P. D. and Phillips, D. H. (1996) DNA adducts from chemotherapeutic agents. *Mutation Res.* **355,** 13–40.
2. Kohn, K. W. (1996) Beyond DNA cross-linking: history and prospects of DNA-targeted cancer treatment. 15th Bruce F. Cain Memorial Award Lecture. *Cancer Res.* **56,** 5533–5546.
3. Tilby, M. J., Styles, J. M., and Dean, C. J. (1987) Immunological detection of DNA damage caused by melphalan using monoclonal antibodies. *Cancer Res.* **47,** 1542–1546.
4. Tilby, M. J., Newell, D. R., Viner, C., Selby, P. J., and Dean, C. J. (1993) Application of a sensitive immunoassay to the study of DNA adducts formed in peripheral blood mononuclear cells of patients undergoing high-dose melphalan therapy. *Eur. J. Cancer* **29A(5),** 681–686.

5. Den Engelse, L., Van Benthem, J., and Scherer, E. (1990) Immunolocytochemical analysis of in vivo DNA modifications. *Mutation Res.* **233,** 265–287.
6. Blommaert, F. A., Michael, C., Terheggen, P. M. A. B., Muggiam, F. M., Kortes, V., Chomagel, J. H., Hart, A. A. M., and Den Engelse, L. (1993) Drug-induced DNA modification of buccal cells of cancer patients receiving carboplatin and cisplatin combination chemotherapy, as determined by an immunocytochemical method: inter-individual variation and correlation with disease response. *Cancer Res.* **53,** 5669.
7. Motykiewic,z G., Malusecka, E., Grzybowska, E., Chorazy, M., Zhang, Y.-J., Perera, F. P., and Santella, R. M. (1995) Immunohistochemical quantification of polycyclic aromatic hydrocarbon-DNA adducts in human lymphocytes. *Cancer Res.* **55,** 1417.
8. Seiler, F., Kirstein, U., Eberle, G., Hochleitner, K., and Rajewsky, M. F. (1993) Quantification of specific DNA-alkylation products in individual cells by monoclonal antibodies and digital imaging of intensified nuclear fluorescence. *Carcinogenesis* **14,** 1907.
9. Frank, A. J., Proctor, S. J., and Tilby, M. J. (1996) Detection and quantification of melphalan-DNA adducts at the single cell level in hemopoietic tumor cells. *Blood* **88(3),** 977–984.
10. Haugland, R. P. (1997) *Handbook of Fluorescence Probes and Research Chemicals.* Molecular Probes, Inc., pp. 608–614.

14

Measurement of Drug-Induced DNA Interstrand Crosslinking Using the Single-Cell Gel Electrophoresis (Comet) Assay

Victoria J. Spanswick, Janet M. Hartley, Timothy H. Ward, and John A. Hartley

1. Introduction

DNA damaging agents have been widely used in cancer chemotherapy for many years and have proved successful in the treatment of both solid tissue and haematological malignancies. Many commonly used clinical agents, such as members of the nitrogen mustard, chloroethylnitrosourea, dimethane-sulphonate and platinum classes, are bifunctional. DNA interstrand crosslinks (ISC) formed in cells are clearly critical cytotoxic lesions and the formation of DNA ISC has been shown to correlate with cytotoxicity in vitro *(1–5)*. Acquired resistance in vitro to such agents can occur by a number of mechanisms, for example altered drug transport *(6)*, intracellular detoxification via enhanced glutathione and glutathione-S-transferase activity *(7)*, but enhanced DNA repair capacity can also play an important role *(3)*. Clinically the mechanisms of acquired resistance to DNA damaging agents are less clear but enhanced repair of ISC has been suggested to play a role in the acquired resistance of some cancers, e.g., chronic lymphocytic leukaemia to nitrogen mustards *(8)*. In addition, the inherent sensitivity (and curability) of some tumors, e.g., testicular cancer, to DNA damaging agents may result in part from their inability to repair critical DNA lesions *(9)*.

DNA ISC formation can be measured relatively easily in plasmid DNA using an agarose gel based assay *(10)* and ISC formation and its repair can be measured in intact cells using the technique of alkaline elution *(11)*. Although sensitive enough to measure ISC at pharmacologically relevant doses, alkaline

From: *Methods in Molecular Medicine, Vol. 28: Cytotoxic Drug Resistance Mechanisms*
Edited by: R. Brown and U. Böger-Brown © Humana Press Inc., Totowa, NJ

elution requires a relatively large number of cells and the prior radiolabelling of cellular DNA. As a result it cannot be easily adapted for in vivo studies.

The single-cell gel electrophoresis or comet assay was originally developed by Ostling and Johanson *(12)* as a method which allows visualization of DNA damage in individual cells. Used extensively to detect single strand breaks in a range of applications *(13)*, it was also suggested that adaptation to measure DNA ISC was possible *(14,15)*. Subsequently a number of groups have performed this successfully *(16–19)*.

In order to detect DNA ISC cells are irradiated immediately prior to analysis to deliver a fixed level of random DNA strand breakage. Cells are then embedded in agarose on a microscope slide and lysed to remove cellular proteins. The DNA is then denatured under alkaline conditions and subjected to electrophoresis. During electrophoresis any relaxed or broken DNA fragments migrate further than supercoiled undamaged DNA. After appropriate staining the DNA resembles a comet with a brightly fluorescent head and a tail whose length and intensity is determined by the level of DNA strand breakage produced within the cells (**Fig. 1A,B**). The tail moment is used as a measure of damage and is defined as the product of the percentage of DNA in the comet tail, and the distance between the means of the head and tail distributions, based on the definition by Olive et al. *(20)* (**Fig. 1C**). The presence of DNA ISC will retard the migration of the irradiated DNA during electrophoresis hence giving a reduced tail moment compared to the non-crosslinked irradiated control. Removal of DNA ISC can also be assessed as an increase in tail moment with time following a drug-free incubation period.

The technique is reproducible, more sensitive than methods such as alkaline elution, requires fewer cells and has the important advantage that analysis can be made at the single cell level. It is therefore possible to determine heterogeneity of ISC formation and its repair in a cell population. The method is applicable to studies with cultured cell lines, human lymphocytes and solid tumor tissue. Correlations can therefore be made between both the level of ISCs and the efficiency of their repair with both inherent and acquired resistance to DNA crosslinking agents in vitro and in vivo.

2. Materials

2.1. Cell Preparation and Drug Exposure

2.1.1. Suspension Cell Lines

1. Appropriate tissue culture medium.
2. Glutamine (Sigma, Poole, UK).
3. Fetal calf serum (FCS) (Gibco Life Technologies, Paisley, UK).

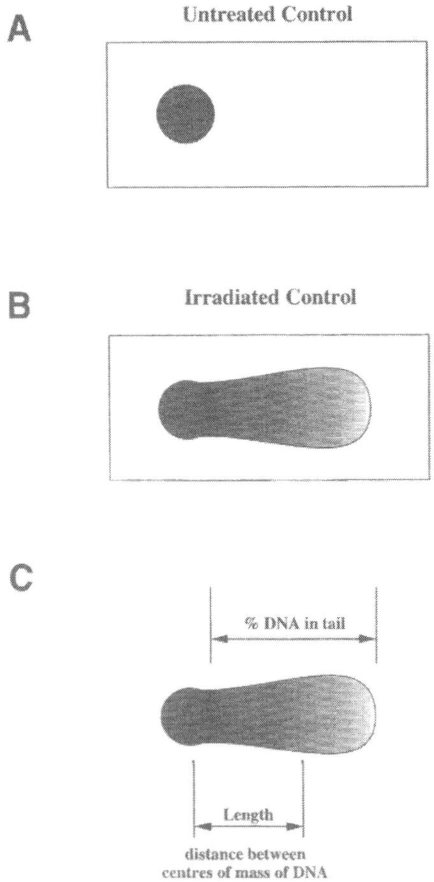

Fig. 1. Diagramatic representation of typical results from the Comet assay. **(A)** Untreated control. **(B)** Irradiated control. **(C)** Calculation of tail moment.

2.1.2. Adherent Cell Lines

1. Appropriate tissue culture medium.
2. Glutamine (Sigma).
3. FCS (Gibco Life Technologies).
4. Trypsin (0.05%) (Gibco Life Technologies).
5. Versene: 1 m*M* disodium ethylenediaminetetraacetic acid (EDTA), 0.5% phenol red.

2.1.3. Human Lymphocytes

1. Ficoll-Paque (Pharmacia Biotech, St. Albans, UK).
2. RPMI 1640 tissue culture medium (Sigma).
3. Glutamine (Sigma).
4. FCS (Gibco Life Technologies).

2.1.4. Solid Tumor Tissue

1. M6 tissue culture medium: RPMI 1640 (Sigma): L15 medium (Sigma), 50:50.
2. FCS (Gibco Life Technologies).
3. Selenium, pyruvate, insulin, and transferrin (SPIT) solution (Sigma).
4. Penicillin:streptomycin solution (Sigma) (*see* **Note 1**).
5. Tissue disassociation solution: collagenase (500 μg/mL) (Sigma), hyluronidase (500 μg/mL) (Sigma) in phosphate buffered saline (PBS), pH 7.4.
6. 40-μm and 100-μm mesh cell strainers (Becton Dickinson, Oxford UK).
7. PBS, pH 7.4.

2.2. Single-Cell Gel Electrophoresis (Comet) Assay

1. Single-frosted glass microscope slides and 24 × 40 mm coverslips.
2. Agarose, Type 1-A (Sigma).
3. Agarose, Type VII: low gelling temperature (LGT) (Sigma).
4. Lysis buffer: 100 m*M* disodium EDTA, 2.5 *M* NaCl, 10 m*M* Tris-HCl, pH to 10.5 with sodium hydroxide pellets. 1% triton X-100 to be added immediately before use. Store at 4°C.
5. Alkali buffer: 50 m*M* NaOH, 1 m*M* disodium EDTA, pH 12.5. Caution: corrosive. Store at 4°C.
6. Neutralization buffer: 0.5 *M* Tris-HCl, pH 7.5. Store at 4°C.
7. PBS, pH 7.4. Store at 4°C.
8. Flat-bed electrophoresis. This should be of sufficient size to hold a large number of slides, e.g., 30 × 25 cm gel tank from Flowgen Instruments, Lichfield, UK which holds up to 36 slides.

2.3. Staining and Visualization

1. Propidium iodide (Sigma), 2.5 μg/mL. Make up fresh before use. Caution: Toxic and light sensitive.
2. Glass coverslips, 24 × 40 mm.
3. Double-distilled water.
4. Epi-fluorescence microscope equipped with high pressure mercury light source using a 580 nm dichromic mirror, 510–560 nm excitation filter and 590 nm barrier filter for propidium iodide staining (e.g., Nikon inverted microscope Diaphot model TMD).
5. Images are visualized, captured, and analyzed using a suitable image analysis system. Our laboratory uses Kinetic Imaging Komet assay software (Kinetic Imaging, Liverpool, UK).

3. Methods

3.1. Cell Preparation and Drug Exposure

3.1.1. Suspension Cell Lines

1. Exponentially growing cells should be used at a density of 2.5×10^4 cells/mL in the appropriate medium containing 1 m*M* glutamine and 10% FCS.

2. Cells are treated with the crosslinking agent in duplicate and incubated for the appropriate time at 37°C in a humidified atmosphere with 5% carbon dioxide (*see* **Note 2**).
3. Pellet cells by centrifugation at 200*g* for 5 min at room temperature.
4. Remove supernatant and resuspend cells in fresh drug-free medium containing 1 m*M* glutamine and 10% FCS maintained at 37°C.
5. Incubate cells using the aforementioned conditions for the required post-treatment time (*see* **Note 3**).

3.1.2. Adherent Cell Lines

1. Exponentially growing cells are treated in duplicate and incubated as described in **Subheading 3.1.1.**
2. After the appropriate incubation, carefully remove the media and replace with fresh drug-free medium containing 1 m*M* glutamine and 10% FCS maintained at 37°C.
3. Incubate cells for the required post-treatment time using conditions described in **Subheading 3.1.1.**
4. Remove media and trypsinize cells with 0.05% trypsin:versene (1:1) until all cells have rounded up and detached (*see* **Note 4**).
5. Neutralize trypsinization by the addition of fresh media containing 1 m*M* glutamine and 10% FCS.
6. Transfer cells to a universal tube, wash twice with media containing 1 m*M* glutamine and 10% FCS maintained at 4°C

3.1.3. Human Lymphocytes

1. Collect whole blood using heparin or sodium citrate as the anticoagulant.
2. Carefully layer the whole blood onto an equal volume of Ficoll-Paque (*see* **Note 5**).
3. Centrifuge at 450*g* for 25 min at room temperature.
4. Remove layer of lymphocytes at the interface and wash twice with fresh media maintained at 37°C.
5. For in vitro experiments dose and incubate lymphocytes as described in **Subheading 3.1.1.**
6. Alternatively for in vivo investigations, (i.e., where ISC are to be detected in patients treated with DNA crosslinking drugs) isolate lymphocytes as quickly as possible after sampling. Wash lymphocytes twice with RPMI 1640 containing 1 m*M* glutamine and 10% FCS maintained at 4°C. Continue assay from **Subheading 3.2., step 3**.

3.1.4. Solid Tumor Tissue

1. Solid tumor samples (5–10 mm diameter) should be placed in 10 mL serum free M6 medium maintained at 4°C immediately after collection (*see* **Note 6**).
2. Place the tumor material in a 10 cm Petri dish and cover with medium. This should be carried out in a class II biological safety cabinet.

3. Carefully remove all blood vessels, clots, and necrotic areas from the tissue using sterile scalpel and forceps.
4. Mince the tissue roughly using with two sterile scalpels, transfer the suspension to a universal tube, and centrifuge at 200*g* for 5 min at room temperature.
5. Carefully remove the supernatant and resuspend the pellet in 5 mL tissue disassociation medium.
6. Incubate at 37°C for a minimum of 30 min and a maximum of 1 h.
7. Place the digested mince onto a 100-μm mesh filter and gently rub through collecting the slurry in a Petri dish.
8. Pass the slurry through a 40-μm mesh filter several times to achieve a single cell suspension.
9. Centrifuge and resuspend the sample as described in **steps 4** and **5** respectively. This should be repeated twice.
10. Resuspend the final pellet in approximately 20 mL M6 medium containing 10% FCS, SPIT, and penicillin/streptomycin to achieve a final concentration of 10^4 cells/mL or greater (*see* **Note 7**).
11. Plate the cells at the above concentration and incubate for 72 h at 37°C in a humidified atmosphere with 5% carbon dioxide to allow the cells to attach to the culture vessel.
12. Culture the cells for approximately 14–28 d, changing the media as necessary, until sufficient cells have been obtained and are free of debris, erythrocytes, and lymphocytes.
13. Drug exposure is carried out as detailed in **Subheading 3.1.2.** using the appropriate supplemented M6 medium (*see* **Note 8**).
14. In vivo investigations can also be carried out using solid tumor tissue from patients treated with DNA crosslinking drugs. Prepare a single-cell suspension (2.5×10^4 cells/mL) as quickly as possible from isolated tumor sample as described in aforementioned **steps 1–9**. Continue the assay from **Subheading 3.2., step 3**.

3.2. Single-Cell Gel Electrophoresis (Comet) Assay

Important: all stages of this assay should be carried out on ice, solutions maintained at 4°C, and incubations performed in the dark where indicated (*see* **Note 9**).

1. Precoat microscope slides with 1% type 1-A agarose in water by pipetting 1 mL of molten agarose onto the center of the slide and place a coverslip on top. Allow to set and remove the coverslip. Slides are then allowed to dry overnight at room temperature. The slides must be dry before use (*see* **Note 10**).
2. After required drug exposure/repair time, pellet cells by centrifuging at 200*g* for 5 min at 4°C. Remove supernatant and resuspend cells to a final concentration of 2.5×10^4 cells/mL in the appropriate tissue culture media maintained at 4°C ensuring that a single-cell suspension has been achieved (*see* **Note 11**).
3. Irradiate samples on ice at the appropriate dose except for the untreated unirradiated control (*see* **Notes 12** and **13**).

4. Take 0.5 mL of resuspended cells and put in a 24-well plate on ice. Add 1 mL of molten 1% LGT agarose in water cooled to 40°C, mix, pipet onto the center of the slide and place a coverslip on top. Once set, remove coverslip and place in a tray on ice. Duplicate slides should be prepared per dose (*see* **Note 14**).
5. Add ice-cold lysis buffer containing 1% triton X-100 ensuring that all slides are sufficiently covered.
6. Incubate on ice for 1 h in the dark.
7. Carefully remove lysis buffer ensuring that the gels are intact and remain on the slides (*see* **Note 15**).
8. Add ice-cold double distilled water to completely cover the slides. Incubate on ice for 15 min in the dark. This should then be repeated a further three times.
9. Remove slides from tray and transfer carefully to an electrophoresis tank (*see* **Note 16**).
10. Cover slides with ice-cold alkali buffer and incubate for 45 min in the dark (*see* **Note 17**).
11. Electrophorese for 25 min at 18 V (0.6 V/cm), 250 mA. This must be carried out in the dark (*see* **Note 18**).
12. Carefully remove slides from the buffer and place on a horizontal slide rack.
13. Flood each slide twice with 1 mL neutralization buffer and incubate for 10 min.
14. Rinse slides twice with 1 mL PBS and incubate for 10 min.
15. Remove all excess liquid from slides and allow to dry overnight at room temperature.

3.3. Staining and Visualization

1. Re-hydrate slides in double distilled water for 30 min.
2. Flood each slide twice with 1 mL of 2.5 μg/mL propidium iodide (PI) solution and incubate for at least 30 min at room temperature in the dark (*see* **Note 19**).
3. Rinse slides twice with double-distilled water for 10 min and once for 30 min.
4. Allow slides to dry at room temperature in the dark (*see* **Note 20**).
5. Place a few drops of distilled water onto the slide and cover with a coverslip (*see* **Note 21**).
6. Examine individual cells and comets at 20 × magnification analyzing a minimum of 25 images per slide (50/dose) (*see* **Note 22**).
7. Percentage decrease in tail moment is calculated using the following formula:

$$\% \text{ decrease in tail moment} = [1 - (\text{TMdi} - \text{TMcu})/(\text{TMci} - \text{TMcu})] \times 100$$

   where TMdi; tail moment of drug treated irradiated sample; TMcu; tail moment of untreated unirradiated control; and TMci; tail moment of untreated irradiated control.
8. The percentage decrease in tail moment is proportional to the level of DNA crosslinking (*see* **Note 23**).

3.4. Examples

Figure 2 illustrates DNA interstrand crosslinking in human lymphocytes. In the first example **(A)** lymphocytes were isolated from a healthy individual and

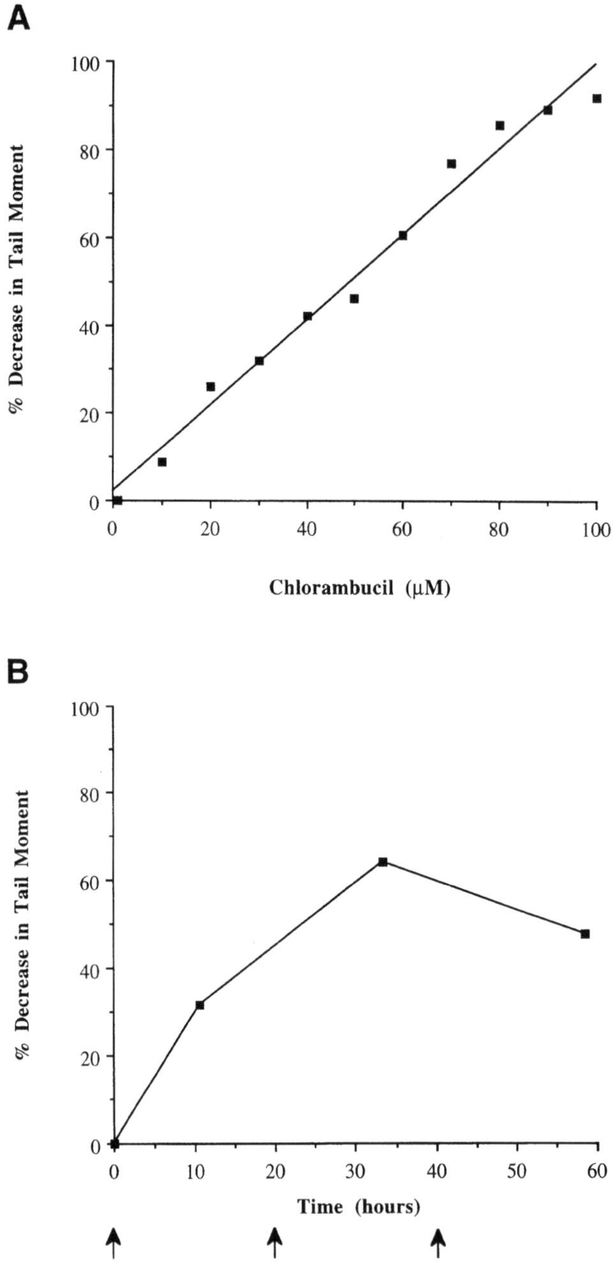

Fig. 2. DNA interstrand crosslinking in human lymphocytes as represented by percentage decrease in tail moment. **(A)** In vitro formation of DNA ISC with the nitrogen mustard Chlorambucil in normal lymphocytes taken from a healthy donor. Lympho-

exposed to the clinically used crosslinking drug chlorambucil in vitro. Levels of ISC increase linearly with dose of chlorambucil over a wide dose range. The second example (**B**) shows the analysis of lymphocytes taken from a patient treated with Ifosfamide. Crosslinks are clearly observed in vivo following chemotherapy.

4. Notes

1. Supplementation of tissue culture media with penicillin/streptomycin is optional and our laboratory does not use it in the maintenance of suspension and adherent cell lines.
2. If the chosen drug is to be reconstituted in solvents such as dimethylsulphoxide, the final concentration of solvent added to the cells should be no greater than 0.01%. This is to avoid any additional DNA damage and cell death.
3. The length of the post-treatment time is dependent on the type of crosslinking agent used and the peak of ISC formation. A time-course experiment should be performed to ascertain this. For example, following a 1-h treatment the peak of ISC for chlorambucil is reached following a 3-h post-incubation, while cisplatin requires a post-incubation of 6–12 h. For repair experiments, the post-treatment time can be further extended.
4. Trypsinize cells at room temperature as quickly as possible to avoid any additional DNA damage and to prevent crosslink repair. Alternatively a nonenzymatic preparation can be used such as cell disassociation solution (Sigma). It is imperative that a single-cell suspension is achieved. If several cells migrate together through the gel, an overestimated comet tail moment will result.
5. Vacutainer® CPT™ cell preparation tubes (Becton Dickinson) can be used as an alternative to the standard Ficoll-Paque protocol for lymphocyte isolation. This allows for sterile blood collection and cell separation using a single centrifugation step.
6. Tumors may be stored overnight in M6 medium. The pH should be carefully monitored and maintained between pH 6.5–7.0.
7. The number of cells plated should be as high as possible and 10^4 cells/mL should be regarded as a minimum. If less than 10^4 cells/mL are obtained, the time required to achieve confluency will be longer and care must be taken to avoid invasion by normal fibroblasts. Viability may be determined using trypan blue

---

cytes were incubated for 1 h in the presence of Chlorambucil followed by a 3-h post incubation in the absence of drug. (**B**) In vivo formation of DNA ISC in lymphocytes taken from a patient with a soft tissue sarcoma treated with Ifosfamide at 4.5 g × 3. Arrows indicate the start of each drug infusion. The results are from single representative experiments and each point is the mean percentage decrease in tail moment calculated from 50 cells. No significant formation of DNA strand breakage was observed in either example as determined from matched samples analysed without the 10 Gy irradiation step.

exclusion. However, owing to the large number of differing cell types, the percent viability refers to the whole population and not tumor cells exclusively.

8. Alternatively, cells may be cultured in 24-well plates at a concentration of 2.5×10^4 cells/well to reduce the total cell number required.
9. It is imperative that the comet assay should be performed on ice and in the dark where indicated throughout the text. This is to prevent any crosslink repair. All solutions should be ice-cold and maintained at 4°C.
10. Precoated slides should be prepared and dried in advance. Slides can be stored dry at room temperature for a number of weeks in an airtight container.
11. Cells can be used from frozen if stored at –80°C in the appropriate tissue culture medium containing 10% FCS and 10% dimethylsulphoxide. Sample should be rapidly thawed to 4°C and washed with tissue culture medium. Drug treatments and the comet assay are then performed as usual.
12. Each experiment should include an untreated unirradiated control. In addition an untreated irradiated control should also be included with every group of irradiated samples. This is to allow for any change in irradiation exposure between sequential irradiation steps.
13. An irradiated standard curve should be performed to establish the radiation dose required as different cell types may produce different results. Ideally the dose should give a head to tail DNA ratio of approximately 50:50. Our laboratory finds 10 Gy optimum for most cell lines and lymphocytes.
14. Molten 1% LGT agarose should be maintained at 40°C to aid uniform gel preparation. The thickness of the gel should be consistent between different slides to ensure uniform DNA migration. The gel should not flood the entire slide and the frosted section should be avoided. Ideally all gels should have the parameters of the coverslip.
15. A number of protocols have stated that following lysis the slides can be kept overnight or even days in this solution prior to alkali DNA unwinding and electrophoresis. We advise that this should not be carried out as the gels tend to break up and slip off the slide. It is therefore recommended that all steps of the comet assay should be processed in a single day.
16. Slides should be placed in a flat-bed electrophoresis tank lengthways with the frosted end towards the anode. It is essential that the tank is level and all slides face the same direction.
17. The level of alkali buffer should be consistent from one experiment to the next. It is advisable to measure the volume of buffer required ensuring that all slides are covered by at least 5-mm buffer.
18. These electrophoresis parameters are optimal for our equipment. The current can be adjusted to suit an individuals requirement.
19. The most commonly used fluorescent stains are PI and ethidium bromide. The highly sensitive fluorochrome SYBR Green (Flowgen Instruments) has also been used successfully. It has the advantage of being far more sensitive that propidium iodide and produces no background fluorescence. However, it fades much more rapidly under intense ultraviolet (UV) light.

20. Visualizing the slides dry produces optimum results as all the cells are in the same plane giving clear cellular definition *(21)*. This is favored instead of the traditional wet slide method which can cause difficulties in focusing and quantitation.
21. Slides should be analyzed as quickly as possible. If the coverslip is left on for a considerable length of time, it will become permanently stuck.
22. Each slides should be scored blind to avoid any prejudgement, taking care to ensure that comets are measured from the entire gel area and no part of the slide is analyzed more than once.
23. It is important to determine in the first instance if the drug under test will produce detectable single strand breaks as well as crosslinks. This may be achieved by performing the comet assay on drug treated cells but excluding the irradiation step.

References

1. Sunters, A., Springer, C. J., Bagshawe, K. D., Souhami, R. L., and Hartley, J. A. (1992) The cytotoxicity, DNA crosslinking ability and DNA sequence selectivity of the aniline mustards melphalan, chlorambucil and 4-[bis(2-chloroethyl) amino]benzoic acid. *Biochem. Pharmacol.* **44,** 59–64.
2. O'Connor, P. M. and Kohn, K. W. (1990) Comparative pharmacokinetics of DNA lesion formation and removal following treatment of L1210 cells with nitrogen mustards. *Cancer Commun.* **2,** 387–394.
3. Zwelling, L. A., Michaels, S., Schwartz, H., Dobson, P. P., and Kohn, K. W. (1981) DNA crosslinking as an indicator of sensitivity and resistance of mouse L1210 leukaemia to cis-diamminedichloroplatinum (II) and L-phenylalanine mustard. *Cancer Res.* **41,** 640–649.
4. Erickson, L. C., Laurent, G., Sharkey, N. A., and Kohn, K. W. (1980) DNA crosslinking and monoadduct repair in nitrosourea-treated human tumour cells. *Nature* **288,** 727–729.
5. Bedford, P. and Fox, B. W. (1983) DNA-DNA interstrand crosslinking by dimethanesulphonic acid esters. *Biochem. Pharmacol.* **32,** 2297–2301.
6. Rutman, R. J., Chun, E. H. L., and Lewis, F. S. (1968) Permeability difference as a source of resistance to alkylating agents in Ehrlich tumour cells. *Biochem. Biophys. Res. Commun.* **32,** 650–657.
7. Yang, W. Z., Begleiter, A., Johnston, J. B., Israels L. G., and Mowat, M. R. A. (1992) Role of glutathione and glutathione S-transferase in chlorambucil resistance. *Mol. Pharmacol.* **41,** 625–630.
8. Torres-Garcia, S. J., Cousineau, L., Caplan, S., and Panasci, L. (1989) Correlation of resistance to nitrogen mustards in chronic lymphocytic leukaemia with enhanced removal of melphalan-induced DNA crosslinks. *Biochem. Pharmacol.* **38,** 3122–3123.
9. Koberle, B., Grimaldi, K. A., Sunters, A., Hartley, J. A., Kelland, L. R., and Masters, J. R. W. (1997) DNA repair capacity and cisplatin sensitivity of human testis tumour cells. *Int. J. Cancer* **70,** 551–555.

10. Hartley, J. A., Berardini, M. D., and Souhami, R. L. (1991) An agarose gel method for the determination of DNA interstrand crosslinking applicable to the measurement of the rate of total and "second-arm" crosslink reactions. *Anal. Biochem.* **193,** 131–134.
11. Kohn, K. W., Ewig, R. A. G., Erickson, L. C., and Zwelling, L. A. (1981) Measurement of strand breaks and crosslinks by alkaline elution, in *DNA Repair* (Friedberg, E. C. and Hanawalt, P. C., eds.), Dekker, New York, pp. 379–408.
12. Ostling, O. and Johanson, K. J. (1984) Microelectrophoretic study of radiation-induced DNA damages in individual mammalian cells. *Biochem. Biophys. Res. Commun.* **123,** 291–298.
13. Fairbain, D. W., Olive, P. L., and O'Neill, K. L. (1995) The comet assay: a comprehensive review. *Mutat. Res.* **339,** 37–59.
14. Tice R. R., Strauss, G. H., and Peters, W. P. (1992) High-dose combination alkylating agents with autologous bone marrow support in patients with breast cancer: preliminary assessment of DNA damage in individual peripheral blood lymphocytes using the single cell gel electrophoresis assay. *Mutat. Res.* **271,** 101–113.
15. Hartmann, A. and Speit, G. (1994) Comparative investigations of the genotoxic effects of metals in the single cell gel (SCG) assay and the sister chromatid exchanges (SCE). *Mutat. Res.* **346,** 49–56.
16. Olive, P. L., Wlodek, D., Durand, R. E., and Banath, J. P. (1992) Factors influencing DNA migration from individual cells subjected to gel electrophoresis. *Exp. Cell. Res.* **198,** 259–267.
17. Olive, P. L. and Banath, J. P. (1995) Sizing highly fragmented DNA in individual apoptotic cells using the comet assay and a DNA crosslinking agent. *Exp. Cell. Res.* **221,** 19–26.
18. Pfuhler, S. and Wolf, H. W. (1996) Detection of DNA crosslinking with the alkaline comet assay. *Environ. Mol. Mutagen.* **27,** 196–201.
19. Ward, T. H., Butler J., Shahbakhi, H., and Richards, J. T. (1997) Comet assay studies on the activation of two diaziridinylbenzoquinones in K562 cells. *Biochem. Pharmacol.* **53,** 1115–1121.
20. Olive, P. L., Banath, J. P., and Durand, R. E. (1990) Heterogeneity in radiation-induced DNA damage and repair in tumour and normal cells measured using the "comet" assay. *Radiat. Res.* **122,** 86–94.
21. Klaude, M., Erikkson, S., Nygren, J., and Ahnstrom, G. (1996) The comet assay: mechanisms and technical considerations. *Mutat. Res.* **363,** 89–96.

15

PCR Analysis of Microsatellite Instability

Gillian L. Hirst

1. Introduction

Microsatellites are simple, tandemly repeated DNA sequences which are abundantly distributed throughout the human genome, and because of their polymorphic nature have been widely utilized as genetic markers *(1)*. They consist of a repeating unit of 1–5 base pairs, averaging 25–60 bases in length, and are commonly found in the form d(CA)n : d(GT)n *(2)*. It has been estimated that there are approximately 100,000 CA/GT repeat sequences in the human genome *(3)*. Studies in colorectal tumors first reported the appearance of instability at microsatellites sequences involving either an expansion or contraction of the repeat sequence *(4–6)*. Such microsatellite instability has now been reported in a variety of different tumor types including lung, breast, stomach, endometrium, and bladder (*7–11*, reviewed in ***12***). In addition, a number of other diseases are associated with instability in trinucleotide repeats, such as fragile X syndrome *(13)*, myotonic dystrophy *(14)* and Huntington's Disease *(15)*.

Microsatellite instability is found to be a common feature of nearly all tumors from patients with hereditary nonpolyposis colorectal cancer (HNPCC) *(4,16)*. The majority of HNPCC cases arise through germline mutations in two genes, hMSH2 and hMLH1 on chromosomes 2 and 3, which encode the human homologs of bacterial mismatch repair genes, MutS and MutL *(17,18)*. Cells which display microsatellite instability are termed as having an RER+ phenotype, which stands for replication error *(5)*. Such RER+ tumor cells have been shown to have defects in mismatch repair and possess a mutator phenotype *(19)*.

Work initially linking the loss of mismatch repair with drug resistance was noted in repair deficient bacteria which are hypersensitive to the methylating agent MNNG *(20)*. Later work showed that a number of tumor cell lines tolerant

From: *Methods in Molecular Medicine, Vol. 28: Cytotoxic Drug Resistance Mechanisms*
Edited by: R. Brown and U. Böger-Brown © Humana Press Inc., Totowa, NJ

to methylating agents are also mismatch repair defective and demonstrate an RER+ phenotype *(19,21)*. In addition, more recent studies have implicated the loss of mismatch repair in the tolerance of tumor cells to a number of other classes of cytotoxic drugs including cisplatin and doxorubicin *(22–26)*, and it is becoming apparent that mismatch repair may play an important role in the cytotoxic nature of certain drugs.

The most common way of analyzing microsatellites is by PCR, using PCR primers, one of which is end-labelled with ^{32}P or ^{35}S γATP, or an internal radiolabel is added with [α-^{32}P]dCTP in the PCR reaction. Dye-labeled primers have also become available which may be detected on fluorescent detection apparatus, e.g., 373A DNA fragment analyzer (Applied Biosystems). Sequences and/or information relating to microsatellite primers for a variety of species can be obtained from the GenBank database or published maps (e.g., *27–29*), or in the literature. The PCR products are then usually run on denaturing polyacrylamide gels so that single stranded DNA can be separated and the two alleles resolved. The sizes of the alleles on the autoradiograph are determined by referring to an M13 sequencing ladder run alongside samples as a molecular-weight marker. Theoretically, one allele should produce one band on a gel but in practice several bands are seen (**Fig. 1**), which is thought to be owing to events such as mispriming, strand slippage, and the terminal transferase activity of Taq DNA polymerase *(30,31)*. This can make interpretation of gels difficult. In addition, extra bands may arise if PCR products are internally radiolabeled using [α-^{32}P]dCTP due to separation of the CA and TG strands on the gel *(32)*. If these products differ sufficiently in their nucleotide content, then one strand will be preferentially labeled compared to the other and will cause little interference in scoring gels. This is usually the case when primers are located close to the repeat sequence, but problems may arise if primers are located further upstream and downstream, producing a lot of flanking sequence in the PCR product. Use of a 'touchdown' protocol *(30)* which utilizes the exponential nature of PCR can greatly improve the quality of microsatellite profiles *(33)* by decreasing the chance for mispriming. The early rounds of the PCR reaction use annealing temperatures several degrees above the theoretical annealing temperature of the primers, and each subsequent round drops the annealing temperature by one or two degrees until the touchdown temperature is reached. Another technique to combat the problem of anomalous PCR products which involves two or three stages of linear amplification has also been described *(34)*.

Below is given a protocol for PCR amplification of microsatellite sequences using internal radiolabelling and a touchdown protocol which has been successfully used to analyze microsatellite instability in human, mouse and canine DNA.

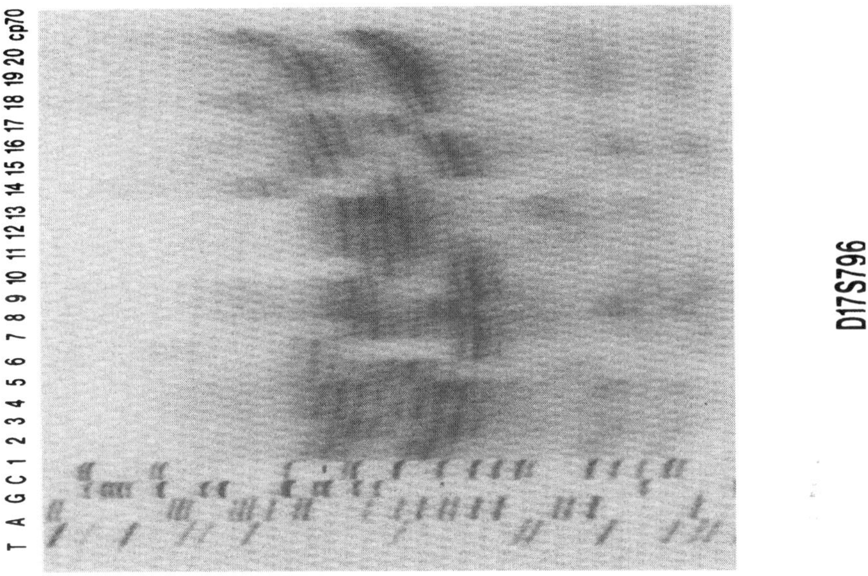

Fig 1. Example of microsatellite instability at the locus D17S796 in twenty subclones of the cisplatin resistant cell line A2780/cp70. The PCR products were fractionated on a 6% denaturing polyacrylamide gel and detected by autoradiography. The first four lanes show the M13 sequencing ladder used as a molecular-weight marker. Reproduced with authors permission.

2. Materials

2.1. Polymerase Chain Reaction

1. Taq DNA polymerase, 5U/µL supplied with 10x PCR buffer: 100 m*M* Tris-HCl, 15 m*M* $MgCl_2$, 500 m*M* KCl, pH 8.3 (20°C) (Boehringer Mannheim, Mannheim, Germany).
2. PCR dNTP Mixture containing premixed dATP, dCTP, dGTP, and dTTP, 10 m*M* each (Boehringer Mannheim).
3. Microsatellite primers (e.g., MapPairs™ from Research Genetics, Huntsville, Alabama, USA).
4. Autoclaved thin walled PCR microfuge tubes suitable for use in a thermal cycler (Eppendorf, BDH, Poole, UK).
5. Mineral Oil (Sigma, Poole, UK).
6. α^{32}P-CTP (Redivue) ~ 110TBq/mL (Amersham International, Amersham, UK).
7. Autoclaved ddH_2O.
8. Thermal cycler for DNA amplification, e.g., Hybaid Omnigene II (Hybaid, Teddington, UK).
9. Genomic DNA samples of between 50–100 ng/µL.

2.2. Agarose Gel Electrophoresis

1. Running buffer: 1X TBE buffer diluted from 10X stock: 0.89 *M* Tris, 0.89 *M* boric acid, 2 m*M* EDTA, pH 8.0.
2. 1.8% agarose minigel.
3. Ethidium bromide, 10 mg/mL, light sensitive (Sigma).
4. 5X sample loading buffer: 30% v/v glycerol, 0.25% w/v bromophenol blue, 0.25% w/v xylene cyanol FF.
5. DNA molecular weight markers, e.g., 123 base pair ladder (Gibco, Paisley, UK).

2.3. Polyacrylamide Gel Electrophoresis

1. Repelcote (VS) silicone treatment (BDH, Poole, UK).
2. Sequencing gel apparatus with 0.4 mm spacers and shark tooth combs, e.g., Model S2 (Gibco) produces a 30 × 40 cm gel.
3. Electrical tape (3M).
4. Large bulldog clips.
5. Polyacrylamide-Easigel polyacrylamide gel mixture: 6% w/v acrylamide, 0.3% w/v bisacrylamide, 7 *M* urea, 1X TBE, ratio 19.1 (Scotlab, Coatbridge, Scotland).
6. Temed (N,N,N'-tetramethylethylene-diamine) (Sigma).
7. 10% Ammonium persulphate; make fresh as required.
8. M13 DNA sequencing ladder, e.g., Sequenase 2.0 (United States Biochemical, Cleveland, Ohio) for use as a molecular weight marker.
9. ^{35}S dATP (Redivue) ~ 22Tbq/mL (Amersham) to label the M13 sequencing ladder.
10. Formamide sample loading buffer: 10 mL formamide, 10 mg xylene cyanol FF, 10 mg bromophenol blue, 200 μL 0.5 *M* EDTA.
11. Water bath at 94°C.
12. 3MM Whatmann paper (Whatmann, Maistone, UK).
13. Gel drier, e.g., BioRad.
14. X-ray film, e.g., Kodak XAR film.
15. Autoradiograph cassette with tungstate intensifying screens.

3. Method

3.1. PCR

Remember to observe local laboratory rules and use appropriate caution when handling any radioactivity.

1. Thaw samples and PCR reagents except the DNA polymerase on wet ice (*see* **Note 1**). Determine the quantity of PCR master mix required for the number of samples + 1 using the following PCR set up for a reaction of 25 μL total volume: 2.5 μL 10X PCR buffer including $MgCl_2$ at 15 m*M*, 0.8 μL dNTP mix, 0.1 μL α^{32}P CTP, 0.1 μL *Taq* polymerase, 18.5 μL autoclaved dH_2O. Remember to include a negative control consisting of all the PCR reagents minus the template DNA, for each different set of primers. Another useful control is a reaction containing all the reagents minus primers (**Note 2**).

Table 1
Example of a Typical Touchdown PCR Protocol for Primers whose Optimal Annealing Temperature (Tm) is 56°C

Stage number	Temperature	Number of cycles to be performed at each stage
Stage 1	Denature DNA for 5 min at 94°C	1 cycle
Stage 2	94°C, 1 min 60°C, 1 min 72°C 1 min	2 cycles
Stage 3	94°C, 1 min 59°C, 1 min 72°C, 1 min	2 cycles Reduce annealing temperature by 1°C every 2 cycles until Tm is reached
Stage 6	94°C 1 min 56°C 1 min 72°C 1 min	25 cycles
Stage 7	72°C, 5 min	1 cycle
Stage 8	4°C	Hold

[a]The initial annealing temperature starts several degrees above the optimal annealing temperature of the primers and drops by one degree every two cycles of PCR until the desired 'touchdown' annealing temperature is achieved, at which point 10–25 rounds of cycling are performed.

2. Add 1 μL (50–100 ng) of DNA and 1 μL of each primer (4 μ*M*) to PCR tubes and keep on ice. Make up the PCR master mix, adding the 1 μL *Taq* DNA polymerase last, straight from –20°C. Vortex and briefly pulse the master mix in a benchtop minifuge (*see* **Note 3**). Add 22 μL to each reaction, vortex, and pulse briefly again. Overlay reactions with 30 μL of mineral oil.
3. Having calculated the theoretical annealing temperature (Tm) of the primers (*see* **Note 4**), perform a suitable PCR touchdown protocol following the parameters given in **Table 1**, which uses an example where the theoretical Tm of the primers is 56°C, and the touchdown goes from 60°–56°C.
4. To check for a successful PCR, visualize products on a 1.8% TBE agarose minigel. For a 100 mL gel, 1.8g agarose in 100 mL 1X TBE. Ethidium bromide can be added to the gel (5 μL of 10 mg/mL in 100 mL gel) which we usually find to be sufficient. Load approximately 8 μL of sample mixed with 2 μL 5X sample loading buffer, and run at 180V for approximately 30 min in 1X TBE buffer (An alternative option is to add ethidium bromide solution to the running buffer at 0.5 mg/mL). Alternatively, the gel can be stained afterwards in a solution of ethidium bromide (0.5 mg/mL in 1X TBE). Detect bands using a UV transilluminator. Products may be stored at 4°C or –20°C until use, however it is expedient to run them within a few days if they are radiolabelled with ^{32}P.

3.2. Polyacrylamide Gel Electrophoresis

Remember to wear gloves when using acrylamide.

1. Following successful PCR, samples are visualized on a 6% denaturing polyacrylamide gel to separate alleles and determine size (*see* **Note 5**). Clean sequencing gel plates, combs and spacers with hot water and detergent, and rinse with dH_2O. If necessary, plates can be cleaned with a solution of KOH/methanol, made by adding approx 5g KOH in 100 mL methanol. Spray clean plates with alcohol and allow to dry. One plate can be coated with silicone treatment such as Repelcote to ensure that the gel remains attached to only one of the glass plates when they are separated after electrophoresis (*see* **Note 5**).
2. Insert spaces and seal the sides and bottom of the two glass plates together tightly with electrical tape. First prepare a sealing gel: 2 mL polyacrylamide, 2 µL Temed, 30 µL 10% ammonium persulphate. Mix by swirling. Immediately pour in between glass plates using a 10 mL glass pipet, or a plastic syringe and allow to coat the bottom of the plates. Whilst this is setting, prepare the main gel: 70 mL polyacrylamide gel mixture, 27.6 µL Temed, 554 µL 10% ammonium persulphate. Mix by swirling and draw up into a pipet or 50 mL plastic syringe barrel. Immediately pour in a continuous stream between the glass plates, holding the plates at a 45° angle on one bottom corner so that the gel flows evenly along the lower part of the side spacer. Make sure that no air bubbles are trapped (*see* **Note 5**). Lie plates horizontally but raise the loading end slightly, at an angle of approximately 10° to the bench to ensure polyacrylamide does not leak out. Insert a 0.4 mm sharks tooth comb between the two gel plates, straight edge first in order to create a trough the width of the comb in the top of the gel, and clamp in place with a large bulldog clip. Clamp further bulldog clips on the sides of the gel plates to prevent leakage. Don't clamp clips on the bottom edge without a spacer as this will distort the gel. Then allow the gel to set at room temperature for approximately 1 h.
3. Remove the bulldog clips and electrical tape from the bottom edge of the plates with a scalpel, and fit into sequencing gel apparatus. Fill tanks with 1X TBE and pre-run the gel, for 30–60 min at approximately 35–40mA/1500–1900V, 60W for a 0.4 mm gel.
4. Mix 4 µL of labeled PCR product with 4 µL of formamide sample loading buffer. Denature samples and pre-made molecular weight markers in a water bath at 94°C for 5 min. Remove and place on ice for 2–5 min.
5. Meanwhile switch off gel apparatus and remove shark tooth comb. Clean the comb, and the trough formed in the gel with buffer to remove unpolymerized polyacrylamide. Re-insert the comb with teeth in first into the pre-formed trough, allowing teeth to touch the top surface of the gel causing a slight indentation. Do not allow teeth to pierce the gel.
6. Load approximately 7 µL of sample into each well using flat edged pipet tips. Add 4 µL of molecular weight markers to each well (*see* **Note 6**).

7. Run the gel at 35–40mA/1500–1900V for about 2 h until the xylene cyanol FF marker dye (light blue) reaches the bottom of the gel.
8. Switch off electrical supply and remove glass plates. Watch they may be hot! Remove the electrical tape from the two sides of the gel with a scalpel and place the plates flat onto the laboratory bench. Also remove the comb. Gently separate the glass plates with a palette knife or large flat spatula, taking care not to wrinkle or rip the gel. (Do not use a scalpel blade as this can be extremely dangerous). Start by inserting the knife into one corner and prise the plates apart slowly. Make sure the gel sticks to the bottom plate, otherwise turn the plates around so the other plate is bottom. Once separated, the gel should be totally stuck to one of the glass plates. Remove the spacers. Place 3MM Whatmann paper cut to size on top of the gel and gently smooth out any air bubbles. Slowly remove the paper with the gel attached and cover with Saran wrap.
9. Dry the gel under vacuum for 30–60 min at 80°C.
10. Place gel in an autoradiograph cassette with intensifying screens and expose to X-ray film at –70°C for 24–72 h.

4. Notes

1. In order to prevent cross contamination when performing PCR it is important to separate your PCR reactions from previous DNA preparations. Try to perform PCR reactions in a bench area apart from other laboratory work, or if this is not possible use a tray to keep work isolated. It is also good practice to keep a separate set of pipettes for pre-PCR work. Keep your own stocks of PCR reagents, and in small aliquots frozen at –20°C. Use sterile techniques and autoclaved equipment. Exposure to UV irradiation in a UV DNA crosslinker (e.g., Stratagene) can sterilize pipettes and other equipment from contaminating DNA.
2. It is useful and less costly to optimize the PCR conditions for each primers conditions without radiolabel first. In the event of PCR not working there are a number of trouble shooting approaches which can be taken and there are several excellent review chapters ***(35,36)***. One of the most critical factors influencing PCR is the magnesium (Mg^{2+}) concentration which may vary from 0.5 m*M* to 5 m*M* depending on the influence of components in the reaction mixture including dNTP's, free pyrophosphate (PPi) and EDTA. The sequence of the primers will influence the success of a PCR greatly. However, commercially available and published primers should already be optimally designed. Primer concentration may also affect a PCR reaction, as high primer concentration may promote mispriming, and low primer concentrations affect yield, but generally a concentration of between 0.1 and 0.5 μ*M* is optimal. Other factors which may be altered are the cycling conditions, template concentration and the Taq polymerase concentration which is usually optimal between 0.5 and 2.5 units. There are now a number of commercially available PCR trouble shooting kits, e.g., Boehringher Mannheim which includes buffers of different pH and magnesium content, and may be of use in determining the PCR correct conditions.
3. Remember to vortex all solutions before pipetting, and briefly pulse in a microcentrifuge to bring reagents down from the sides and underneath the lid.

4. The theoretical annealing temperature of the primers may be calculated from the following simplified formula: 2°C × (A + T) + 4°C × (G + C) *(37)*. It is probably the most crucial factor in the design of a high specific PCR, as too high an annealing temperature will result in no product and too low an annealing temperature may result in non-specific products. A standard PCR protocol, each cycle or round of PCR consists of three steps: a DNA denaturation step at 94°C, a primer annealing step, and a primer extension step at 72°C. When calculating a touchdown protocol, start cycles using an initial annealing temperature several degrees higher than actual Tm, e.g., For primers with a Tm of 56°C, 60°C would be a suitable initial annealing temperature. Reduce by one degree every second cycle until reach 56°C, and then perform 25 cycles at this temperature. In optimizing a PCR protocol it may be necessary to try several "theoretical" Tm.
5. Denaturing polyacrylamide gels can be made in advance e.g. the day before kept at 4°C, ensuring the exposed edges are kept covered in Saran wrap and moist paper towels. The M13 sequencing ladder used as a molecular weight marker can also be made in advance and stored at 4°C. To silicone-treat the sequencing plates, pour a small amount of silicone solution onto one of the glass plates, wipe over with a paper towel pad ensuring all the surface is covered with the silicone and rinse with dH_2O. Allow the plate to dry. If air bubbles do appear while pouring the gel, they can be sometimes eliminated by gently squeezing the plates together just below the bubble. If the bubble persists, the gel can be poured out, and re-poured, or failing that, the plates re-cleaned and a new gel solution made. Additionally, bubble-getters are now available commercially, which are the width of a spacer and can be inserted in between the plates to remove the bubble!
6. To conserve time it may be possible to load several samples in one lane on a polyacrylamide gel, providing there is sufficient separation between the expected sizes of the products. It is useful to load molecular weight markers in the first and/or last lanes of the gel and note position. This will help to orientate the gel once processed.

References

1. Hearne, C. M., Ghosh, S., and Todd, J. A. (1992) Microsatellites for linkage analysis of genetic traits. *Trends Genet.* **8,** 288–294.
2. Beckmann, J. S. and Weber, J. L. (1992) Survey of human and rat microsatellites. *Genomics* **12,** 627–631.
3. Loeb, L. (1994) Microsatellite instability: marker of a mutator phenotype in cancer. *Cancer Res.* **54,** 5059–5063.
4. Aaltonen, L. A., Peltomaki, P., Leach, F. S., Sistonen, P., Pylkkanen, L., Meckline, J. P., Jarvinen, H., Powell, S. M., Jen, J., Hamilton, S. R., Petersen, G. M., Kinzler, K. W., Vogelstein, B., and de la Chapelle, A. (1993) Clue to the pathogenesis of familial colorectal cancer. *Science* (Washington D.C.) **260,** 812–816.
5. Thibodeau, S. N., Bren, G., and Schaid, D. (1993) Microsatellite instability in cancer of the proximal colon. *Science* **260,** 816–819.

6. Ionov, Y., Peinado, M. A., Malkhosyan, S., Shibata, D., and Perucho, M. (1993) Ubiquitous somatic mutations in simple repeated sequences reveal a new mechanism for colonic carcinogenesis. *Nature* **363,** 558–561.
7. Shridhar, V., Siegfried, J., Hunt, J., del Mar Alonso, M., and Smith, D. I. (1994) Genetic instability of microsatellite sequences in many non-small cell lung carcinomas. *Cancer Res.* **54,** 2084–2087.
8. Patel, U., Grundfest-Broniatowski, S., Gupta, M., and Banerjee, S. (1994) Microsatellite instabilities at five chromosomes in primary breast tumors. *Oncogene* **9,** 3695–3700.
9. Miranov, N. M., Aguelon, A. M., Potapova, G. I., Omori, Y., Gorbunov, O. V., Klimenkov, A. A., and Yamasaki, H. (1994) Alterations of (CA)n DNA repeats and tumor suppressor genes in human gastric cancer. *Cancer Res.* **54,** 41–44.
10. Risinger, J. L., Berchuck A., Kohler, M. F., Watson, P., Lynch, H. T., and Biyd, J. (1993) Genetic instability of microsatellites in endometrial carcinoma. *Cancer Res.* **53,** 5100–5103.
11. Gonzalez-Zulueta, M., Ruppert, J. M., Tokino, K., Tsai, Y. C., Spruck, C. H., Miyao, N., Nichols, P. W., Hermann, G. G., Horn, T., Steven, K., Summerhayes, I. C., Sidransky, D., and Jones, P. A. (1993) Microsatellite instability in bladder cancer. *Cancer Res.* **53,** 5620–5623.
12. Eshleman, J. R. and Markowitz, S. D. (1995) Microsatellite instability in inherited and sporadic neoplasms. *Curr. Opin. Oncol.* **7,** 83–89.
13. Kremer, E. J., Pritchard , M., Lynch, M., Yu, S., Holman, K., Baker, E., Warren, S. T., Schlessinger, D., Sutherland, G. R., and Richards, R. I. (1991) Mapping of DNA instability at the fragile X to a trinucleotide repeat sequence p(CCG)n. *Science* (Washington, DC) **252,** 1711–1714.
14. Mahadevan, M., Tsilfidis, C., Sabourin, L., Shutler, G., Amemiya, C., Jausen, G., Neville, C., Narang, M., and Barcelo, J. (1992) Myotonic dystrophy mutation: an unstable CTG repeat in the 3' untranslated region of the gene. *Science* (Washington, DC) **255,** 1253–1255.
15. The Huntington's Disease Collaborative Research Group. (1993) A novel gene containing a trinucleotide repeat that is expanded and unstable on Huntington's disease chromosomes. *Cell* **72,** 371–383.
16. Aaltonen, L. A., Peltomaki, P., Mecklin, J-P., Jarvinen, H., Jass, J. R., Green, J. R., Lynch, H. T., Watson, R., Tallqvist, G., Juhola, M., Sistonen, P., Hamilton, S. R., Kinzler, K., Vogelstein, B., and de la Chapelle, A. (1994) Replication errors in benign and malignant tumors from hereditary nonpolyposis colorectal cancer patients. *Cancer Res.* **54,** 1645–1648.
17. Fishel R., Lescoe, M. K., Rao, M. R. S., Copeland, N. G., Jenkins, N. A., Garber, J., Kane, M., and Kolodner, R. (1993) The human mutator gene homolog MSH2 and its association with hereditary nonpolyposis colon cancer. *Cell* **75,** 1027–1038.
18. Leach, F. S., Nicolaides, N. C., Papodopoulos, N., Liu, B., Jen, J., Parsons, R., Peltomaki, R., Sistonen, P., Aaltonen, L. A., Nystrom-Lahti, M., Guan, X-Y., Zhang, J., Meltzer, P. S., Yu, J-W. (1993) Mutations of a *mutS* homolog in hereditary nonpolyposis colorectal cancer. *Cell* **75,** 1215–1225.

19. Parsons, R., Li, Gi-M, Longley, M. J., Fang, W-H., Papadopoulos, N., Jen, J., de la Chapelle, A., Kinzler, K. W., Vogelstein, B., and Modrich, P. (1993) Hypermutability and mismatch repair deficiency in RER+ tumor cells. *Cell* **75,** 1227–1236.
20. Karran, P. and Marinus, M. G. (1982) Mismatch correction at O^6-methylguanine residues in *E. coli. Nature* **296,** 868–869.
21. Koi, M., Umar, A., Chauhan, D. P., Cherian, S. P., and Carethers, J. M., (1994) Human chromosome 3 corrects mismatch repair deficiency and reduces *N*-methyl-*N'*-nitro-*N*-nitrosoguanidine tolerance in colon tumor cells with homozygous *hMLH1* mutation. *Cancer Res.* **54,** 4308–4312.
22. Anthoney, D. A., McIlwrath, A. J., Gallagher, W. M., Edlin, A. R. M., and Brown, R. (1996) Microsatellite instability, apoptosis and loss of p53 function in drug resistant tumor cells. *Cancer Res.* **56,** 1374–1381.
23. Drummond, J. T., Anthoney, A., Brown, R., and Modrich, P. (1996) Cisplatin and adriamycin resistance are associated with MutLalpha and mismatch repair deficiency in an ovarian tumor cell line. *J. Biol. Chem.* **16,** 19,645–19,648.
24. Aebi, S., Kurdi-Haidar, B., Gordon, R., Cenni, B., Zheng, H., Fink. D., Christen, R. D., Boland, C. R., Koi M., Fishel, R., and Howell, S. B. (1996) Loss of DNA mismatch repair in acquired resistance to cisplatin. *Cancer Res.* **56,** 3087–3090.
25. Fink, D., Nebel, S., Aebi, S., Zheng, H., Cenni, B., Nehme, A., Christen, R. D., and Howell, S. B. (1996) The role of DNA mismatch repair in platinum drug resistance. *Cancer Res.* **56,** 4881–4886
26. Brown, R., Hirst, G. L., Gallagher, W. M., McIlwrath, A. J., Margison, G. P., van der Zee, A. G., and Anthoney, D. A. (1997) hMLH1 expression and cellular responses of ovarian tumour cells to treatment with cytotoxic anticancer agents. *Oncogene.* **15,** 45–52.
27. Gyapay, G., Morisette, J., Vignell, A., Dib, C., Fizames, C., Millasseau, P., Marc, S., Bernardi, G., Lathrop, M., and Weissenbach, J. (1994) The 1993–94 Genethon human genetic linkage map. *Nature Genet.* **7,** 246–339.
28. Ostrander, E. A., Mapa, F. A., Yee, M., and Rine, J., (1995) One hundred and one new simple sequence repeat-based markers for the canine genome. *Mammalian Genome* **6,** 192–195.
29. Dietrich, W. F., Miller, J. C., Steen, R. G., Merchant, M., Damron, D., Nahf, R., Gross, A., Joyce, D. C., Wessel, M., Dredge, R. D., Marquis, A., Stein, L. D., Goodman, N., Page, D. C., and Lander, E. S. (1994) A genetic map of the mouse with 4,006 simple sequence length polymorphisms. *Nature Genet.* **7,** 220–245.
30. Don R. H., Cox, P. T., Wainwright, B. J., Baker, K., and Mattick, J. S. (1991) Touchdown PCR to circumvent spurious priming during gene amplification. *Nucleic Acids Res.* **19,** 4008.
31. Clark, J. M. (1988) Novel non-template nucleotide addition reactions catalysed by procaryotic and eucaryotic DNA polymerases. *Nucleic Acids Res.* **16,** 9677–9686.
32. Litt, M. (1991) PCR of TG microsatellites, in *PCR: A Practical Approach* (McPherson, M. J., Quirke, P., and Taylor, G. R., eds.), IRL Press, Oxford, UK, pp. 85–100.

33. Mellersh, C. and Sampson, J. (1993) Simplifying detection of microsatellite length polymorphisms. *Biotechniques* **15,** 582–584.
34. Odelberg, S. J. and White, R. (1993) A method for accurate amplification of polymorphic CA-repeat sequences. *PCR Methods Appl.* **3,** 7–12.
35. Kidd. K. K. and Ruano, G. (1995) Optimizing PCR, in *PCR 2: A Practical Approach* (Mcpherson, M. J., Hames, B. D., and Taylor, G. R., eds.), IRL Press, Oxford, UK, pp. 1–22.
36. Saiki, R. K. (1989) The design and optimization of the PCR, in *PCR Technology: Principles and Applications for DNA Amplification* (Erlich, H. A., ed.), Stockton Press, NY, pp.7–16.
37. Thein, S. L. and Wallace, R. B. (1986) The use of synthetic oligonucleotides as specific hybridisation probes in the diagnosis of genetic disorders, in *Human Genetic Diseases: A Practical Approach* (Davis, K. E. and Herndon, V. A., eds.), IRL Press, Oxford, UK, pp. 33–50.

16

O^6-Alkylguanine-DNA Alkyltransferase Assay

Amanda J. Watson and Geoffrey P. Margison

1. Introduction

Alkylating agents exert a wide range of biological effects in both pro- and eukaryotes and there is ever increasing evidence that these effects are mediated *via* alkylation at the O^6position of guanine in DNA *(1–4)*. Repair of such adducts can be mediated by O^6-alkylguanine-DNA alkyltransferase (ATase) *(3,4)*. Both pro- and eukaryote ATases transfer alkyl groups from the O^6-position of guanine in alkylated DNA (or from other low molecular weight substrates); *(5)* to a cysteine residue located at the active site of the protein: the reaction is stoichiometric and the protein is autoinactivated *(6)*. This mechanism has been exploited in the design of several different radioactivity-based assays for the enzyme. These involve either measurement of methyl group transfer to protein or the analysis (e.g., by HPLC) of methylated substrate DNA before and after exposure to cell or tissue extracts or restriction endonuclease (RE) site deprotection of synthetic oligonucleotide substrates containing O^6-methylguanine.

The most common method of assaying ATase activity in cell or tissue extracts, which we have used successfully and propagated to a number of other laboratories over a number of years (e.g., *7*), involves measuring [^{3}H] methyl group transfer to ATase protein. Essentially, high specific radioactivity [^{3}H]-methylated DNA substrate is incubated with extract under protein-limiting conditions until the transfer reaction is complete. Excess substrate DNA is hydrolyzed to acid solubility and radioactivity in the residual protein is measured by liquid scintillation counting.

The availability of very high specific activity ^{32}P- and ^{35}S-labeled deoxynucleoside triphosphates has encouraged the development of more sensitive ATase assays based on end-labeled fragments of oligonucleotides containing

From: *Methods in Molecular Medicine, Vol. 28: Cytotoxic Drug Resistance Mechanisms*
Edited by: R. Brown and U. Böger-Brown © Humana Press Inc., Totowa, NJ

O^6-alkylguanine sometimes in a RE site. A number of different methods have been devised *(8–12)* but a convenient, highly sensitive alternative to the standard methyl transfer method is not, as yet, in widespread use.

2. Materials

2.1. Preparation of Substrate DNA

2.1.1. Deproteinization of DNA

1. Calf thymus DNA (*see* **Note 1**).
2. Duran (or other wide-necked glass) bottles. Due to the hazards associated with this procedure (*see* **Note 2**) minimize the possibility of leakage by ensuring that the bottles have a good seal.
3. Proteinase K.
4. Phenol equilibrated with 1 *M* Tris-HCl, pH 8.0. Prepare fresh as required. Add an equal volume of 1 *M* Tris, pH 8.0, to the phenol. Shake, allow to settle, and aspirate off as much of aqueous phase as possible. Extreme caution must be exercised when handling and disposing of phenol (*see* **Note 2**).
5. 3 *M* NaAc, pH 4.0.
6. Absolute ethanol.
7. Ether.
8. N_2.
9. Water-bath set at 55°C.
10. 5 mL plastic syringe.
11. Water-pump aspirator.
12. 50-mL Falcon tubes (conical bottom).

2.1.2. Methylation of DNA

1. Duran (or other wide-necked glass) bottles (*see* **Subheading 2.1.1.**).
2. 0.02 *M* Ammediol, pH 10.0 (pH adjustment is not necessary).
3. 5 mCi [^{3}H] MNU. Preferably ~20 Ci/mmol (Amersham International, 1 mCi/mL in ethanol). Use immediately on delivery.
4. Absolute ethanol.
5. Pasteur pipets.
6. Water vacuum aspirator.
7. Ether.
8. Ethanol: Ether (1:1)
9. N_2.
10. Chemical fume cupboard.

2.1.3. Checking New Substrate

1. Buffer I : 50 m*M* Tris-HCl, pH 8.3, 1 m*M* EDTA, 3 m*M* DTT. This buffer, prepared without DTT, may be stored for several months at 4°C and used for up to 1 wk following the addition of DTT.

2. 5 mL Syringes.
3. 21G Syringe needles.
4. Ecoscint (National Diagnostics/Mensura).
5. Scintillation counter.

2.2. Preparation of Cell/Tissue-Free Extracts

1. Buffer I (*see* **Subheading 2.1.3.**).
2. Phosphate buffered saline (PBS) : 0.8% NaCl, 0.02% KCl, 0.15% $Na_2H_2PO_4$, 0.02% KH_2PO_4, pH 7.4.
3. Phenylmethylsulphonyl Fluoride (PMSF); (Sigma): 50 m*M* in 100% ethanol. Store at –20°C. Stable for at least 3 mo.
4. Leupeptin (Sigma), 10 mg/mL in ddH_2O. Store at 4°C. Stable for at least 1 mo.
5. Sonicator fitted with microtip probe suitable for 1.5-mL Eppendorf tubes (*see* **Note 3**).

2.3. Protein Estimation

1. CBG (Coomassie brilliant blue G250) dye reagent concentrated stock : 780 m*M* CBG (Sigma, 75% dye content), 25% (v/v) ethanol (BDH analar), 7.4 *M* orthophosphoric acid, 0.01% Triton X-100 (v/v), 0.01% SDS (w/v). Store at 4°C in the dark for up to one year. Before use, dilute to 1 in 5 in ddH_2O, leave at 4°C overnight then filter through 3 mm filter paper. Store at 4°C in the dark for up to 3 mo. Commercial reagents are available (*see* **Note 4**).
2. IBSA: 1 mg/mL bovine serum albumin (BSA) in buffer I. Store at 4°C.
3. BSA protein standards: standards of 0.1, 0.2, 0.3, 0.4, 0.5, 0.6, 0.8, 1.0 mg/mL BSA in buffer I are prepared from IBSA. Standards are filtered (0.2 μm) and stored for up to 6 mo at 4°C.
4. Scintillation minivials.
5. Plastic spectrophotometer cuvets.
6. Multi-dispense pipet (*see* **Note 5**).
7. Spectrophotometer set to read at absorbance 595 nm.

2.4. DNA Estimation

1. 10X TNE Buffer : 100 m*M* Tris base, 10 m*M* EDTA, 2 m*M* NaCl, pH 7.4. Filter before use (0.45 μm) and store at 4°C for up to 3 mo.
2. Calf thymus DNA standard (Pharmacia biotech, ultrapure), 100 μg/mL in TNE. Store at 4°C for up to 3 mo.
3. Hoechst 33258 (bisbenzamide) stock dye solution, 1 mg/mL in ddH_2O. Store at 4°C in the dark for up to 6 mo.
4. TKO 100 mini-fluorometer and fluorometer cuvet (Hoefer; *see* **Note 6**) .

2.5. Assay

1. [^{3}H] Methylated calf thymus DNA (*see* **Subheading 2.1.**).
2. IBSA (*see* **Subheading 2.3.**).
3. BSA, 10 mg/mL in ddH_2O. Store at 4°C.

4. Perchloric acid (PCA): 1 *M* and 4 *M* in ddH_2O.
5. NaOH, 10 m*M* in ddH_2O.
6. Ecoscint (National Diagnostics/Mensura).
7. Scintillation minivials.
8. Dry heat blocks set at 37°C and 75°C.
9. Multi-dispense pipet (*see* **Note 5**).
10. Scintillation counter.

3. Methods

3.1. Preparation of Substrate DNA

3.1.1. Deproteinization of DNA

1. Dissolve CT DNA at 2 mg/mL in TE (up to 300 mL) on a stirrer overnight in a IL Duran bottle. There will be some insoluble bits but it is not necessary to remove them.
2. Place bottle in 55°C water bath for 5 min then add solid proteinase K (30 mg). The bits should disappear quickly, but leave for 1 h, swirling occasionally before adding another 30 mg of proteinase K.
3. After a further 1 h at 55°C move to fume cupboard on tray, cool under running tap water and add equal volume of phenol equilibrated to pH8.0 using 1 *M* Tris (*see* **Subheading 2.1.1.**). Cap and shake vigorously for 5 min—be aware of the possibility of leakage.
4. Allow to stand for about 1 1/2 h at room temperature: the phenol should settle out and can be almost completely removed by aspiration.
5. Decant supernatant into 50 mL falcon tubes (conical bottom) and spin at 1000*g* room temperature, 10 min.
6. Observe interface carefully: if clear, re-extraction is not necessary (*see* **Note 7**). Remove phenol from bottom of tube using glass 5-mL pipet or Pasteur pipet and rubber pipet bulb or pipet pump. Do not worry about taking some of the aqueous layer. Pour off supernatants into Duran bottle of appropriate capacity.
7. Add 1/10 volume of 3 *M* NaAc pH 4.0 to pooled aqueous phases, mix well, and add 2 volumes cold ethanol. Cap and mix by inversion.
8. Lift out DNA on glass pipet and transfer to smaller Duran. Wash 3 times with ethanol at room temperature by vigorous shaking and water vacuum pump aspiration of the ethanol. Make sure DNA spreads out in ethanol to ensure complete penetration of ethanol.
9. Wash at room temperature three times with ethanol:ether (1:1) and then three times with ether alone. Each time, pour off the washes into a tray in a fume cupboard. (Keep away from naked flames/electrical appliances.)
10. Dry DNA in stream of N_2 to remove the ether, teasing apart fibrous DNA with Pasteur pipets. Dry to constant weight.

3.1.2. Methylation of DNA

Owing to the radiochemical hazard involved, the following procedure should be carried out in a fume cupboard set at maximum flow rate. Handling and disposal of [^{3}H] must be performed in accordance with local rules pertaining to radioactive substances. We advise monitoring for [^{3}H] contamination of the work area before starting and, of course, on completion.

1. For 5 mCi [^{3}H]-MNU in 1 mL ethanol: dissolve 40 mg DNA on a stirrer plate overnight at 8 mg/mL in 0.02 *M* Ammediol, pH 10.0 in a 25-mL Duran bottle. Transfer 2 mL of this solution to a separate container. (This is to be used for rinsing [^{3}H] vial—*see* **step 3**.)
2. In tray in fume cupboard, CAREFULLY remove seals from [^{3}H]MNU vial using blunt forceps. Use a twisting rather than pulling action and put aluminium ring and sealing disc directly into beaker in tray. Recap vial with black plastic cap provided—avoid shaking.
3. Put Duran on stirrer in tray, and using 5-mL plastic syringe, carefully transfer MNU solution into stirring DNA solution. Rinse out vial with two 1-mL aliquots of DNA solution by serial transfer. Put syringe and empty vial in sink for careful rinsing.
4. Continue stirring DNA for 5 h at room temperature. Carefully remove stirrer bar then add 1/10 vol 3 *M* NaAc, pH 4.0 and 2 volumes of cold ethanol. Form DNA precipitate by swirling and inversion being very careful of leakage—any spills will contain [^{3}H]-methanol which will blow off rapidly.
5. When DNA has formed a tight ball, carefully remove supernatant using a Pasteur pipet attached to a water vacuum pump the outflow of which is piped directly into the sink drain hole to avoid splashing. Do not be concerned about tiny fragments of DNA being sucked down the sink but do avoid the bulk of the DNA! It is possible to remove all of the supernatant safely in this way.
6. Wash the DNA with ethanol (about 20–30 mL per wash) making sure pellet is "fluffed" out each time. After 10 washes check [^{3}H] radioactivity counts in 500 μL of wash (+3 mL scintillant) to monitor the washing efficiency. Ideally the last wash should be close to background, but as small fragments of DNA may be present, two consecutive washes with similar cpm is acceptable.
7. Dry DNA by washing in ethanol:ether (1:1) twice and ether twice. DO NOT aspirate supernatants down sink! Pour them carefully into a stainless steel tray for evaporation and thorough washing down sink.
8. Blow off residual ether in a slow stream of nitrogen, teasing apart DNA with Pasteur pipets if necessary. Transfer to preweighed clean glass vial and dry to constant weight.

3.1.3. Checking New Substrate

1. Weigh about 8 mg DNA and dissolve at 2 mg/mL in buffer I in a clean glass vial. Pass DNA 10 times through 21G needle into 5 mL syringe to ensure homogeneity of DNA (*see* **Note 8**).
2. Count (in duplicate at least) 10-μL aliquots of DNA solution in 3 mL Ecoscint.
3. Assume O^6-MeG content to be 6% of total cpm and set up ATase assay using up to 10-fold excess of ATase (*see* **Subheading 3.5.**). The plateau level will give an accurate measure of O^6-MeG content (calculate from specific activity

of [^{3}H]MNU used). Plateau levels between 600 and 1200 cpm are appropriate for assaying most cells and tissues (*see* **Note 9**). DNA methylated using the above conditions gave 25 pmoles O^6-MeG/mg DNA: 2 ug DNA was found to contain 580 cpm as ATase-repairable radioactivity (at 30% counting efficiency).

4. Carry out a kinetic experiment (i.e., incubate substrate and extract for increasing times) using the amount of extract giving 50% of the plateau level. This will determine the time for the reaction to go to completion.

3.2. Preparation of Extracts

Samples must be stored on ice throughout the procedure to conserve ATase activity.

1. Preparation and storage of cells/tissues/lymphocytes.
   Cells : harvest, wash with PBS, store cell pellet at –20°C.
   Tissue: snap-freeze (dry-ice or liquid nitrogen) and store at –20°C or –70°C.
   Lymphocytes: collect whole blood into universal containing EDTA (final concentration 25 m*M*). Isolate lymphocytes by density centrifugation *(12)*, wash with PBS and store cell pellet at –20°C.
   The number of cells or weight of tissue required for the assay will depend upon the level of ATase activity (e.g., *see* **Note 10**).
2. Transfer tissue or cell pellet to 1.5 mL Eppendorf tube in ice and add cold Buffer I (500–1000 µL) containing 5 µg/mL leupeptin (*see* **Note 11**).
3. Sonicate sample (*see* **Note 3**) within a MSC class I cabinet to minimize exposure to aerosols. It may be necessary to mince with fine scissors or add glass beads to the sample to aid sonication (*see* **Note 12**).
4. Add PMSF to the sample immediately following sonication so that the final concentration is 0.5 m*M* (i.e., 1/100 of volume).
5. Centrifuge at 15,000–20,000*g* for 10 min at 4°C (*see* **Note 13**).
6. Transfer supernatent to a clean Eppendorf in ice. Extracts are now ready for use. For short-term storage (≤48 h), in ice preferably in cold room/cabinet, is recommended. If for longer periods, extracts should be snap-frozen (dry-ice or liquid nitrogen) and stored at –20°C. Activity may be lost on freeze-thawing but we have not systematically investigated this.

3.3. Protein Estimation (13; see Note 14)

1. Add, in duplicate, 40 µL of each standard or unknown (*see* **Note 15**) to the bottom of a scintillation minivial. Blank tubes contain buffer I only.
2. Add 2 mL of CBG/ Biorad reagent to each tube and gently mix (*see* **Note 5**).
3. Transfer 1 mL of blank sample to the cuvet and zero the machine at 595 nm. Repeat with duplicate blank sample to check reproducibility and stability of readings (*see* **Note 16**).
4. Transfer 1 mL of the unknown sample to the cuvet, record the reading, drain the cuvette thoroughly and repeat with the next sample.

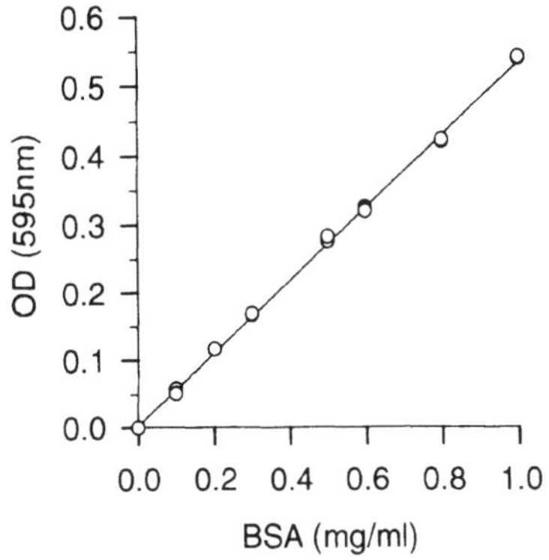

Fig. 1. Protein standard curve. Duplicate or triplicate sample readings are averaged and concentration is extrapolated from the standard curve. Standard deviation of protein estimations should be ≤5%.

5. Construct standard curve by plotting absorbance of standards versus protein concentration (mg/mL). Calculate protein concentration (mg/mL) of samples by reference to the standard curve (*see* **Fig. 1**; *see* **Note 17**).

3.4. DNA Estimation (13; see Note 6)

1. Switch on the TKO 100 at least 15 min before taking measurements so that the lamp is ready and the temperature in the chamber stabilizes.
2. Freshly prepare working solution of Hoechst 33258 by diluting to 1 µg/mL in 1× TNE, wrap in foil to protect from light and allow to warm to room temperature before use.
3. Set the sensitivity of the detector monitor to about 50% by turning the scale knob approximately five full clockwise turns from the fully counter position.
4. Add 2 mL of dye solution to the cuvet, if necessary wipe the sides of the cuvet with a low lint tissue and place in the sample chamber.
5. Zero the instrument.
6. Deliver 2 µL of DNA standard into the 2 mL dye solution and mix by pipetting the solution into and out of a disposable pipette several times without introducing bubbles.
7. Close the sample chamber and adjust the scale control knob until the display reads "100." This one-point standardization sets the machine to read the DNA concentration directly in µg/mL. However, it is advisable to run a calibration curve every few weeks to ensure that the standard has not degraded, the instrument is running properly, and that a consistent technique is being applied (*see* **Note 18**).
8. Remove the cuvette from the sample chamber. Empty and drain the cuvette thoroughly by blotting it upside down on a paper towel between readings.

9. Repeat **steps 4–8** at least once to verify that results are reproducible (*see* **Note 19**).
10. Read the DNA concentration (μg/mL) of your sample by repeating **steps 4–6**. Read the display immediately and record the value (*see* **Note 20**). Duplicate or triplicate reading are taken and averaged (*see* **Note 17**).

3.5. ATase Assay

1. Dilute substrate DNA to 200 cpm/μL in Buffer I (see **Subheading 3.1.3.**). At room temperature:
2. Dispense 100 μL (i.e., 20,000 cpm) of substrate into scintillation minivials, taking care not to touch the sides (*see* **Note 21**).
3. Add appropriate volume of extract to the bottom of the tube, avoiding the substrate if possible. At least two "blank" tubes containing substrate only should be included to determine background counts (*see* **Note 21**).
4. Mix extract and substrate by gently shaking the tube taking care to avoid splashing the walls.
5. Add IBSA to the bottom of the tube to give a final volume of 300 μL (*see* **Note 22**).
6. Incubate at 37°C until the reaction is complete (*see* **Note 23**). Reaction time will depend upon the particular substrate (see **Subheading 3.1.3.**) and tissue/cells used and should be established by experiment.
7. After incubation add 100 μL BSA, 100 μL 4 *M* PCA, 2 mL 1 *M* PCA. If reaction volume has been increased to 1.1 mL (*see* **Note 22**) add 400 μL 4 *M* PCA instead of 100 μL.
8. Heat at 75°C for 50 min to ensure complete hydrolysis of the DNA substrate (*see* **Note 21**).
9. Centrifuge at 2100*g* for 10 min.
10. Aspirate the supernatant (*see* **Note 24**) taking care not to disturb the pellet and add 4 mL PCA.
11. Repeat centrifugation and aspiration.
12. Add 300 μL 10 m*M* NaOH to each tube and shake to disperse the protein pellet, followed by 3 mL Ecoscint.
13. Cap tubes and shake thoroughly before scintillation counting.
14. Calculate the cpm for each tube by averaging two 5-min counts. Unusually high counts particularly in the first few tubes may indicate chemiluminescence and these tubes should be re-counted to constant cpm.

3.6. Calculation of ATase Specific Activity

1. Plot cpm versus volume of extract for each sample and from the linear part of the curve calculate cpm/μL (*see* **Fig. 2**).
2. Multiply cpm/μL by conversion factor (*see* **Note 25**) to give fmoles/mL.
3. Divide fmoles/mL by either protein (in mg/mL) or DNA (in μg/mL) concentration to give ATase specific activity in fmoles/mg protein or fmoles/μg DNA respectively (*see* **Note 26**).

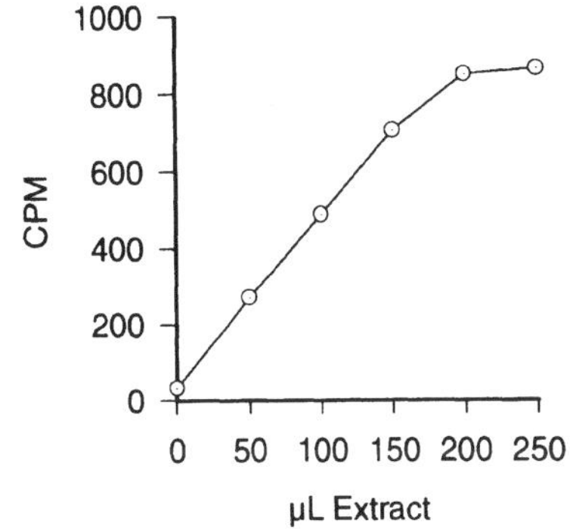

Fig. 2. Results of a typical ATase assay plotted as cpm vs volume of extract. Critical analysis of the data is important to ensure reliable results:

1. Background cpm should be within the range acceptable for the substrate (usually 20–50 cpm).
2. Minimum of 3 points must be linear (i.e., assay under protein limiting conditions).
3. Cpm at maximum volume must be at least twice background cpm.
4. Standard deviation of assay ≤10%.
5. Plateau level of curve (in this case 900 cpm) should correspond to the maximum number of cpm transferrable from substrate to protein (usually 6% of total cpm; *see* **Subheading 3.1.3.**). In some tissues (e.g., rat GIT) where protease activity is high, plateau levels may be lower than expected presumably owing to proteolytic degradation of the ATase. However, providing that specific activities are calculated based on the protein limiting (i.e., linear) part of the curve and all the above criteria are followed, reliable results may be obtained.
6. ATase specific activity of positive control sample (where used, *see* **Note 11**) is within acceptable range.

Assuming compliance with the above, limit of sensitivity of this method ≥2fmoles ATase.

4. Notes

1. We routinely use Sigma calf thymus DNA (<3% protein).
2. Phenol is a powerful systemic poison, which is readily absorbed through the skin causing chemical burns on contact. Phenol should be neutralized with an equal volume of 4 *M* NaOH before disposal down the sink in high dilution.
3. We routinely use a Heatmaster Sonicator fitted with a microtip probe (standard tapered with 3.2 mm diameter) and sonicate for 10 s at 216 µm (peak to peak amplitude). Appropriate sonication conditions will depend upon the particular machine and probe used and should be established by experiment.
4. Biorad dye reagent (Biorad) supplied as a 5× stock may be used as an alternative to CBG. Standard curves using CBG are linear up to 1 mg/mL compared to those using Biorad which plateau around 0.6–0.8 mg/mL.

5. We recommend using an Eppendorf multipette plus (Eppendorf) or similar positive displacement machine to repeat dispense quickly and accurately.
6. Hoechst 33258 binds to the minor groove of DNA. When 365 nm light (long UV) excites this dye, fluorescence results and can be measured by mini-fluorometer (as described here), fluorescence spectrophotometer ***(14)*** or fluorescence microtiter plate-reader. We have also used a microtiter (96-well) based assay ; 10 µL sample or standard (range 0–50 µg/mL DNA) and 100 µL Hoechst (1 µg/mL) per well.
7. If the interface is not clear re-extraction is necessary. Remove upper aqueous layer from each tube and combine in a Duran. Repeat **steps 3–5**.
8. It is important to ensure homogeneity of DNA by syringing since, quite often, the DNA forms small gelatinous "blobs" which are very difficult to see. If not dispersed these manifest themselves as highly variable counts on the plateau (substrate limiting conditions) of the assay.
9. It may be appropriate to use less substrate when trying to detect very low levels of ATase since less substrate will produce lower background counts. It is important that ATase specific activity calculations are based on the linear part of the protein dependence curves.
10. Cells and tissues vary greatly in ATase activity and therefore the amount of extract required to detect activity will also vary. The following may be used as a starting guide if ATase activity is unknown.

    Cells: Bacterial—pelleted from 1.5 mL of stationary culture
    Mammalian—10^7 cells
    Lymphocytes—10 mL whole blood

    Tissue: 1–10 mg

    More (or less) cells or tissue may be used providing sonication is effective without compromising ATase activity.

    Inclusion of a positive control (i.e., ATase expressing cell line or tissue) in both extraction and assay procedures is strongly advised particularly when assaying samples with very low or unknown ATase activity.

    Occasionally, substrate-limiting conditions are attained at the lowest volume of extract used. In this case, repeat the assay using appropriate dilutions of extract in IBSA.
11. A minimum buffer volume of 500 µL is needed to avoid heating of the sample during sonication. If smaller extract volumes (300–500 µL) are required it may be necessary to sonicate the sample for shorter times or on ice. Establish appropriate conditions by experiment.
12. Some tissues (e.g., gut and tumour) are more difficult to disrupt and therefore require the addition of 0.1–0.2g glass beads (100 mesh, BDH) and/or mincing before sonication.
13. It may be possible to omit this step if very few cells are used but this should be checked by experiment.
14. If a platereader with appropriate filter is available this procedure may be adapted as a microtitre (96-well) plate assay. We have successfully used 40 µL of sample or standard (linear range 0–0.1 mg/mL protein) and 200 µL of dye reagent per well.

15. Samples (e.g., liver or tumour tissue) may need to be diluted in buffer I to achieve absorbance within linear range of standard curve (*see* **Fig. 1**).
16. Re-zero the machine where necessary; frequency will depend upon the particular machine.
17. Replicate protein and DNA estimations should be within 5%.
18. The DNA standard (100 µg/mL) is set to read 100, therefore a sample reading 35 has a concentration of 35 µg/mL. To generate a standard curve, follow **steps 1–9** (**Subheading 3.4.**), then measure (in duplicate) 4, 6, 8, 10 µL of the DNA standard. Plot sample concentration versus the averaged reading. The data should yield a linear graph.
19. Once reproducible readings have been produced, do not touch the scale knob again until all measurements have been completed. Do zero the instrument after every reading.
20. The observed fluorescence stabilizes after a few seconds and then begins to drop as the chamber warms.
21. High background counts (≥ twice normal background) usually indicate a problem with sample hydrolysis. Check hydrolysis incubation time and temperature, and PCA concentration. Ensure that substrate is added to the bottom of the tube and is therefore effectively hydrolyzed.
22. The final volume is not critical providing the reaction goes to completion and the substrate is hydrolysed in 1.0 *M* ± 5% PCA. For example, it may, occasionally be necessary to assay larger volumes (up to 500 µL) of cell or tissue extract in order to detect activity. In this case the total assay volume may be increased to 1.1 mL with Buffer I.
23. ATase is not a true enzyme, i.e., the reaction is stoichiometric and autoinactivating. Reaction should go to completion in all cases.
24. Dispose of waste in accordance with local rules for handling [^{3}H].
25. Calculation of conversion factor (CF). The conversion factor is calculated from the counting efficiency and substrate specific activity:
    a. dpm = cpm CE
       where CE = counting efficiency of scintillation counter (e.g., 30%)
    b. $1\text{Ci} = 2.22 \times 10^{12}$ dpm $\therefore$ 1 pCi = 2.22 dpm
    c. Substrate specific activity (SA) in Ci/mmol (= pCi/fmol).
       Re-calculate monthly by reference to decay chart.

    From (a), (b), and (c)

    $$\text{fmol/ µL} = \text{cpm/µL} \times 1\ (\text{SA} \times 2.22 \times \text{CE})$$
    $$\text{fmol/mL} = \text{cpm/µL} \times 1000\ (\text{SA} \times 2.22 \times \text{CE})$$
    $$\text{fmol/mL} = \text{cpm/µL} \times \text{CF}$$
    $$\therefore \quad \text{CF} = 1000\ (\text{SA} \times 2.22 \times \text{CE})$$
26. Lymphocyte specific activities should be expressed in terms of fmoles/µg DNA since in this way contaminating erythrocytes (which do not contain DNA) will not have a significant impact on the measurement. Although for most other purposes either expression of activity is acceptable, there is a growing tendency to use fmoles/µg DNA because from this value the number of ATase molecules per cell may be calculated.

References

1. Singer, B. (1979) *N*-nitroso alkylating agents: formation and persistence of alkyl derivatives in mammalian nucleic acids as contributing factors in carcinogenesis. *J. Natl. Cancer Inst.* **62,** 1329–1339.
2. Saffhill, R., Margison, G. P., and O'Connor, G. P. (1985) Mechanisms of carcinogenesis induced by alkylating agents. *Biochim. Biophys. Acta* **823,** 111–145.
3. Yarosh, D. B. (1985) The role of O^6-methylguanine-DNA methyltransferase in cell survival, mutagenesis and carcinogenesis. *Mut. Res.* **145,** 1–16.
4. Margison, G. P. and O'Connor, P. J. (1990) Biological consequences of reactions with DNA: role of specific lesions, in *Handbook of Experimental Pharmacology* (Grover, C. S. and Grover, P. L., eds.), pp. 547–571.
5. Dolan, M. E., Moschel, R. C., and Pegg, A. E. (1990) Depletion of mammalian O^6-alkylguanine-DNA alkyltransferase activity by O^6-benzylguanine provides a means to evaluate the role of this protein in protection against carcinogenic and therapeutic alkylating agents. *Proc. Natl. Acad. Sci. USA* **87,** 5368–5372.
6. Lindahl, T., Demple, B., and Robbins, P. (1982) Suicide inactivation of the E. coli O^6-methylguanine-DNA methyltransferase. *Embo J.* **1,** 1359–1363.
7. Fan, C. Y., Potter, P. M., Rafferty, J., Watson, A. J., Cawkwell, L., Searle, P. F., O'Connor, P. J., and Margison G. P. (1990) Expression of a human O^6-alkylguanine-DNA- alkyltransferase cDNA in human cells and transgenic mice. *Nucleic Acids Res.* **18,** 5723- 5727.
8. Margison, G. P., Cooper, D. P., and Brennand, J. (1985) Cloning of the E. coli O^6-methylguanine and methylphosphotriester methyltransferase gene using a functional DNA repair assay. *Nucleic Acids Res.* **13,** 1939–1952.
9. Wilkinson, M. C., Potter, P. M., Cawkwell, L. C., Georgiadis, P., Patel, D., Swann, P. F., and Margison, G. P. (1989) Purification of the E.coli ogt gene product to homogeneity and its rate of action on O^6-methylguanine, O^6-ethylguanine and O^4-methylguanine in dodecadeoxyribonucleotides. *Nucleic Acids Res.* **17,** 8475–8484.
10. Wu, R. S., Hurst-Calderone, S., and Kohn, K. W. (1987) Measurement of O^6-alkylguanine-DNA-alkyltransferase activity in human cells and tumour tissues by restriction endonuclease inhibition. *Cancer Res.* **47,** 6229–6235.
11. Brent, T. P. and Remack, J. S. (1988) Formation of covalent complexes between human O^6-alkylguanine-DNA alkyltransferase and BCNU-treated defined length synthetic oligonucleotides. *Nucleic Acids Res.* **16,** 6779–6788.
12. Coutinho, L. H., Gilleece, M. H., Dewynter, E. A., Will, A., and Testa, N. G. (1993) Clonal and long-term culture using human bone-marrow, in *Haemopoesis: A Practical Approach,* vol. 288. (Testa, N. G. and Molyneux, G. M., eds.).
13. Bradford, M. M. (1976) A rapid and sensitive method for the quantitation of microgram quantities of protein utilising the principle of protein-dye binding. *Anal. Biochem.* **72,** 248–272.
13. Instructions - TKO 102 Standards Kit (Hoefer Scientific Instruments, Newcastle-under-Lyme, UK).
14. Cesarone, C. F., Bolognesi L., and Santi L. (1979) Improved microfluorimetric DNA determination in biological material using 33258 Hoechst. *Anal. Biol.* **100,** 188.

17

Analysis of the p53 Status of Tumors

An Overview of Methods

Jonas Bergh

1. Introduction

1.1. Background on p53

The tumor suppressor gene TP53, encoding the p53 protein, has its gene locus on the short arm of chromosome 17 p13.1 *(1,2)*. p53 has been denoted "guardian of the genome" *(3)* owing to its essential cellular functions in apoptosis control, cell-cycle control, chromosomal segregation, gene transcription, and genomic stability *(4)*. The gene encodes a protein of 393 amino acids *(5)*. The tertiary structure of the p53 protein is known to a relatively large extent; the DNA binding region has been localized to amino acids 102 to 292. Murine double minute-2 (MDM2) binds to the amino terminal of the p53 protein and is a negative regulator of p53 *(6)*. p53 is normally activated by ultraviolet (UV)-light, radiation, cytostatics, and carcinogens. The activation by these may involve interaction with the ataxia telangiectasia gene (ATM). The p53 gene can be inactivated by somatic or germ-line mutations. Somatic mutations in the p53 gene is the most common genetic abnormality so far described in human cancer *(7)*. Patients with germ-line p53 mutation's are part of the Li-Fraumeni syndrome. These patients have an increased risk of developing adrenocortical, breast, gastrointestinal tract, and lung carcinoma, as well as soft-tissue sarcoma and malignant melanoma *(8,9)*. Studies on mice have revealed that induced deficiency of both alleles of the p53 gene is associated within an increased risk of lymphomas and sarcomas *(10)*. p53 can also be inactivated by certain viral oncoproteins, such as human papilloma virus protein E6, SV40 large T-antigen, hepatitis B viral X protein, and adenovirus protein E1B *(4)*. Cells with abnormal p53 function have been described as having

From: *Methods in Molecular Medicine, Vol. 28: Cytotoxic Drug Resistance Mechanisms*
Edited by: R. Brown and U. Böger-Brown © Humana Press Inc., Totowa, NJ

a selective growth advantage, as well as different response to radiotherapy, tamoxifen, and cytostatics *(5,11–15)*. Normal activation of the p53 gene can either lead to induction of apoptosis or growth control via its major downstream mediator, CIP1 (p21), which is a major regulator of different cell-cycle regulatory proteins, such as cyclin-dependent kinases and DNA polymerase.

1.2. p53 Status of Human Cancer

Fifty percent or more of the tumors from patients with lung carcinoma and colon carcinoma have been described to have p53 abnormalities in their tumors *(16)*. However, these figures must be interpreted with some caution, as the majority of these studies have used immunohistochemical positivity as a surrogate endpoint for a mutant p53. At the other end of the p53 mutation frequency spectrum, testicular teratomas and patients with nephroblastomas (Wilms' tumors) only have p53 mutations in a low percentage of the studied cases *(17,18)*. This latter finding is interesting because these tumors generally are considered to be very sensitive to different cytotoxic agents, and patients with these tumors are cured at a very high rate. Animal models of testicular teratomas have demonstrated increased p53 protein levels *(19)*. The protein was transcriptionally inactive, but differentiation of the tumor cells with retinoic acid decreased the p53-levels, which was simultaneously coupled to an increase of the p53 related transcriptional activity *(19)*. Furthermore, the topoisomerase II (TOPOII) cytotoxic agent etoposide—sometimes used in the therapy of testicular teratomas—could also activate p53 and induce apoptosis *(19,20)*.

Analyses of the p53 status in tumor biopsies have revealed that patients with tumors with increased protein expression of p53 or a mutant p53 have a worse prognosis. This has been demonstrated for patients with bladder, breast, colon, gastric, nonsmall cell lung, oesophagus, ovarian and prostate carcinoma and the group of soft-tissue sarcomas *(11,21–37)*.

The mutation sites in p53 may be different between dissimilar histopathological entities, which may reflect the differences in etiology for the various malignant tumors in humans. Hepatocellular carcinoma (in many parts of the world coupled to aflatoxin B exposure or hepatitis B infections), has a relative dominance of mutations in amino acid 249, whereas colon carcinomas frequently have mutations in codon 175 *(38–40)*. Furthermore, a more detailed analyses of the p53 status in relation to mutation sites strongly indicate that different mutations have quite different functional and clinical implications. 119 breast cancer tumors with previously demonstrated p53 mutations were further analyzed *(36)*. Patients with tumors with p53 mutations in the L2 and L3 regions had a significantly worse survival rate, statistically *(36)*. The L2 and L3 regions are part of the zinc-binding domain, involved in direct DNA contact and claimed to be of importance for protein stabilization *(41)*. Similarly mutations in the L3 region in colo-rectal carcinomas resulted in significantly shorter survival for these patients, statistically *(42)*.

We have previously demonstrated that the mutation sites were partly dissimilar between lymph node-positive and lymph node-negative breast cancer patients *(11)*. Furthermore, patients with tumors with mutations in the evolutionarily conserved regions II and V had significantly shorter survival, statistically, compared with patients with mutations outside the evolutionarily conserved regions *(11)*. More interestingly, patients with breast cancers with mutations outside the evolutionarily conserved region had a similar prognosis compared with those without proven mutations *(11)*. Taken together these data underline the importance of obtaining the exact nature of the p53 mutation, whereas one type of p53 mutation may result in a completely different functional alterations leading to different clinical behavior compared with another p53 mutation at a different site.

1.3. p53 as Predictive Factor

As well as its independent prognostic value, in some studies p53 has also been claimed to have a predictive value, i.e., the p53 pattern has been claimed to be a determinant of the response to certain therapeutic treatments in experimental models. Initial preclinical studies disclosed that a mutant p53 was associated with worse response to chemotherapy and radiation *(5,13,14)*. Later studies have disclosed that the pattern may be more complex. Inactivation of the wild-type p53 gene has been described to increase the sensitivity to paclitaxel with a factor 7–9 *(43)*. Furthermore, another research group disclosed that inactivation of the wild-type p53 gene also resulted an increased sensitivity to carboplatin, cisplatin, and melphalan *(44)*. Both of these studies were carried out on human foreskin fibroblasts and mouse embryo fibroblasts, respectively *(43,44)*. In a further study on human lymphoblastoid cell lines from probands of Li-Fraumeni families with heterozygous germ-line mutations (p53 wt/mut) of the p53 gene *(45)*, no difference could be detected between the two different heterozygous mutations and normal cells in the response to paclitaxel *(45)*. The response to radiation on the other hand was impaired for the two study lines with two different heterozygous mutations *(45)*.

Clinical studies on breast cancer patients have disclosed that an increased p53 protein expression or mutant p53 seem to be associated with an improved effect by adjuvant postoperative radiotherapy *(12,15)*. The latter clinical findings are partly supported by radiotherapy studies on lymphoblastoid human cell lines *(46)*. In this study radiation was capable of inducing apoptosis at an equivalent frequency in both mutant and wild-type p53, but with delayed kinetics *(46)*.

Missense mutation and positive immunohistochemistry for the p53 protein have been demonstrated in resistant ovarian carcinomas treated by cisplatin-based chemotherapy *(47)*. This observation is essentially concordant with another study on Bcl-2 and p53 demonstrating enhanced levels of Bcl-2 and/or p53 during the progression of in vitro sensitivity of resistant cells *(48)*. In locally advanced and metastatic breast cancer, patients with specific p53 mutations have been described to be associated with primary resistance to weekly doxorubicin *(49)*.

2. How to Examine the p53 Status

As previously indicated, p53 has several important regulatory cellular functions. Abnormalities of p53 have been associated with worse prognosis and dissimilar response to different oncological therapeutical modalities. Accordingly, the following section will discuss the different methods used for detection of p53 abnormalities. These methods could be molecular biological strategies focused on alteration of genomic DNA or RNA; alternatively, they could be focused on the p53 protein expression, most commonly mirrored by immunohistochemistry. From a theoretical point of view, protein analysis may be the best choice, because the p53 protein is responsible for the function. However, as will be discussed, this method has thus far proved to have some shortcomings.

2.1. Protein Determination

2.1.2. Immunohistochemistry

Immunohistochemistry is a quick, relatively inexpensive, and potentially suitable method for protein detection, including determination of the p53 protein. The different steps using the anti-p53 monoclonal antibody (mAb), pAb 1801, are outlined in **Table 1**. Normal cells have the capacity to normally express the wild-type, normal p53 protein. The wild-type protein has a half-life of 15–20 min *(50)* whereas the mutated p53 gene will give rise to a protein with a half-life of 4–20 h *(51–54)*. This prolonged half-life of the mutated protein is the basis for the immunohistochemical detection of mutant p53 protein, which will be retained for a longer time in the cell. Immunohistochemistry has the capacity to reveal the p53 localization on the cellular and subcellular level, which is an advantage. This may give important insight into the questions of antigen distribution and heterogeneity among the cancer cells, and to disclose the expression in tumor cells vs the normal surrounding stroma. For these reasons, immunohistochemistry has been the method of choice for many laboratories for p53 determinations (**Table 1**). Recently, flow cytometry has been described as "a more sensitive and objective" method for the evaluation of the

Table 1
Immunohistochemical Procedure for the Monoclonal Antibody pAb 1801

1. Fixation of the biopsy in buffered formalin; fixative penetration time is approximately 1 mm/h. Alternatively, fixed frozen sections from frozen tumors can be used.
2. Make 5-µm histological sections.
3. Deparaffinize according to standard protocols (not valid for frozen sections).
4. Block endogenous peroxidase (50 mL PBS + 0.5 mL 30% H_20_2, for 10 min).
5. Wash 3 × 5 min in PBS.
6. Antigen retrieval in microwave oven; Wash for 5 min in distilled water, put the slides in cyvetts containing 0.01 *M* citrate buffer at pH 6.0, run three times at 850 W for 3 min × 5. Let the slides cool for 20 min.
7. Wash 3 times in PBS, 3 × 5 min.
8. Block unspecific antigens in 2% BSA for 20 min in a humid chamber.
9. Add the primary antibody for pAb 1801 in the dilution 1/100 containing 2% bovine serum albumin (BSA) for 30 min (Optimal antibody concentration has to be determined on a section with a proven p53 mutation and positive immunohistochemistry.)
10. Wash 3 times in PBS 5–10 min.
11. Secondary antibody: in this case, a biotinylated goat antimouse/rabbit antibody diluted 1/200 in 1% BSA for 30 min.
12. Wash three times in PBS.
13. Add the streptavidin-avidin-biotin complex containing horseradish peroxidase (DUET®; Dako, Glostrup, Denmark) diluted 1/200 in 1% BSA for 30 min.
14. Wash 3 × 5 to 10 min in PBS.
15. Develop in DAB (50 mL PBS + 1 mL 3,3 diaminobenzidine tetrahydrochloride [DAB] + 8 µL H_20_2) for 5 min.
16. Wash in PBS for 5 min.
17. Counterstain with Mayer's hematoxylin for 1 min, tap water for 10 min "to blue it."
18. Dehydration—mount.

p53 status compared with immunohistochemistry ***(55)***. However, this conclusion was only on 23 bladder carcinoma samples. More importantly, flow cytometry as compared to immunohistochemistry lacks the morphological confirmation of the measured cells, i.e., p53 expression in normal cells will not be discriminated from the expression in cancer cells by the use of flow cytometry.

A wide range of different antibodies have been used for immunohistochemical detection of mutant p53 protein. These different p53 antibodies recognize different epitopes and the majority of the antibodies are unable to discriminate between mutant p53 protein and the wild-type protein. However, that may not be a problem owing to the described discrepancy in half-life between the variants of p53, wild-type, and mutant proteins.

A marked degree of variability in the immunohistochemical results has been demonstrated in different breast cancer studies *(56–58)*. The degree of positivity varied from 15.5–54% in 14 breast cancer studies *(57)*. The number of immunohistochemically positive cells varied from 29–54% with four different p53 antibodies *(59)*. Dissimilar fixation procedures and different paraffin temperature may provide explanation for the partly different immunohistochemical results *(60)*. The importance of these issues have been underlined in a pilot study on 22 breast cancer biopsies using the mAb pAb 1801 for p53 determination. Formalin was compared with Bouins fixative, with no difference in the results obtained *(37,60)*. However, the fixation time was of importance. Six h formalin fixation was compared with 24 h fixation. Fifteen of 22 samples fixed for 24 h completely lost their immunoreactivity. Interestingly, microwave treatment retrieved the p53 antigen in all cases but one *(60)*.

Two hundred and forty-five breast cancer patients were investigated in a comparative study using the p53 antibodies pAb 1801, p53-BP-12, DO7, and CM1. These authors concluded that pAb 1801 and DO7 gave the best antigen localization after microwave antigen retrieval *(61)*. Furthermore, these authors concluded that pAb 1801 gave the best prognostic information. In another comparative study, six p53 antibodies (Bp53-12, pAb 1801, DO7, pAb240, CM1, and Signet) were investigated on a paraffin-embedded colo-rectal carcinoma material *(62)*. These authors claimed that using a "target unmasking fluid" resulted in the p53 antibody DO7 as best, with sensitivity and specificity of 57% and 90%, respectively. Furthermore, 33 human lung cancer cell lines, 17 small cell, and 16 nonsmall cell with p53 mutations were investigated for the immunohistochemical expression using two different antibodies, pAb 421 and pAb 1801, compared with p53 sequencing data *(63)*. Eight and 12 of the lung cancer cell lines were negative using the antibodies pAb 1801 and pAb 421, respectively *(63)*. The negative immunohistochemistry was mainly seen in cell lines with deletions, nonsense, and splicing mutations *(63)*. On the other hand, missense mutations localized to exons 5–8 were almost always identified with the immunohistochemical technique *(63)*. In support of these findings, 54 operated primary nonsmall lung carcinomas were investigated for their p53 status *(64)*. One of 8 p53 nonsense mutation were detectable with the mAbs BP53-12 and DO7, whereas the missense mutations were detected in 15 of 17 cases, supporting the findings from the cell line study *(64)*. Similar results were obtained by the authors in a study comparing the immunohistochemical p53 protein expression with cDNA-based sequencing of the p53 gene on more than 300 primary breast cancer biopsies *(65)*. Forty out of 45 point mutations were identified with immunohistochemistry, whereas only 2 out of 13 deletions, 2 out of 3 insertions, and no one of the 6 stop codons were identified with the mAb pAb 1801 compared with eDNA sequencing (**Table 2**). Furthermore,

Table 2
Comparison Between Immunohistochemical Detection of p53 Using the Monoclonal Antibody pAb 1801 with Sequencing of cDNA

		Deletions		Insertions			
	Point Mutations	In frame	Out of frame	In frame	Out of frame	Stops	Total
IHC[a] +	40	2	0	1	1	0	44
IHC –	5	3	8	0	1	6	23
Unknown	0	0	0	0	1	1	2
Total	45	5	8	1	3	7	69

[a]Adapted from ref. ***65***.

patients with positive immunohistochemistry but wild-type p53 according to cDNA-based sequencing had a trend for improved survival, which was statistically significant in the relapse-free survival analysis compared with the group of patients who had tumors that were positive with both techniques ***(65)***. Similar data have been presented by another research group ***(66)***. This finding may be owing to the fact that pAb 1801 detected enhanced wild-type p53 protein levels, which may be associated with a better prognosis owing to an increased normal p53 function.

In conclusion immunohistochemistry is a quick method for p53 determination. This seems to be very suitable for detection of the majority of point mutations, whereas deletions and stop codons to a large extent will be missed. The pros and cons have been discussed recently elsewhere and sequencing was still considered to be the gold standard ***(67)***.

2.2.2. Luminometric Immunoassay (LIA) for p53 Protein Determination

The p53 protein can also been measured by other methods. The LIA method is intended for measurement of the p53 protein in tumor cytosols normally prepared for the routine biochemical measurement of the oestrogen and progesteron receptor status. The LIA method has been demonstrated to be useful and to give prognostic information in a breast cancer material ***(34)***. The principal laboratory steps are outlined in **Table 3**. The LIA measurement of the p53 protein has been compared with immunohistochemical expression and cDNA-based sequencing on more than 200 primary breast cancers (Norberg et al., unpublished data). In brief, the LIA technique seems to have the same principal limitations as the immunohistochemical determination, and the sensitivity and specificity is no better than with immunohistochemical determination.

Table 3
Luminometric Immunoassay (LIA) for p53 Protein Determination

1. Add 10 µL of either the cytosol or a standard sample (containing a defined amount of p53 protein), mix with 100 µL of the tracer (ABEI—conjugated p53 monoclonal antibody DO1), to a precoated (p53 pAb 1801) test tube.
2. Incubate 16–22 h at room temperature.
3. Wash three times with 2 mL of 0.15 *M* NaCI.
4. Measure the chemoluminescence with the LIA-mat starter service kit (Byk-Sangtec Diagnostica, Dietzenbach, Germany) as integrals for a periods of 5 s in a luminometer.
5. Measure the total protein content separately, for example using the BIO-RAD Protein assay system.
6. Correlate the p53 LIA protein value to the total protein value.

2.2.3. p53 Antibodies in Patient Sera

Serum p53 auto-antibodies have been reported from patients with breast, colon, head and neck, liver, lung, ovarian, and pancreatic carcinoma, as well as in Burkitt's lymphoma, myclodysplastic syndromes, and acute myeloid leukemia *(7,68–83)*. The auto-antibodies in the patient sera have been analyzed with different techniques, such as enzyme-linked immunosorbent assay (ELISA), immunoprecipitation and Western blot. In lung cancer, 8% to 30% of the patients have been described to have p53 auto-antibodies, whereas the corresponding figure for breast cancer patients has been in the range 5–15%. A general comment is that the presence of auto-antibodies seems to be considerably lower compared with described mutation frequencies/enhanced protein levels in the corresponding primary cancers. The mechanism for the immune response to p53 has been indicated by the involvement of the 70-kDa heat-shock protein in the antigenic presentation of protein from the p53 tumor suppressor gene *(72)*. The potential relevance of these p53 auto-antibodies is not known. However, some authors have indicated the potential that serum p53 antibodies may serve as an early marker for lung cancer *(75)*. This has to be interpreted with some caution owing to the minimal patient number in their study *(75)*. Furthermore, patients with circulating p53 auto-antibodies with loco-regional breast cancer have been claimed to have statistically significantly shorter overall survival, not to be confirmed in the relapse-free survival figures *(77)*. In accordance with this, patients with primary head and neck cancer with squamous-cell carcinoma morphology had a significantly increased risk of relapse and shortened survival if they had serum p53 auto-antibodies *(69)*.

Thus, one may conclude that a variable proportion of patients with p53 abnormalities in their cancers also have a humoral response that can be detected in serum. The possible clinical relevance and use of this method for early detection is still to be proven.

2.2. Molecular Biological Techniques

2.2.1. Screening for p53 Mutations

Various techniques have been described to screen for mutations. The interest in this area is motivated by the fact that the present sequencing techniques are technically complicated, expensive, and time-consuming to run. The aim in this area is to establish additional rapid and readily available screening techniques coupled with confirmatory methods. The following screening methods could be considered for p53 detection: RNase protection assays ***(84)***, loss of heterozygosity (LOH), single-strand conformational polymorphism (SSCP), denaturing gradient gel electrophoresis (DGGE) ***(85,86)***, constant denaturant gel electrophoresis (CDGE) ***(87)***, dideoxy fingerprinting, and detection of base-pair mismatch using hydroxylamine and osmium tetroxide ***(88)***. The RNase protection assays and the osmium tetroxide method will not be described further in this chapter ***(84,88)***.

An important comment relevant for all screening techniques is that they must have high sensitivity in order to diminish the risk of false-negative samples and high specificity to avoid false-positivity. Data on sensitivity and specificity ideally should be presented for each method and when needed, information on the potential clinical relevance should also be presented.

2.2.2. LOH

Approximately 60% of breast cancer samples have been demonstrated to have LOH in the 17p13 region; 50% or less of the remaining alleles have a p53 mutation ***(89–91)***. The principle for the LOH analysis is to examine the potential difference between the paternal and the maternal allele for defined di-, tri-, and tetra repeats for the region of interest, in this case 17p13. In the heterozygous situation, the disappearance in the tumor of one allele compared with normal tissue is a demonstration of LOH. For natural reasons, a homozygous signal pattern, identical paternal and maternal alleles, will not be informative with this technique. The LOH technique is of major interest for screening of samples for multiple regions of interest.

2.2.3. SSCP

The use of polymerase chain reaction (PCR) in combination with SSCP is so far the most common molecular biological screening technique for p53 mutations. Different temperatures must be used in combination with different glycerol concentrations in order to optimize an eventual migration shift, and thus increase the sensitivity of SSCP. The sensitivity of the SSCP has been published as varying from 58–100% in samples with known p53 mutations *(92,93)*. The sensitivity seems to be higher for small segments compared with large segments, and the low figure of 58% refers to a segment with the size of 307 base pairs *(94)*. Accordingly, a negative SSCP result can not *per se* exclude a mutation. We have performed a SSCP study and our results were in the lower range of previously published data, and the inter-observer variability was marked (Norberg et al., unpublished data). The principal requirement of optimization for each mutation may require a rather tedious procedure and thus one may ask whether up-front sequencing sometimes may be more cost-effective.

2.2.4. CDGE

CDGE is intended for mutation screening and is a modification of the DGGE method *(85,87)*. The basic principal for both these methods is that the DNA base-pair guanine-cytosine is kept together with three hydrogen bounds, whereas adenine-thymidine is kept together only with two hydrogen bounds in a semi-denaturating environment, thus giving different melting behavior of the double-stranded DNA (dcDNA). This separation of the DNA strands can be performed on a acrylamide gel containing a chemical denaturant of an urea formamide gradient; 100% denaturation corresponds to 7 *M* urea and 40% formamide *(87,95)*. The CDGE technique uses a predetermined optimal urea-formamide concentration for optimal DNA strand separation to allow screening of multiple samples for a given fragment.

In a comparative study on samples with p53 mutations, the CDGE technique detected 15 of 17 abnormalities, whereas the corresponding value in this study for SSCP was 18 of 20 samples *(96)*. The CDGE technique has been described to have a very high sensitivity in being able to detect 1% mutated cells in a cell population *(41)*.

2.2.5. Dideoxy Fingerprinting (ddF)

The dideoxy fingerprinting (ddF) is described by Sarkar et al. *(92)* to be a "hybrid between dideoxy sequencing and SSCP." The method is rapid, large and small regions can be amplified and screened. In the initial publication, Sarkar et al. detected 84 out of 84 known mutations. The frequency of false positivity has been described to be low—in the order of 5% *(92,97)*. The ddF technique has been explored on 73 primary breast cancers *(97)*. Sarkar et al. claimed that this technique detected 100% of the gene mutations, but compared with SSCP, ddF technique requires 50% more effort *(97)*.

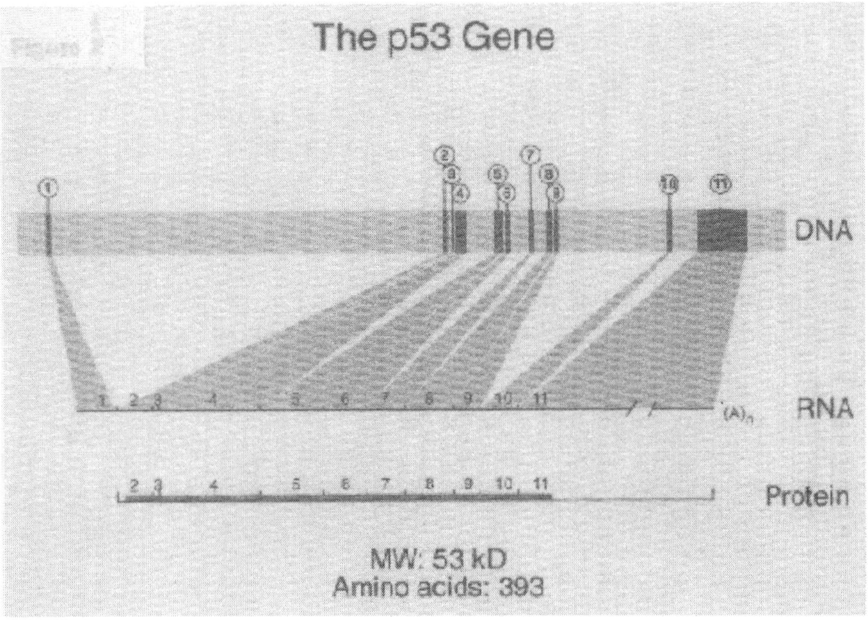

Fig. 1. The tumor-suppressor gene p53:(TP53)-activation of the gene and downstream effects, with focus on cell-cycle regulation and apoptosis.

2.2.6. Sequencing

The p53 gene consist of 11 exons. Large introns are located between exons 1 and 2 at 9 and 10. Furthermore, fairly large introns are located between exons 4 and 5, 10 and 11, followed by 6–7 and 7–8 (**Fig. 1**). Owing to the large introns combined with the location of the mutations, most studies have been focused on mutation analysis of exon 4/5–8. Thus, one should remember this potential shortcoming when the p53 mutation frequency in relation to site is discussed.

Sequencing of genomic DNA is recommended to include a microdissection step, whereas the common solid tumors in many cases are characterized by a marked tumor stroma surrounding the cancer cells (**Table 4**). The addition of the microdissection is supported by the fact that 2 of 16 mutations were missed in a small pilot experiment comparing cDNA sequencing with genomic DNA from human breast cancer samples containing known mutations *(97a)*. The potential advantage in using genomic sequencing is, of course, that information on the p53 status will be obtained from the introns, including the splice regions (**Tables 5** and **6**). In a comparative study on 95 breast cancer samples,

Table 4
DNA Preparation and Isolation from Paraffin Blocks

1. Make 16-µm histological sections.
2. Counter stain with methylene blue for morphological orientation.
3. Microdissection of the tumor cell nests, removal of the tumor stroma. After microscopical confirmation, the surrounding normal tissue may be taken for control.
4. Add the microdissected material to 50 µL 1X TE (10 m*M* Tris HCl, pH 7.5, 1 m*M* EDTA), can be frozen.
5. Add 150 µL of 1.33X sample buffer (63 m*M* Tris HCl, pH 8.4, 133 m*M* EDTA, 133 m*M* NaCl, 1.33% sodium dodecyl sulfate [SDS]) and 7 µL Proteinase K (20 mg/mL).
6. Incubate overnight at 55°C.
7. Add two wax pellets.
8. Add 200 µL Phenol and 400 µL Chloroform.
9. Mix by tilting the tubes for 20 min in a "blood cradle;" check the covers.
10. Short centrifugation; 10,000*g* for approx 1–3 s.
11. Incubate for 5 min at 65°C to allow the wax to melt.
12. Centrifuge 10,000*g* for 10 s.
13. Place on wet ice until the wax has solidified.
14. Pour out the DNA phase. Should be on top of the solidified wax/chloroform/ phenol phase, to 1.5 mL Eppendorf tubes.
15. Add 500 µL of 99.5% ethanol (+4°C); tilt the tubes.
16. Centrifuge at 14,000*g* for 3 min.
17. Pour away the ethanol.
18. Add 500 µL of 70% ethanol.
19. Centrifuge at 14,000*g* for 1 min.
20. Remove the ethanol by a pipet.
21. Let airdry in a sterile hood.
22. Dissolve in 50 µL TE-buffer (10 m*M* Tris-HCl, 1 m*M* EDTA) overnight at 4°C.
23. Heat the samples at 90 C for a few minutes; be careful with the covers.
24. Store in fridge or in a freezer depending on time until use.

one further mutation was detected using genomic sequencing (microdissected material) vs cDNA not counting intron and splice-site mutations ***(97a)***. The eventual functional implications of intron and splice-site mutations of the p53 gene so far is not known. Accordingly possible clinical implications are even more far-fetched. Our findings indicate the possibility of enhanced RNA levels, at least in breast cancers, which may be the explanation for the comparable result using cDNA based sequencing with genomic sequencing on microdissected material.

Table 5
RNA Preparation and Isolation

1. Frozen tumor; sample size approximately 5 × 2 × 2 mm; remove in frozen condition. Remember to wear gloves for prevention of RNA degradation. Perform the dissection with a disposable scalpel in a sterile Petri dish on dry ice to avoid thawing.
2. Add the tumor section to a 1.5-mL polypropylene microcentrifuge tube containing 300 μL of extraction solution (RNAzole, Cinna Biotec, Houston, TX) on wet ice.
3. Grind the tissue using a disposable micropestle.
4. Add 300 μL of RNAzole and 400 μL of a mixture of chloroform and isoamyl alcohol (24:1) to the tube.
5. Mix for 10 s on a vortex mixer.
6. Return to wet ice for 10 min to allow the RNA to phase-separate from tissue and other cellular components.
7. Spin on a microcentrifuge for 10 min at 14,000*g*.
8. Remove 350 μL of the upper phase and transfer to a new tube containing 400 μL isopropanol.
9. Brief vortex mixing of the new tube on wet ice for 30 min.
10. Microcentrifuge at 14,000*g* for 20 min.
11. Discard the supernatant.
12. Wash the pelleted RNA twice with 70% ethanol.
13. Dry briefly.
14. Dissolve in 100 μL diethyl pyrocarbonate-(DEPC)-treated water and 1 μL of RNA guard (25U, Pharmacia Biotech, Uppsala, Sweden).

Table 6
cDNA Synthesis

1. Heat the RNA at 90°C for 3 min for denaturation.
2. Chill on wet ice for 3 min.
3. 25 μL RNA transferred to a microcentrifuge containing 10 μL of Moloney murine leukaemia virus (MMLV) reverse transcriptase (200 U; Pharmacia Biotech), 2.5 μL RNA guard 62,5 U, 37.5 μL of 2 × "cDNA mix" (90 m*M* Tris-HCl, pH 8.3, 138 m*M* KCl, 18 m*M* $MgCl_2$, 30 m*M* dithiothreitol [DTT], 3.6 m*M* deoxycytidine triphosphate [dCTP], 3.6 m*M* deoxyadenosine triphosphate [dATP], 3.6 m*M* deoxythymidine triphosphate [dTTP], 3.6 m*M* deoxyinosine triphosphate [dITP], 0.9 m*M* deoxyguanosine triphosphate [dGTP], and 0.152 A_{260} U of pd[N]$_6$ random primers [approximately 2.5 pmol of primers]), final volume of 75 μL.
4. Incubate at 37°C for 1 h.
5. Heat denaturate at 90°C for 3 min.
6. Store at –20°C.

The most important advantage with genomic-based sequencing is that paraffin-embedded samples can be analyzed. This means that it should be possible to analyze the large histopathological archives at pathology departments with reference to DNA alterations.

2.2.7. Investigational Molecular-Biology Techniques

Minisequencing may be used for detection of a single base-pair mutation in a predefined region. The ship technology is utilizing multiple primers simultaneously. Furthermore, attempts are done using the endonuclease enzymes for detection of mismatch cleavage. These techniques may be used for rapid screening of mutations in the future.

3. Conclusions

p53 is an important gene responsible for key cellular functions like apoptosis and cell-cycle control. Mutated p53 or more commonly enhanced p53 protein levels have been described to be associated with worse prognosis for many human malignancies. This may partly be owing to the fact that the effect by cytostatics, radiation, and tamoxifen seem to be closely linked to the p53 status in a complex fashion. Certain sites of the p53 gene seem to more essential for some of the p53 functions. The p53 status can be monitored either by protein determination or with molecular-biology methods. Methods for p53 mutation determination should have information on sensitivity specificity. The protein methods may miss a high proportion of stop codons and deletions, and detect enhanced protein levels from the wild-type p53. Molecular-biology screening methods may be useful, but today the degree of sensitivity and specificity for p53 mutation detection seems to be variable. Sequenced-based diagnosis is tedious, but probably the most accurate method for evaluation of the p53 status. Ideally, this should be coupled to functional p53 protein analysis and relevant clinical end-points like relapse-free-and overall survival.

Acknowledgments

Our p53 studies have been supported by grants from the Swedish Cancer Society and from Pharmacia Biotech. For the different methods, I am especially grateful to Torbjörn Norberg, Hans Nordgren, and Gunilla Kärf. The excellent secretarial assistance by Marléne Forslund is highly appreciated.

References

1. McBride, O., Merry, D., and Givol, D. (1986) The gene for human p53 cellular tumor antigen is located on chromosome 17 short arm (17p13). *Proc. Natl. Acad. Sci. USA* **83,** 130–134.
2. Miller, C., Mohandas, T., Wolf, D., Prokocimer, M., Rotter, V., and Koeffler, H. (1986) Human p53 gene localized to short arm of chromosome 17. *Nature* **319,** 783–784.

3. Lane, D. (1992) p53, guardian of the genome. *Nature* **358,** 15–16.
4. Harris, C. (1996) Structure and function of the p53 tumor suppressor gene: clues for rational cancer therapeutic strategies. *J. Natl. Cancer. Inst.* **88,** 1442–1455.
5. Zambetti, G. and Levin, A. (1993) A comparison of the biological activities of wild-type and mutant p53. *FASEB J.* **7,** 855–865.
6. Kussie, P., Gorina, S., Marechal, V., Elenbaas, B., Moreau, J., Levine, A., and Pavietich, N. (1996) Structure of the MDM2 oncoprotein bound to the p53 tumor suppressor transactivation domain. *Science* **274,** 948–953.
7. Schhchtholz, B., Legros, Y., Gillet, D., Gaillard, C., Marty, M., Lane, D., Calvo, F., and Soussi, T. (1992) The immune response to p53 in breast cancer patients is directed against immunodominant epitopes unrelated to the mutational hot spots. *Cancer Res.* **52,** 6380–6384.
8. Malkin, D., Li, F., Strong, L., Fraumeni Jr, J., Nelson, C., Kim, D., Kassel, J., Gryka, M., Bischoff, F., Tainsky, M. and Friend, S. (1990) Germ line p53 mutations in a familial syndrome of breast cancer, sarcomas, and other neoplasms. *Science* **250,** 1233–1238.
9. Srivastava, S., Zou, Z., Pirollo, K., Blattner, W., and Chang, E. (1990) Germ-line transmission of a mutated p53 gene in a cancer-prone family with Li-Fraumeni syndrome. *Nature* **348,** 747–749.
10. Donehower, L., Harvey, M., Slagle, B., McArthur, M., Montogomery Jr., C., Butel, J., and Bradley, A. (1992) Mice deficient for p53 are developmentally normal but susceptible to spontaneous tumours. *Nature* **356,** 215–221.
11. Bergh, J., Norberg, T., Sjögren, S., Lindgren, A. and Holmberg, L. (1995) Complete sequencing of the p53 gene provides prognostic information in breast cancer patients, particularly in relation to adjuvant systemic therapy and radiotherapy. *Nature Med.* **1,** 1029–1034.
12. Jansson, T., Inganäs, M., Sjögren, S., Norberg, T., Lindgren, A., Holmberg, L. and Bergh, J. (1995) p53 status predicts survival in breast cancer patients treated with or without postoperative radiotherapy: a novel hypothesis based on clinical findings. *J. Clin. Oncol.* **13,** 2745–2751.
13. Lowe, S., Ruley, H., Jacks, T. and Housman, D. (1993) p53–dependent apoptosis modulates the cytotoxicity of anticancer agents. *Cell* **74,** 957–967.
14. Lowe, S., Bodis, S., McClatchey, A., Remington, L., Ruley, H., Fisher, D., Housman, D. and Jacks, T. (1994) p53 status and the efficacy of cancer therapy in vivo. *Science* **266,** 807–810.
15. Silvestrini, R., Veneroni, S., Benini, E., Daidone, M., Luisi, A., Leutner, M., Maucione, A., Kenda, R., Zucali, R., and Veronesi, U. (1997) Expression of p53, glutathione S-transferase-π, and bcl-2 proteins and benefit from adjuvant radiotherapy in breast cancer. *J. Natl. Cancer Inst.* **89,** 639–645.
16. Carson, D. and Lois, A. (1995) Cancer progression and p53. *Lancet* **346,** 1009–1011.
17 Velculescu, V. and El-Deiry, W. (1996) Biological and clinical importance of the p53 tumor suppressor gene. *Clin. Chem.* **42,** 858–868.
18. Greenblatt, M., Bennett, W., Hollstein, M., and Harris, C. (1994) Mutations in the p53 tumor suppressor gene: clues to cancer etiology and molecular pathogenesis. *Cancer Res.* **54,** 4855–4878.

19. Lutzker, S. and Levine, A. (1996) A functionally inactive p53 protein in teratocarcinoma cells is activated by either DNA damage or cellular differentiation. *Nature Medicine* **2,** 804–810.
20. Chresta, C. and Hickman, J. (1996) Oddball p53 in testicular tumors. *Nature Med.* **2,** 745–746.
21. Chang, F., Syrjänen, S., and Syrjänen, K. (1995) Implications of the p53 tumorsuppressor gene in clinical oncology. *J. Clin. Oncol.* **13,** 1009–1022.
22. Sarkis, A., Dalbagni, G., Cordon-Cardo, C., Zhang, Z.-F., Sheinfeld, J., Fair, W., Herr, H., and Reuter, V. (1993) Nuclear overexpression of p53 protein in transitional cell bladder carcinoma: a marker for disease progression. *J. Natl. Cancer Inst.* **85,** 53–59.
23. Remvikos, Y., Tominaga, 0., Hammel, P., Laurent-Puig, P., Salmon, R., Dutrillaux, B., and Thomas, G. (1992) Increased p53 protein content of colorectal tumours correlates with poor survival. *Br. J. Cancer* **66,** 758–764.
24. Starzynska, T., Bromley, M., Ghosh, A., and Stern, P. (1992) Prognostic significance of p53 overexpression in gastric and colorectal carcinoma. *Br. J. Cancer* **66,** 558–562.
25. Martin, H., Filipe, M., Morris, R., Lane, D., and Silvestre, F. (1992) p53 expression and prognosis in gastric carcinoma. *Int. J. Cancer* **50,** 859–862.
26. Mitsudomi, T., Oyama, T., Kusano, T., Osaki, T., Nakanishi, R., and Shirakusa, T. (1993) Mutations of the p53 gene as a predictor of poor prognosis in patients with non-small-cell lung cancer. *J. Natl. Cancer Inst.* **85,** 2018–2023.
27. Bosan, S., Viale, G., Radaelli, U., Bossi, P., Bonoldi, E., and Coggi, G. (J993) p53 accumulation in ovarian carcinomas and its prognostic implications. *Human Pathol.* **24,** 1175–1179.
28. Visakorpi, T., Kallioniemi, O.-P., Heikkinen, A., Koivula, T., and Isola, J. (1992) Small subgroup of aggressive, highly proliferative prostatic carcinomas defined by p53 accumulation. *J. Natl. Cancer. Inst.* **84,** 883–887.
29. Drobnjak, M., Latres, E., Pollack, D., Karpeh, M., Dudas, M., Woodruff, J., Brennan, M., and Cordon-Cardo, C. (1994) Prognostic implications of p53 nuclear overexpression and high proliferation index of Ki-67 and adult soft-tissue sarcomas. *J. Natl. Cancer. Inst.* **86,** 549–554.
30. Thor, A., Moore II, D., Edgerton, S., Kawasaki, E., Reibsaus, E., Lynch, H., Marcus, J., Schwartz, L., Chen, L.-C., Mayall, B., and Smith, H. (1992) Accumulation of p53 tumor suppressor gene protein: an independent marker of prognosis in breast cancers. *J. Natl. Cancer. Inst.* **84,** 845–855.
31. Andersen, T., Holm, Nesland, J., Heimdal, K., Ottestad, L., and Børresen, A.-L. (1993) Prognostic significance of TP53 alterations in breast carcinoma. *Br. J. Cancer* **68,** 540–548.
32. Elledge, R., Fuqua, S., Clark, G., Pujol, P., Allred, D., and McGuire, W. (1993) Prognostic significance of p53 gene alterations in node-negative breast cancer. *Br. Cancer Res. Treat.* **26,** 225–235.
33. Thorlacius, S., Børresen, A., and Eyfjord, J. (1993) Somatic p53 mutations in human breast carcinomas in an Icelandic population: a prognostic factor. *Cancer Res.* **53,** 1637–1641.

34. Borg, A., Lennerstrand, J., Stenmark-Askmalm, M., Fernö, M., Brisfors, A., Öhrvik, A., Stål, O., Killander, D., Lane, D., and Brundell, J. (1995) Prognostic significance of p53 overexpression in primary breast cancer; a novel luminometric immunoassay applicable on steroid receptor cytosols. *Br. J. Cancer* **71,** 1013–1017.
35. Elledge, R., Clark, G., Fuqua, S., Yu, Y.-Y., and Alired, D. (1994) p53 protein accumulation detected by five different antibodies: relationship to prognosis and heat shock protein 70 in breast cancer. *Cancer Res.* **54,** 3752–3757.
36. Børresen, A.-L., Ikdahl Andersen, T., Eyfjord, J., Cornelis, R., Thorlacius, S., Borg, A., Johanson, U., Theillet, C., Scherneck, S., S, H., Cornelisse, C., Hovig, E., and Devilee, P. (1995) TP53 mutations and breast cancer prognosis: particularly poor survival rates for cases with mutations in the zinc-binding domains. *Genes Chromosom. Cancer.* **14,** 71–75.
37. Silvestrini, R., Benini, E., Daidone, M., Veneroni, S., Boracchi, P., Cappelletti, V., Di Fronzo, G., and Veronesi, U. (1993) p53 as an independent prognostic marker in lymph node-negative breast cancer patients. *J. Natl. Cancer. Inst.* **85,** 965–970.
38. Levine, A., Momand, J., and Finlay, C. (1991) The p53 tumor suppressor gene. *Nature* **351,** 453–456.
39. Hsu, I., Metcalf, R., Sun, T., Welsh, J., Wang, N., and Harris, C. (1991) Mutational hotspot in the p53 gene in human hepatocellular carcinoma. *Nature* **350,** 427–428.
40. Bressac, B., Kew, M., Wands, J., and Ozturk, M. (1991) Selective G to T mutations of p53 gene in hepatocellular carcinoma from Southern Africa. *Nature* **350,** 429–431.
41. Børresen-Dale, A.-L. (1997) Subgroups of p53 mutations may predict the clinical behaviour of cancers in the breast and colon and contribute to therapy response, in *Prognostic and Predictive Value of p53* (Klijn, J., ed.), Elsevier Science BV, Amsterdam, pp. 23–33.
42. Børresen-Dale, A.-L., Lothe, R., Meling, G., Hainaut, P., Rognum, T., and Skovlund, E. (1997) TP53 and long-term prognosis in colorectal cancer; mutations in the L3 Zn-binding domain predict poor survival. *Clin. Cancer Res.* **4,** 203–210.
43. Wahl, A., Donaldson, K., Fairchild, C., Lee, F., Foster, S., Demers, W., and Galloway, D. (1996) Loss of normal p53 function confers sensitization to Taxol by increasing G2/M arrest and apoptosis. *Nature Med.* **2,** 72–79.
44. Hawkins, D., Demers, G., and Galloway, D. (1996) Inactivation of p53 enhances sensitivity to multiple chemotherapeutic agents. *Cancer Res.* **56,** 892–898.
45. Delia, D., Mizutani, S., Lamorte, G., Goi, K., Iwata, S., and Pierotti, M. (1996) p53 activity and chemotherapy. *Nature Med.* **2,** 724–725.
46. Xia, F., Wang, X., Wang, Y.-H., Tsang, N.-M., Yandell, D., Kelsey, K., and Liber, H. (1995) Altered p53 status correlates with differences in sensitivity to radiation-induced mutation and apoptosis in two closely related human lymphoblast lines. *Cancer Res.* **55,** 12–15.
47. Righetti, S., Della Torre, G., Pilotti, S., Menard, S., Ottone, F., Colnaghi, M., Pierotti, M., Lavarino, C., Comarotti, M., Oriana, S., Bohm, S., Bresciani, G.,

Spatti, G., and Zunino, F. (1996) A comparative study of p53 gene mutations, protein accumulation, and response to cisplatin-based chemotherapy in advanced ovarian carcinoma. *Cancer Res.* **56,** 689–693.

48. Eliopoulos, A., Kerr, D., Herod, J., Hodgkins, L., Krajewski, S., Reed, J., and Young, L. (1995) The control of apoptosis and drug resistance in ovarian cancer: influence of p53 and Bcl-2. *Oncogene* **11,** 1217–1228.
49. Aas, T., Børresen, A.-L., Geisler, S., Smith-Sorensen, B., Johansen, H., Varhaug, J., Akslen, L., and Lonning, P. (1996) Specific p53 mutations are associated with de novo resistance to doxorubicin in breast cancer patients. *Nature Med.* **2,** 811–814.
50. Gronostajski, R., Goldberg, A., and Pardee, A. (1984) Energy requirement for degradation of tumor-associated protein p53. *Mol. Cell Biol.* **4,** 442–448.
51. Reich, N. and Levine, A. (1984) Growth regulation of a cellular tumour antigen, p53, in nontransformed cells. *Nature* **308,** 199–201.
52. Finlay, C., Hinds, P., Tan, T.-H., Eliyahu, D., Oren, M., and Levine, A. (1988) Activating mutations for transformation by p53 produce a gene product that forms an hsc70–p53 complex with an altered half-life. *Mol. Cell Biol.* **8,** 531–539.
53. Iggo, R., Gatter, K., Bartek, J., Lane, D., and Harris, A. (1990) Increased expression of mutant forms of p53 oncogene in primary lung cancer. *Lancet* **35,** 675–679.
54. Hinds, P., Finlay, C., Quartin, R., Baker, S., Fearon, E., Vogelstein, B., and Levine, A. (1990) Mutant p53 cDNAs from human colorectal carcinomas can cooperate with ras in transformation of primary rat cells: a comparins of the [19]hot spot" mutant phenotypes. *Cell Growth Diff.* **1,** 571–580.
55. Kraggerud, S., Dolven Jacobsen, K., Beern, A., Stokke, T., Holm, R., Smedsharnmer, L., Børresen-Dale, A.-L., and Fossa, 5. (1997) A comparison of different modes for the detection of p53 protein accumulation. *Pathol. Res. Pract.* **193,** 1–8.
56. Elledge, R. and Aflred, D. (1994) The p53 tumor suppressor gene in breast cancer. *Br. Cancer Res. Treat.* **32,** 39–47.
57. Bhargava, V., Thor, A., Deng, G., Ljung, B.-M., Morre II, D., Waldman, F., Benz, C., Goodson III, W., Mayall, B., Chew, K., and Smith, H. (1994) The association of p53 immunopositivity with tumor proliferation and other prognostic indicators in breast cancer. *Modern Pathol.* **7,** 361–368.
58. Ikdahl Andersen, T. and Børresen, A.-L. (1995) Alterations of the TP53 gene as a potential prognostic marker in breast carcinomas. *Diag. Mol. Pathol.* **4,** 03–211.
59. Jacquemier, J., Moles, J., Penault-Llorca, F., Adelaide, J., Torrente, M., Viens, P., Bimbaum, D., and Theillet, C. (1994) p53 immunohistochemical analysis in breast cancer with four monoclonal antibodies: comparison of staining and PCR-SSCP results. *Br. J. Cancer* **69,** 846–852.
60. Silvestrini, R., Rao, S., Benini, E., Gracia Daidone, M., and Pilotti, S. (1995) Immunohistochemical detection of p53 in clinical breast cancers: A look at methodologic approaches. *J. Natl. Cancer. Inst.* **87,** 1020.
61. Home, G., Anderson, J., Tiniakos, D., McIntosh, G., Thomas, M., Angus, B., Henry, J., Lennard, T., and Home, C. (1996) p53 protein as a prognostic indicator in breast carcinoma: a comparison of four antibodies for immunohistochemistry. *Br. J. Cancer* **73,** 29–35.

62. Baas, I., Mulder, J., Offerhaus, G., Vogelstein, B., and Hamilton, 5. (1994) An evaluation of six antibodies for immunohistochemistry of mutant p53 gene product in archival colorectal neoplasmas. *J. Pathol.* **172,** 5–12.
63. Bodner, S., Minna, J., Jensen, S., DAmico, D., Carbone, D., Mitsudomi, T., Fedorko, I., Buchhagen, D., Nau, M., Gazdar, A., and Linnoila, R. (1992) Expression of mutant p53 proteins in lung cancer correlates with the class of p53 gene mutation. *Oncogene* **7,** 743–749.
64. Top, B., Mooi, W., Kiaver, S., Boerrigter, L., Wisman, P., Elbers, U., Visser, S., and Rodenhuis, S. (1995) Comparative analysis of p53 gene mutations and protein accumulation in human non-small-cell lung cancer. *Int. J. Cancer.* **64,** 83–91.
65. Sjogren, S., Inganas, M., Norberg, T., Lindgren, A., Nordgren, H., Holmberg, L., and Bergh, J. (1996) The p53 gene in breast cancer: prognostic value of complementary DNA sequencing versus immunohistochemistry. *J. Natl. Cancer. Inst.* **88,** 173–182.
66. Kovach, J., Hartmann, A., Blaszyk, H., Cunningham, J., Schaid, D., and Sommer, S. (1996) Mutation detection by highly sensitive methods indicates that p53 gene mutations in breast cancer can have important prognostic value. *Proc. Natl. Acad. Sci. USA* **93,** 1093–1096.
67. Elledge, R. (1996) Assessing p53 status in breast cancer prognosis: where should you put the thermometer if you think your p53 is sick? *J. Natl. Cancer. Inst.* **88,** 141–143.
68. Angelopoulou, K., Diamandis, E., Sutherland, D., Kellen, J., and Buntings, P. (1994) Prevalence of serum antibodies against the p53 tumor suppressor gene protein in various cancers. *Int. J. Cancer.* **58,** 480–487.
69. Bourhis, J., Lubin, R., Roche, B., Koscielny, S., Bosq, J., Dubois, I., Talbot, M., Marandas, P., Scbwaab, G., Wibault, P., Luboinski, B., Eschwege, F., and Soussi, T. (1996) Analysis of p53 serum antibodies in patients with head and neck squamous cell carcinoma. *J. Natl. Cancer. Inst.* **88,** 1228–1233.
70. Caron de Fromentel, C., May-Levin, F., Mouriesse, H., Leinerle, J., Chandrasekaran, K., and May, P. (1987) Presence of circulating antibodies against cellular protein p53 in a notable proportion of children with B-cell lymphoma. *Int. J. Cancer.* **39,** 185–189.
71. Crawford, L., Pim, D., and Bulbrook, R. (1982) Detection of antibodies against the cellular protein p53 in sera from patients with breast cancer. *Int. J. Cancer.* **30,** 403–408.
72. Davidoff, A., Iglehart, J., and Marks, J. (1992) Immune response to p53 is dependent upon p53/HSP70 complexes in breast cancers. *Proc. Natl. Acad. Sci. USA* **89,** 3439–3442.
73. Labrecque, S., Naor, N., Thomson, D., and Matlashewski, G. (1993) Analysis of the anti-p53 antibody response in cancer patients. *Cancer Res.* **53,** 3468–3471.
74. Laurent-Puig, P., Lubin, R., Semhoun-Ducloux, S., Pelletier, G., Fourre, C., Ducreux, M., Briantais, M., Buffet, C., and Soussi, T. (1995) Antibodies against p53 protein in serum of patients with benign or malignant pancreatic and biliary diseases. *Gut* **36,** 455–458.

75. Lubin, R., Zalcman, G., Bouchet, L., Tre'daniel, J., Legros, Y., Caxals, D., Hirsch, A., and Soussi, T. (1995) Serum p53 antibodies as early markers of lung cancer. *Nature Med.* **1,** 701–702.
76. Marxsen, J., Schmiegel, W., Roder, C., Harder, R., Juhl, H., Henne-Bruns, D., Kremer, B., and Kaithoff, H. (1994) Detection of the anti-p53 antibody response in malignant and benign pancreatic disease. *Br. J. Cancer* **70,** 1031–1034.
77. Peyrat, J.-P., Bonneterre, J., Lubin, R., Vanlemmens, L., Fournier, J., and Soussi, T. (1995) Prognostic significance of circulating p53 antibodies in patients undergoing surgery for locoregional breast cancer. *Lancet* **345,** 621–622.
78. Porzsolt, F., Schmid, M., Ho~her, D., Muche, R., Gaus, W., and Montenarh, M. (1994) Biologic relevance of auto-antibodies against p53 in patients with metastatic breast cancer. *Onkologie.* **17,** 402–408.
79. Preudhomme, C., Lubin, R., Lepelley, P., Vannimbeke, M., and Fenaux, P. (1994) Detection of serum anti p53 antibodies and their correlation with p53 mutations in myelodysplastic syndromes and acute mycloid leukemia. *Leukemia* **8,** 1589–1591.
80. Schlichtholz, B., Tredaniel, J., Lubin, R., Zalcman, G., Hirsch, A. and Soussi, T. (1994) Analyses of p53 antibodies in sera of patients with lung carcinoma define immunodominant regions in the p53 protein. *Br. J. Cancer* **69,** 809–816.
81. Volkmann, M., Muller, M., Hofmann, W., Meyer, M., Hagelstein, J., Rath, U., Kommerell, B., Zentgraf, H., and Galle, P. (1993) The humoral immune response to p53 in patients with hepatocellular carcinoma is specific for malignancy and independent of the alpha-feto-protein status. *Hepatology* **18,** 559–565.
82. Wild, C., Ridanpää, M., Anttila, S., Lubin, R., Soussi, T., Husgafvel-Pursiainen, K., and Vainio, H. (1995) p53 antibodies in the sera of lung cancer patients: comparison with p53 mutation in the tumour tissue. *Int. J. Cancer.* **64,** 176–181.
83. Winter, S., Minna, J., Johnson, B., Takahashi, T., Gazdar, A., and Carbone, D. (1992) Development of antibodies against p53 in lung cancer patients appears to be dependent on the type of p53 mutation. *Cancer Res.* **52,** 4168–4174.
84. Cotton, R., Rodrigues, N., and Campbell, R. (1988) Reactivity of cytosine and thymine in single-base-pair mismatches with hydroxylamine and osmium tetroxide and its application to the study of mutations. *Proc. Natl. Acad. Sci. USA* **85,** 4397–4401.
85. Fischer, S. and Lerman, L. (1983) DNA fragments differing by single base-pair substitutions are separated in denaturing gradient gels: correspondence with melting theory. *Proc. Natl. Acad. Sci. USA* **80,** 1579–1583.
86. Sheffield, V., Cox, D., Lerman, L., and Myers, R. (1989) Attachment of a 40-base-pair G+C-rich sequence (CC-clamp) to genomic DNA fragments by the polymerase chain reaction results in improved detection of single-base changes. *Proc. Natl. Acad. Sci. USA* **86,** 232–236.
87. Børresen, A.-L., Hovig, E., Smith-Sorensen, B., Malkin, D., Lystad, S., Andersen, T., Nesland, J., Isselbacher, K., and Friend, S. (1991) Constant dena-

turant gel electrophoresis as a rapid screening technique for p53 mutations. *Proc. Natl. Acad. Sci. USA* **88,** 8405–8409.

88. Gibbs, R. and Caskey, C. (1987) Identification and localization of mutations at the Lesch-Nyhan locus by ribonuclease a cleavage. Science., **236,** 303–305.
89. Coles, C., Thompson, A., Elder, P., Cohen, B., Mackenzie, I., Cranston, C., Chetty, U., MacKay, J., MacDonald, M., Nakamura, Y., Hoyheim, B., and Steel, C. (1990) Evidence implicating at least two genes on chromosome 17p in breast carcinogenesis. *Lancet* **336,** 761–763.
90. Davidoff, A., Humphrey, P., Iglehart, J., and Marks, J. (1991) Genetic basis for p53 overexpression in human breast cancer. *Proc. Natl. Acad. Sci. USA* **88,** 5006–5010.
91. Singh, S., Simon, M., Meybohm, I., Jantke, I., Jonat, W., Maass, H., and Coedde, H. (1993) Human breast cancer: frequent p53 allele loss and protein overexpression. *Human Genet.* **90,** 635–640.
92. Sarkar, G., Yoon, H., and Sommer, 5. (1992) Dideoxy fingerprinting (ddF): a rapid and efficient screen for the presence of mutations. *Genomics* **13,** 441–443.
93. Hayashi, K. and Yandell, D. (1993) How sensitive is PCR-SSCP? *Human Mutat.* **2,** 338–346.
94. Sarkar, G., Yoon, H., and Sommer, S. (1992) Screening for mutations by RNA single-strand conformation polymorphism (rSSCP): comparison with DNA-SSCP. *Nucleic Acids Res.* **20,** 871–878.
95. Hovig, E., Smith-Sorensen, B., Brogger, A., and Børresen, A.-L. (1991) Constant denaturant gel electrophoresis, a modification of denaturing gradient gel electrophoresis, in mutation detection. *Mutation Res.* **262,** 63–71.
96. Condie, A., Ecles, R., Børresen, A.-L., Coles, C., Cooper, C., and Prosser, J. (1993) Detection of point mutations in the p53 gene: comparison of single-strand conformation polymorphism, constant denaturant gel electrophoresis, and hydroxylamine and osmium tetroxide techniques. *Human Mutat.* **2,** 58–66.
97. Blaszyk, H., Hartmann, A., Schroeder, J., McGovern, R., Soinmer, S., and Kovach, J. (1995) Rapid and efficient screening for p53 gene mutations by dideoxy fingerprinting. *BioTechniques* **18,** 256–260.

97a. Williams, C., Norberg, T., Ahmadian, A., Pontén, F., Bergh, J., Lundeberg, J., and Uhlén, M. (1998) Assessment of sequence-based p53 analysis in human breast cancer: messenger RNA in comparison with genomic DNA targets. *Clin. Chem.* **44,** 455–462.

98. Stinchcomb, D. (1995) Constraining the cell cycle: Regulating cell division and differentiation by gene therapy. *Nature Med.* **1,** 1004–1006.
99. Norberg, T., Jansson, T., Sjogren, S., Martensson, C., Andreasson, I., Fjallskog, M.-L., Lindman, H., Nordgren, H., Lindgren, A., Holmberg, L., and Bergh, J. (1996) Overview on human breast cancer with focus on prognostic and predictive factors with special attention on the tumour suppressor gene p53. *Acta Oncol.* **(Suppl 5)35,** 96–102.
100. Bergh, J. (1997) Determination and use of p53 in the management of cancer patients with special focus on breast cancer: a review, in *Prognostic and Predictive Value of p53* (Klijn, J., ed.), Elsevier Science BV, Amsterdam, pp. 35–50.

18

Bcl-2 Family Immunohistochemistry

Lloyd R. Kelland and Philip J. Beale

1. Introduction

In recent years, immunohistochemistry as applied to the Bcl-2 family of proteins has represented a burgeoning area of interest to cancer researchers. The majority of studies have focused on the original member Bcl-2, first identified via its involvement in the common t(14;18) chromosomal translocation in B-cell lymphomas *(1)*. However, since this discovery, preclinical and clinical interest in Bcl-2 has dramatically increased owing to (a) its recognition as the first of a new class of oncogene able to prolong survival by inhibiting programmed cell death (apoptosis) and (b) the discovery of many additional related genes/proteins some of which, like Bcl-2, inhibit apoptosis, whereas others, such as Bax, conversely promote cell death *(2)* (**Table 1**).

To date, immunohistochemistry as applied to Bcl-2 family proteins has concentrated mainly on Bcl-2 (e.g., *3–5*) and Bax *(6–8)*, principally because of the lack of commercial availability of high-quality specific antibodies to many of the more recently discovered members. However, as antibodies become available to Mcl-1, Bcl-X, Bak, Bad, Bik, Bcl-w, Bag-1, (as described by Krajewski and colleagues *9–13*), then the methodologies described here may also be applied.

Immunohistochemistry is highly specific, relatively sensitive, quick, and relies on the specific binding of an antibody to the antigen in the tissue. The reaction is localized with respect to cell structure by attaching a microscopically dense marker to the antigen-antibody complex. The antigen, antibody, and microscopically dense probe are linked together by successive incubations. The technique may be applied to cytospin preparations of living cells (tumor continuous cell lines, ascites, peripheral blood), cryostat/frozen sections, or formalin- or alcohol-fixed paraffin-embedded pathological tissue sections *(14)*. Because formalin fixation may mask some tissue antigens, the use of the

From: *Methods in Molecular Medicine, Vol. 28: Cytotoxic Drug Resistance Mechanisms*
Edited by: R. Brown and U. Böger-Brown © Humana Press Inc., Totowa, NJ

Table 1
Bcl-2 Family Members

Pro-apoptotic	Anti-apoptotic
Bax	Bcl-2
Bcl-Xs	Bcl-Xl
Bak	Bcl-w
Bad	Bfl-1
Bid	Brag-1
Bik	Mcl-1
Hrk	A1

nonenzymatic microwave oven or oven-based antigen-retrieval methods for paraffin sections ***(15–18)*** has been particularly useful in conjunction with the most widely available and used anti-Bcl-2 (mouse monoclonal ab-124, Dako, Santa Barbara, CA) and anti-Bax (rabbit polyclonal N20, Santa Cruz Biotechnology, Santa Cruz, CA) antibodies. Following sample preparation and incubation with a primary antibody (which may be monoclonal or polyclonal), microscopic visualization is achieved through secondary signal-amplification processing by a variety of methods; e.g., biotinylated secondary antibody with avidin-(streptavadin)-biotin and horseradish peroxidase (ABC) ***(19)*** or alkaline-phosphatase-antialkaline-phosphatase (APAAP) ***(20)***. Agents such as hydrogen peroxide with 3,3'-diaminobenzidine tetrahydrochloride (DAB) are then used as chromogens with peroxidase to convert the product into a brown insoluble end-product. Counterstains such as hematoxylin or methyl green may also be applied at this stage.

Validation of the result is essential and is achieved through the use of positive and negative controls to assess the method (e.g., labeling with an alternative antibody, using a known positive system as positive controls and determining nonspecific binding as a negative control).

2. Materials

2.1. Sample Preparation

1. Trypsin/ethylenediaminetetraacetic acid (EDTA) sterile solution: 0.05% Trypsin, 0.02% EDTA (Gibco-BRL, Paisley, Scotland).
2. Phosphate-buffered saline (PBS): 120 m*M* sodium chloride, 11.5 m*M* Sodium dihydrogen orthophosphate, 31.3 m*M* potassium dihydrogen orthophosphate, pH 7.4–7.6.
3. Formalin-buffered saline (BDH Laboratory Supplies, Poole, UK), or use 10% formaldehyde (BDH) in PBS.
4. 3-Aminopropyltriethoxysilane (APES)-coated slides for cell pellets (Sigma Chemical Co., St. Louis, MO).
5. APES (Sigma): Working solution of 2–5% APES in acetone (300 mL acetone, 6–15 mL APES). Handle with extreme caution.

Table 2
Availability of Human Reactive Bcl-2 Family Antibodies for Immunohistochemistry

Antibody	Species	Clonality	Source[a]
Bcl-2	Mouse	Monoclonal	Dako, Pharmingen, Oncogene Research Products, Santa Cruz Biotechnology
Bax	Rabbit	Polyclonal	Oncogene Research Products, Pharmingen, Santa Cruz Biotechnology
Bak	Mouse	Monoclonal	Oncogene Research Products
Bak	Goat	Polyclonal	Santa Cruz Biotechnology
Bcl-xS/L	Rabbit	Polyclonal	Oncogene Research Products
Bcl-xL	Goat	Polyclonal	Santa Cruz Biotechnology
Bcl-xS	Rabbit	Polyclonal	Oncogene Research Products
Mcl-1	Rabbit	Polyclonal	Pharmingen, Santa Cruz Biotechnology
A1	Goat	Polyclonal	Santa Cruz Biotechnology
Bcl-w	Goat	Polyclonal	Santa Cruz Biotechnology
NBK (Bik)	Goat	Polyclonal	Santa Cruz Biotechnology
Bfl-1	Goat	Polyclonal	Santa Cruz Biotechnology

[a]Dako (Santa Barbara, CA), Pharmingen (San Diego, CA), Oncogene Research Products (Cambridge, MA), Santa Cruz Biotechnology (Santa Cruz, CA).

2.2. Antigen-Retrieval from Paraffin-Fixed Sections

1. Xylene (low in sulphur) (BDH).
2. Absolute ethanol (BDH).
3. 2% v/v hydrogen peroxide in methanol (BDH).
4. Citric-acid buffer, pH 6.0: 10.5g citric acid (BDH), 130 mL 1 *N* sodium hydroxide, 5 L distilled water. Dissolve citric acid in water, add sodium hydroxide, and mix well.
5. Standard microwave oven (950 W).
6. Hydrophobic marker pen (e.g., Dako Corp., Carpinteria, CA).

2.3. Sample Staining

Use, for example, Vectastain® ABC method (Vector Laboratories, Burlingame, CA), or CSA Dakor (catalyzed signal amplification system for mouse primary antibodies); Dako and APAAP mouse or rat primary antibody kits (Dako).

1. Preblocking buffer: 10–20% normal serum or bovine serum albumin (BSA, Sigma) in PBS.
2. Primary BCL-2 family antibody (**Table 2**).

3. PBST (PBS plus 0.1% Polyoxyethylene sorbitan monolaurate (Tween 20; Sigma).
4. Secondary biotinylated goat anti- (mouse or rabbit) antibody (Vector).
5. Streptavidin-biotin-peroxidase complex (Dako).
6. APAAP (Dako).
7. DAB (BDH, or within kits Vector or Dako) in 0.8% v/v hydrogen peroxide. DAB is a potential carcinogen. Wear rubber gloves, handle with care, do not expose to strong light.
8. Mayers haematoxylin 0.1% (Sigma Diagnostics, Poole, Dorset, UK).
9. Depex-Polystyrene dissolved in xylene (DPX) mountant for microscopy (with xylene); (BDH).
10. 20% acetic acid (AnalaR grade; BDH).

3. Methods

3.1. Sample Preparation

3.1.1. Fixing of Continuous Cell Lines

1. Harvest approximately 5×10^8 cells by incubation for 5–10 min at 37°C in trypsin/EDTA solution.
2. Wash twice in ice-cold PBS by centrifugation (spin at 100*g*, 5 min).
3. Incubate overnight in fridge in formalin-buffered saline or PBS containing 10% v/v formalin.
4. Section and embed in paraffin on APES-coated slides.

3.1.2. Cytospin Preparations

1. Harvest cells as previously noted.
2. Prepare single cell suspension and apply to frosted slides.
3. Air-dry and fix for 2 min with acetone:methanol (1:1).
4. APES-coated slides for cell pellets.
5. Fill racks with clean slides and place in 3% APES solution in acetone for 5 min.
6. Remove and place in running tap water; rinse for 1 min.
7. Place in oven at 60°C to dry completely before storing in slide boxes.

*3.1.3. Antigen Retrieval from Fixed, Paraffin-Embedded Sections (see **Note 1**)*

1. De-wax sections in fresh xylene for 1 min. Repeat with two further 1-min washes in fresh xylene.
2. Wash three times for 1 min in three lots of fresh absolute ethanol.
3. Air-dry and mark each slide with a hydrophobic pen.
4. Place slides in running tap water for 2 min.
5. Pre-heat 600 mL of citric-acid buffer, pH 6.0, in a ventilated, covered plastic bucket in a microwave for 5 min on full power.
6. Place sections widely spaced apart in a plastic rack (to help reduce uneven antigen retrieval owing to bubbles of solution breaking between slides) and place in hot buffer in the microwave.

7. Incubate sections for 10 min on full power (*see* **Note 2**).
8. Remove bucket from microwave and allow sections to stand for a further 10 min in the hot buffer. Use extreme caution when removing lid from bucket of hot buffer; always wear gloves because steam and buffer are very hot.
9. Rinse in fresh tap water for 2 min.

3.1.4. Prestaining

1. Incubate sections in 2% hydrogen peroxide in methanol for 5 min to quench endogenous peroxidase activity.
2. Rinse in fresh running tap water for 5 min.
3. Place in humid chamber and preblock sections in PBS containing 10–20% serum or BSA for 5 min. Usually the serum will be the same as the species in which the secondary biotinylated antibody has been raised.
4. Tip off excess serum, but do not wash.

3.2. Sample Staining (see Notes 3 and 4)

3.2.1. ABC Method

1. Incubate in primary antibody diluted in PBS for 1 h.
2. Wash three times in PBST (0.1% Tween).
3. Incubate with biotinylated secondary (anti-mouse or rabbit as appropriate diluted 1:200) antibody for 1 h.
4. Prepare the streptavidin-biotin complex at least 30 min prior to use.
5. Incubate in ABC reagent containing horseradish peroxidase for 45 min.
6. Wash three times in PBS.
7. Optional step is to amplify the signal with a biotinylated phenolic compound (e.g., biotinyl tyramide) for 15 min followed by a PBST wash. Biotinyl tyramide is included as part of the CSA Dako kit, although our experience with the Bcl-2 family of proteins has shown that this step is not necessary.
8. Expose to DAB/hydrogen peroxide for 5 min. (This solution should be used within 8 h of preparation.)
9. Rinse in tap water.
10. Counter stain with hematoxylin for 5 min.
11. Wash sections in tap water for 2 min.
12. Mount in DPX.
13. Stain positive cells brown and negative cells blue.

3.2.2. APAAP Staining

1. Specimens need to be blocked for 1 min in 20% glacial acetic acid prior to staining to quench endogenous alkaline-phosphatase activity.
2. After incubation with primary antibody and washes, a secondary antibody to the primary antibody species is applied for 1 h followed by PBST washes.
3. APAAP complex is then incubated for 30 min followed by PBST washes.
4. 10–20 Min alkaline-phosphatase substrate, PBST wash, tap-water wash.

5. Counterstain with hematoxylin.
6. Mount in DPX.
7. Positive staining is red.

4. Notes

1. A common drawback of epitope-retrieval methods to unmask antigens in fixed paraffin-embedded sections (either microwave irradiation or enzyme digestion) is that overtreatment may result in damage to the morphology and occasional loss of tissues, whereas undertreatment may produce false-negative results. Thus a series of tests to optimize antigen retrieval should be performed along with establishing positive and negative controls.
2. Only plastic or glass items should be used in the microwave; beware that some plastics may also melt. Because of the high temperatures and times used, evaporation of solutions can be a problem; use large quantities of citric acid buffer so that slides never dry out. A plastic specimen bucket with holes pierced in the lid is ideal.
3. Absent or weak staining may be owing to a number of causes. Problems with the substrate may be owing to deionized water, which can inhibit the peroxidase reaction. This can be overcome by using glass-distilled water for the preparation of the substrate solution. The primary antibody may be inactive owing to potency lost over time, harsh treatment by freeze/thawing, or incorrect pH of the diluent which should be between 7.0–8.2. Inappropriately high dilutions of the biotinylated secondary antibody can result in diminished staining (optimal dilutions are 1:200–1:500). Sodium azide in the buffers will inhibit the peroxidase reaction,
4. Inappropriate staining: excess endogenous peroxidase may be blocked by increasing the incubation time with the hydrogen peroxide. Endogenous protein-bound biotin/lectins/ionic interactions can be eliminated by using an avidin/biotin block and/or adding 0.2 *M* alpha-methyl mannoside (Sigma) to the ABC diluent or making up the ABC reagent in 0.5 *M* NaCl. Impure grades of BSA may cause nonspecific reactions of ABC with tissue; use crystalline grade only. Cross-reactivity between the biotinylated secondary antibody and endogenous immunoglobulins can be overcome by adding 2% normal serum from the tissue species to the biotinylated secondary antibody. Paraffin may have been incompletely removed (use fresh xylene), slides not rinsed properly, or the sections dried out during the procedure.

These points re-emphasize the importance of including appropriate controls with this technique; e.g., a positive control specimen and a negative control specimen to determine nonspecific binding.

References

1. Tsujimoto, Y., Crossman, J., Jaffe, E., and Croce, C. (1985) Involvement of the bcl-2 gene in human follicular lymphoma. *Science* **228,** 1440–1443.
2. Brown, R. (1997) The bcl-2 family of proteins. *Br. Med. Bull.* **53,** 466–477.

3. Gasparini, G., Barbareschi, M., Doglioni, C., Palma, P. D., Mauri, F. A., Boracchi, P., Bevilacqua, P., Caffo, O., Morelli, L., Verderio, P., Pezzella, F., and Harris, A. L. (1995) Expression of bcl-2 protein predicts efficacy of adjuvant treatments in operable node-positive breast cancer. *Clin. Cancer Res.* **1,** 189–198.
4. Henriksen, R., Wilander, E., and Oberg, K. (1995) Expression and prognostic significance of Bcl-2 in ovarian tumours. *Br. J. Cancer* **72,** 1324–1329.
5. Ofner, D., Riehemann, K., Maier, H., Riedmann, B., Nehoda, H., Totsch, M., Bocker, W., Jasani, B., and Schmid, K. W. (1995) Immunohistochemically detectable bcl-2 expression in colorectal carcinoma: correlation with tumour stage and patient survival. *Br. J. Cancer* **72,** 981–985.
6. Krajewski, S., Krajewski, M., Shabaik, A., Miyashita, T., Wang, H. G., and Reed, J. C. (1994) Immunohistochemical determination of in vivo distribution of Bax, a dominant inhibitor of Bcl-2. *Am. J. Pathol.* **145,** 132–136.
7. Krajewski, S., Blomqvist, C., Franssila, K., Krajewska, M., Wasenius, V-M., Niskanen, E., Nordling, S., and Reed, J. C. (1995) Reduced expression of proapoptotic gene Bax is associated with poor response rates to combination chemotherapy and shorter survival in women with metastatic breast adenocarcinoma. *Cancer Res.* **55,** 4471–4478.
8. Binder, C., Marx, D., Binder, L., Schauer, A., and Hiddemann, W. (1996) Expression of Bax in relation to Bcl-2 and other predictive parameters in breast cancer. *Ann. Oncol.* **7,** 129–133.
9. Krajewski, S., Bodrug, S., Gascoyne, R., Berean, K., Krajewski, M., and Reed, J. C. (1994) Immunohistochemical analysis of Mcl-1 and Bcl-2 proteins in normal and neoplastic lymph nodes. *Am. J. Pathol.* **145,** 515–525.
10. Krajewski, S., Bodrug, S., Krajewski, M., Shabaik, A., Gascoyne, R., Berean, K., and Reed, J. C. (1995) Immunohistochemical analysis of Mcl-1 protein in human tissues. Differential regulation of Mcl-1 and Bcl-2 protein production suggests a unique role for Mcl-1 in control of programmed cell death in vivo. *Am. J. Pathol.* **146,** 1309–1319.
11. Krajewski, S., Krajewski, M., Shabaik, A., Wang, H-G., Irie, S., Fong, L., and Reed, J. C. (1994) Immunohistochemical analysis of in vivo patterns of Bcl-X expression. *Cancer Res.* **54,** 5501–5507.
12. Krajewski, M., Moss, S. F., Krajewski, S., Song, K., Holt, P. R., and Reed, J. C. (1996) Elevated expression of Bcl-X and reduced Bak in primary colorectal adenocarcinomas. *Cancer Res.* **56,** 2422–2427.
13. Krajewski, S., Krajewski, M., and Reed, J. C. (1996) Immunohistochemical analysis of in vivo patterns of Bak expression, a proapoptotic member of the Bcl-2 protein family. *Cancer Res.* **56,** 2849–2855.
14. Brandtzaeg, P. (1982) Tissue preparation methods for immunohistochemistry, in *Techniques in Immunohistochemistry,* vol. 1 (Bullock, G. R. and Perusz, P. eds.), Academic, London, pp. 1–75.
15. Shi, S-R. (1991) Antigen retrieval in formalin-fixed, paraffin-embedded tissues: an enhancement method for immunohistochemical staining based on microwave oven heating of tissue sections. *J. Histochem. Cytochem.* **39,** 741–748.

16. Cattoretti, G., Pileri, S., Parravicini, C., Becker, M. H. G., Poggi, S., Bifulco, C., Key, G., D'Amato, L., Sabattini, E., Feudale, E., Reynolds, F., Gerdes, J., and Rilke, F. (1993) Antigen unmasking on formalin-fixed, paraffin-embedded tissue sections. *J. Pathol.* **171,** 83–98.
17. Munakata, S. and Hendricks, J. B. (1993) Effect of fixation time and microwave oven heating time on retrieval of the Ki-67 antigen from paraffin-embedded tissue. *J. Histochem. Cytochem.* **41,** 1241–1246.
18. Man, Y-G. and Tavassoli, F. A. (1996) A simple epitope retrieval method without the use of microwave oven or enzyme digestion. *Appl. Immunohistochem.* **4,** 139–141.
19. Hsu, S-M., Raine, L., and Fanger, H. (1981) Use of avidin-biotin-peroxidase complex (ABC) in immunoperoxidase techniques: a comparison between ABC and unlabeled antibody (PAP) procedures. *J. Histochem. Cytochem.* **29,** 577–580.
20. Cordell, J. L., Falin, B., Erber, W. N., Gosh, A. K., Abdulaziz, Z., MacDonald, S., Pulford, K. A. F., Stein, H., and Mason, D. Y. (1984). Immunoenzymatic labelling of monoclonal antibodies using immune complexes of alkaline phosphatase and monoclonal anti-alkaline phosphatase (APAAP complexes). *J. Histochem. Cytochem.* **32,** 219–229.

19

Genetic Analysis of Drug Resistance by Fluorescence *In Situ* Hybridization

W. Nicol Keith

1. Introduction

Tumor progression is driven by the accumulation of genetic changes, which, in aggregate, confer the malignant phenotype ***(1)***. Thus, tumor development proceeds via clonal divergence with selection for cells with, for example, a proliferative advantage, metastatic potential, or drug resistance phenotype ***(2–5)***. Although Southern blotting and polymorphic microsatellite markers are invaluable in providing information about the genetic alterations that underlie the development of solid tumors, the spatial relationships between tumor cells are destroyed during tissue processing ***(6–8)***. This leads to a loss of information on genetic heterogeneity and small subpopulations and presents an averaging of the genetic changes. Conventional karyotyping would determine both numerical and structural chromosome anomalies, but is largely impractical for the study of solid tumors, owing to the necessity for cell culture to produce metaphase spreads. Fluorescence *in situ* hybridization (FISH) is a powerful method for the analysis of genetic change in solid tumors ***(7,9–12)***. In particular, it allows the visualization of the genetic makeup of individual cells within their histological context ***(7)***. In general, FISH uses chromosome and region specific probes to assess rapidly copy number and rearrangements of chromosomes and genes. The genetically abnormal cells are detected by their aberrant hybridization pattern in the interphase nuclei. Thus, this method of analysis is generally termed "interphase cytogenetics" ***(9,10,12)***. FISH has been used successfully to study a number of genes implicated in drug resistance; the following references can provide some indication of the tremendous potential for clinical and model system analysis ***(6,10,11,13–23)***.

From: *Methods in Molecular Medicine, Vol. 28: Cytotoxic Drug Resistance Mechanisms*
Edited by: R. Brown and U. Böger-Brown © Humana Press Inc., Totowa, NJ

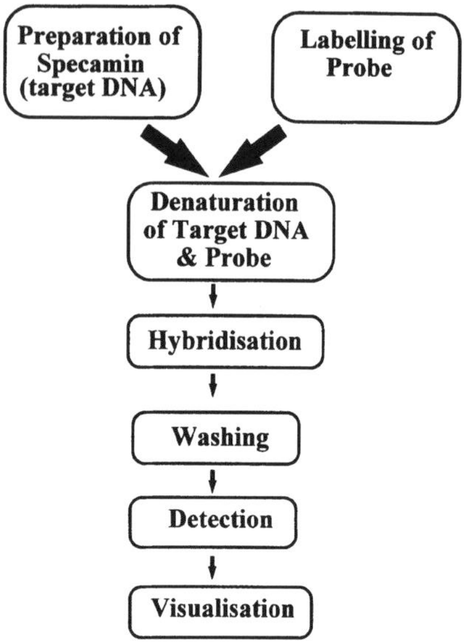

Fig. 1. Overview of FISH.

FISH can be carried out on both frozen sections and sections of formalin-fixed paraffin-embedded material. There is, therefore, the potential to investigate routinely processed pathology specimens. In our experience, frozen sections offer the optimal sensitivity, but retention of good morphology is difficult *(21,22)*. Paraffin sections consistently show good morphology but poorer sensitivity *(7,10,22)*. Thus, the use of paraffin sections is limited largely to the detection of amplified genes, or repetitive sequences such as chromosome-specific centromere sequences *(7,10,22)*. Cell lines are ideally suited to molecular cytogenetic analysis, because chromosomes arrested at metaphase can be prepared and analyzed with high sensitivity *(6,13,14,16,18–20)*. The key steps performed in obtaining high-quality, high-efficiency, quantifiable hybridizations require a balance between the often antagonistic manipulations that reveal the target sequences, yet retain tissue morphology. These include initial tissue fixation, target sequence unmasking with protease followed by re-fixation, and target sequence denaturation. The major steps involved in FISH are shown in **Fig. 1**.

2. Materials (*see* Note 2)

*2.1. General Materials (*see *Note 4)*

1. ANTIFADE + PI +DAPI: Add to antifade (Vector Labs, Burlingame, CA) solution, 0.3 µg/mL Propidium iodide (PI) 0.1 µg/mL 4',6-diamidine-2'-phenylindole dihydrochloride (DAPI).

2. 10% Block: Made up block (Boehringer Mannheim, Darmstadt, Mannheim, Germany) in maleic acid buffer; 100 m*M* maleic acid; 150 m*M* NaCl, pH 7.5, and autoclave.
3. SSC (1X): 0.15 *M* NaCl, 0.015 *M* sodium citrate, pH 7.0.
4. SSC-T (4X): 4X SSC, 0.05% Tween 20.
5. SSC-TB (4X): 4X SSC-T, 0.5% Boehringer block solution.
6. RNase Stock: 10 mg/mL in H_2O. Aliquot and keep at –20°C.
7. Pepsin: 10% in H_2O. Aliquot and keep at –20°C.
8. Methanol/acetic acid (3:1): 75 mL methanol, 25 mL acetic acid. Make fresh just before use.
9. 50% Formamide hybridization mix: For single-copy probes (e.g., cosmids), 2X SSC, 500 µg/mL salmon sperm DNA (SSDNA), 10% dextran sulphate, 50% formamide.
10. 70% Formamide hybridization mix: For repeat sequence probes (e.g., centromeric probes), 2X SSC, 500 ug/mL SSDNA, 10% dextran sulphate, 70% formamide.

2.2. Chromosome Preparation Materials

1. Chromosome medium 1A (Gibco/BRL; Gaithersburg, MD).
2. 5 mL of whole blood, collected in heparinized tube.
3. Hanks' Balanced Salt Solution (HBSS).
4. Thymidine (Sigma Chemical Co., St. Louis, MO): stock concentration at 6 mg/mL, (use at final concentration of 0.35 mg/mL). Make in water, filter, and keep at –20°C.
5. Bromodeoxyuridine (Sigma): stock of 3 mg/mL, (use at final concentration of 0.03 mg/mL). Make in water, filter, and store –20°C.
6. Colcemid (Gibco/BRL): 10 ug/mL = 100X stock, 50 mL/tube containing 5 mL chromosome medium, final concentration of colcemid is 0.1 ug/mL).
7. Hypotonic solution: 0.075 *M* potassium chloride.

2.3. Probe Labeling and Dot-Blot Reagents and Solutions (see Notes 3, 4, and 5)

1. Streptavidin-alkaline phosphatase (AP) conjugate (Gibco-BRL).
2. Digoxigenin (Dig) Detection Kit (Boehringer-Mannheim), containing anti-Dig AP conjugate, X-phosphate, and 4-nitro blue tetrazolium chloride (NBT).
3. To NBT powder add 910 µL dimethylformamide (DMF) + 390 µL water (70% DMF solution).
4. Buffer A: 0.1 *M* Tris, pH 7.5, 1X SSC.
5. Buffer B: 0.1 *M* Tris, pH 7.5, 1X SSC, 3% BSA.
6. Buffer C: 0.1 *M* Tris, pH 9.5, 1X SSC, 50 m*M* $MgCl_2$.
7. STOP Buffer: 0.01 *M* Tris, pH 7.5, 1 m*M* (EDTA).

3. Methods (*see* Note 1)

3.1. Chromosome Preparation from Lymphocytes Using Bromodeoxyuridine and Thymidine

1. Add 200 µL whole blood to 5 mL chromosome medium.
2. Incubate for 72 h, mixing every day at 37°C in 5% CO_2.
3. Add 294 µL of 6 mg/mL Thymidine and incubate at 37°C for 15–17 h in 5% CO_2.

4. Wash 3 times in HBSS; centrifuge at 1.5K for 7 min for each wash. Resuspend in 5 mL fresh chromosome medium containing 50 µL of 3 mg/mL BrdU.
5. Incubate for 7–8 h at 37°C in 5% CO_2 in the dark.
6. Add 50 µL colcemid per tube and incubate 1–3 h.
7. Spin at 500*g* for 5 min.
8. Remove supernatant, and resuspend in 10 mL of Hypotonic solution.
9. Incubate at 37°C for 10–15 min.
10. Add 2–3 mL of methanol/acetic acid (3:1).
11. Centrifuge at 500*g* for 5 min.
12. Remove supernatant. Resuspend in 10 mL methanol/acetic acid.
13. Leave at room temperature for 10–15 min.
14. Repeat **steps 12–14** at least three times.
15. Finally, spin at 500*g* for 5 min and resuspend in a small volume (3–5 mL) of methanol/acetic acid , and store at –20°C.

3.2. Chromosome Preparation from Cell Lines

1. Add colcemid to each flask to 0.1 µg/mL final concentration.
2. Incubate at 37°C for 2–3 h.
3. Trypsinize cells as normal and transfer to a 50-mL falcon tube.
4. Spin at 500*g* for 5 min.
5. Remove supernatant, and resuspend in 10 mL of Hypotonic solution.
6. Incubate at 37°C for 10–15 min.
7. Add 2–3 mL of methanol/acetic acid (3:1).
8. Centrifuge at 500*g* for 5 min.
9. Remove supernatant. Resuspend in 10 mL methanol/acetic acid.
10. Leave at room temperature for 10–15 min.
11. Repeat **steps 8** and **9** at least three times.
12. Finally spin at 500*g* for 5 min and resuspend in a small volume (3–5 mL) of methanol/acetic acid , and store at –20°C.

3.3. Chromosome Preparation

1. Drop a volume of chromosome preparation on to a slide from a height and mark an area of spreads on the slide using a diamond pen.
2. Fix for 1 h in methanol/acetic acid (3:1) at room temperature and air-dry.
3. Incubate for 1 h in 100 µg/mL RNase in 2X SSC at 37°C. Make from frozen RNase stock.
4. Rinse 2X SSC.
5. Digest in pepsin, (0.01% in 10 m*M* HCl) solution for 10 min at 37°C. Make from frozen pepsin stock.
6. Rinse in water.
7. Fix for 10 min in Streck Tissue Fixative (STF) at room temperature. Alternatively use 1% formaldehyde, (add 4 mL of 37% formaldehyde to 146 mL phosphate-buffered saline (PBS), 50 m*M* $MgCl_2$).
8. Dehydrate slides by passing through ethanol series, 70% ethanol for 2 min (twice), 100% ethanol for 2 min (twice).

3.4. Frozen Sections

3.4.1. Cutting and Storage of Sections

1. 5 m*M*-thick frozen sections from tissue blocks stored in liquid nitrogen are placed on aminopropyltriethoxysilane (APES)-treated slides and air-dried.
2. Wrap each slide in parafilm to protect from condensation.
3. Tissue sections are stored at –20°C until use.

3.4.2. Preparation of Sections

1. Allow slides to come to room temperature (this takes a few minutes), and remove parafilm.
2. Mark region of sample with diamond pen.
3. Rinse slides in PBS.
4. Add 100 µL of 10% pepsin stock to 50 mL of 10 mM HCl, and incubate slides in this at 37°C for 5–20 min.
5. Rinse slides in five dip washes with water.
6. Post-fix in STF (Alpha Labs, Eastleigh, Hampshire, UK) for 10 min at room temperature. Alternatively, use 1% formaldehyde (add 4 mL of 37% formaldehyde to 146 mL PBS, 50 m*M* $MgCl_2$).
7. Dehydrate twice in ethanol for 2 min.
8. Air-dry.

3.5. Paraffin Sections

1. Five micron paraffin sections mounted on APES-treated slides (Sigma).
2. Heat slides overnight at 50–60°C.
3. Dewax (in fume hood); xylene, 10 min ×3; methanol, 5 min ×2.
4. Air-dry.
5. Pepsin digestion: (Note that the concentration and incubation times for the pepsin step are quite different from that for frozen sections and chromosomes). Pepsin in 0.2 *N* HCl (add 1 mL of 10% stock to 25 mL of 0.2 *M* HCl). Time variable, 15–60 min, (*see* **Note 9**). Refresh pepsin every 15 min.
6. Rinse five times in water.
7. Post-fix: STF: 10 min at room temperature. Alternatively, use 1% formaldehyde (add 4 mL of 37% formaldehyde to 146 mL PBS, 50 m*M* $MgCl_2$).
8. Dehydrate in 70% EtOH for 2 min, followed by 100% EtOH for 2 min.
9. Air-dry.

3.6. Target and Probe Denaturation (see Note 3)

3.6.1. Target Denaturation (see **Note 9**)

1. Warm 70% formamide (35 mL formamide, 15 mL 2X SSC) to temperature required.
2. Immerse the slide with chromosomes in 70% formamide for time required. Temperature and time are variable. Try: 75°C for 3 min; 75°C for 5 min; 80°C for 3 min; and 80°C for 5 min.

3. Carry out in fume hood and use plastic coplin jars.
2. Rinse in large volume (500 mL) 70% ethanol.
3. Dehydrate: 70% ethanol for 2 min, followed by 100% ethanol for 2 min.
4. Air-dry.

*3.6.2. Probe Denaturation (see **Note 3**)*

3.6.2.1. For Satellite Probes

1. Heat probe (12–15 µL/slide) to 70°C–80°C for 5 min. Place on ice for 5 min.
2. Apply to slide, use 22 × 22 coverslip and seal edges with cow gum.
3. Incubate 37°C overnight (or 42°C, overnight).

3.6.2.2. For Cosmid Probes

1. Heat probe to 70°C for 5 min or to 80°C for 10 min.
2. Place probe at 37°C for 15–60 min to allow for suppression of repetitive sequences in the probe by Cot1 DNA in hybridization mix.
3. Apply to slide (12–15 µL/slide) and seal with rubber cement.
4. Incubate 37°C overnight. **IMPORTANT!** Do not let slides dry out at any stage.

3.7. Wash Steps

1. Remove coverslips by soaking in 2X SSC for 2 min, then peel off the rubber cement.
2. Wash in 50% formamide/1X SSC for 20 min at 42°C.
3. Wash in 2X SSC for 20 min at 42°C.

3.8. Probe Detection (see Notes 3, 6, and 7)

3.8.1. Avidin Detection for Biotinylated Probes (FITC)

All detection steps carried out in humidity chambers in the dark and under parafilm coverslips. Use 100 µL of detection reagent per slide.

1. Rinse in 4X SSC, 0.05% Tween (4X SSC-T) for 3 min.
2. Block slides in 4X SSC-T/0.5% Block (4X SSC-TB) for 10 min at room temperature under parafilm coverslips (in humidity chamber).
3. First layer detection: Add 100 µL to each slide. FITC-Avidin DCS at 1:200 dilution in 4X SSC-TB for 45 min at room temperature.
4. Wash in 4X SSC-T for 10 min at room temperature.
5. Second layer detection: Biotinylated anti-avidin D at 1:100 dilution in 4X SSC-TB for 45 min at room temperature.
6. Wash in 4X SSC-T for 10 min at room temperature.
7. Third layer detection: FITC-avidin DCS at 1:200 dilution in 4X SSC-TB for 45 min at room temperature.
8. Wash in 4X SSC-T for 20 min at room temperature.
9. Dehydrate and mount slides in Antifade with PI and DAPI (*see* **Note 8**).

3.8.2. Digoxigenin Antibody Detection (FITC)

All detection steps carried out in humidity chambers in the dark and under parafilm coverslips. Use 100 µL of detection reagent/slide.

1. Rinse in 4X SSC, 0.05% Tween (4X SSC-T) for 3 min.
2. Block slides in 4X SSC-T/0.5% Block (4X SSC-TB) for 10 min at room temperature under parafilm coverslips (in humidity chamber).
3. First layer detection: Add 100 µL to each slide. Sheep anti-digoxigenin at 1:200 dilution in 4X SSC-TB for 1 h at room temperature.
4. Wash in 4X SSC-T for 10 min at room temperature.
5. Second layer detection: Donkey anti-sheep FITC 1:300 in 4X SSC-TB for 1 h at room temperature.
6. Wash in 4X SSC-T for 20 min at room temperature.
7. Dehydrate and mount slides in Antifade with PI and DAPI (*see* **Note 8**).

3.8.3. Probe Detection Using Avidin and Antibodies for Two Colors (FITC/Texas Red)

All detection steps carried out in humidity chambers in the dark and under parafilm coverslips. Use 100 µL of detection reagent/slide.

1. Rinse in 4X SSC, 0.05% Tween (4 X SSC-T) for 3 min.
2. Block slides in 4X SSC-T/ 0.5% Block (4X SSC-TB) for 10 min at room temperature under parafilm coverslips (in humidity chamber).
3. First layer detection: Add 100 µL to each slide. FITC-Avidin DCS at 1:200 dilution in 4X SSC-TB for 45 min at room temperature.
4. Wash in 4X SSC-T for 10 min at room temperature.
5. Second layer detection: Biotinylated anti-avidin D 1:100 and Sheep anti-digoxigenin 1:200 in 4X SSC-TB for 1 h at room temperature.
6. Wash in 4X SSC-T for 10 min at room temperature.
7. Third layer detection: FITC-Avidin DCS at 1:200 and Donkey anti-sheep Texas Red 1:300 in 4X SSC-TB for 1 h at room temperature.
8. Wash in 4X SSC-T for 20 min at room temperature.
9. Dehydrate and mount slides in *DAPI only* Antifade (*see* **Note 8**).

3.8.4. Two Color Antibody Detection

All detection steps carried out in humidity chambers in the dark and under parafilm coverslips. Use 100 µL of detection reagent/slide.

1. Rinse in 4X SSC, 0.05% Tween (4X SSC-T) for 3 min.
2. Block slides in 4X SSC-T/ 0.5% Block (4X SSC-TB) for 10 min at room temperature under parafilm coverslips (in humidity chamber).
3. First layer detection: Add 100 µL to each slide. Mouse anti-biotin and Sheep anti-digoxigenin at 1:200 dilution in 4X SSC-TB for 1 h at room temperature.
4. Wash in 4X SSC-T for 10 min at room temperature.

5. Second layer detection: Goat anti-mouse Texas Red and Donkey anti-sheep FITC 1:300 in 4X SSC-TB for 1 h at room temperature.
6. Wash in 4X SSC-T for 20 min at room temperature.
7. Dehydrate and mount slides in *DAPI only* Antifade (*see* **Note 8**).

Second Antibody step could also be Goat anti-mouse FITC and Donkey anti-sheep Texas Red 1:300 dilution in 4X SSC-T.

3.9. Probe Labeling

3.9.1. Bionick

1. Incorporation of biotin-16-dUTP by Nick Translation using Biotin-Nick Translation Mix (Boehringer Mannheim)

DNA	X µL (1 µg DNA)
dH_20	(16-X µL)
Biotin-nick mix	4 µL
Final volume	20 µL

2. Mix and centrifuge briefly and incubate at 16°C for 1–4 h.
3. Take out 1 µL of mix to check for incorporation by dot-blot analysis (*see* **Subheading 3.9.3.**).
4. Ethanol precipitate probe.

3.9.2. Dig Nick

Incorporation of dig-11-dUTP by nick translation using Dig-Nick Translation Mix (Boehringer Mannheim). Same procedure as used previously, but use dig-nick mix instead of Biotin.

3.9.3. Dot Blot

This method checks for biotin and dig incorporation in the labeled up probes.

1. After biotin and dig Nick labeling, and after STOP buffer is added, take out 1 µL from each tube. Carry out four serial 1 in 10 dilutions for each (1 + 9 µL water).
2. Dot 1 µL of each of the dilution's onto a nylon membrane in rows (separate membrane for biotin- and dig-labeled probes).
3. Crosslink DNA to membrane with ultraviolet (UV) Stratalinker (autocross link setting).
4. Wash membrane on rocking table in Buffer A for 5 min, pour out, and add Buffer B (kept in cold room) and leave on rocking table for 30 min.
5. Meanwhile, make up the antibody conjugates. To one universal tube, add 5 mL of Buffer B and to another add 5 mL of Buffer C. To the first tube, add 5 µL of streptavidin alkaline phosphatase (for biotin-labeled probes) and 5 µL of anti-dig alkaline phosphatase (for dig-labeled probes).
6. To the second universal add 22 µL of NBT + 17 µL of X-phosphate 5-bromo-4-chloro-3-indolyl-phosphate (BCIP) for both biotin and dig probes. Wrap both universal tubes in tinfoil to keep out the light.

7. Add filter to bag and add alkaline phosphate solution, seal bag, and leave filter wrapped in foil in the dark for 30 min.
8. Take filter out and wash on rocking table in dark for 3 × 5 min with buffer A then 5 min in Buffer C.
9. Add filter to bag and add the developing solution, seal bag, wrap in tinfoil, and leave in the dark for 2 h to overnight.
10. Wash filter in STOP buffer (in dark) for 5 min, then wrap in cling film.

3.9.5. Probe Precipitation

1. Nick Translate 1 µg DNA (biotin nick, dig nick).
2. Add to the 20 µL Nick translation,

5 µL	3 *M* NaA, (pH 8.0)
25–100 µL	Human cot-1 DNA
1 µL	Glycogen
300 µL	100% Ethanol

3. Mix well. Put on dry ice for 30 min, or –20°C overnight.
4. Spin down at 13rpm for 15 min in microfuge. Pour off ethanol carefully.
5. Wash pellet in 100 µL 70% ethanol and centrifuge at 13rpm in a microfuge for 5 min.
6. Carefully pour off ethanol and dry pellet (air dry or rotary evaporate).
7. Resuspend in 60 µL of 50% formamide hybridization mix (for single-copy probes).

4. Notes

1. Starting FISH. If your lab has no experience in FISH, the best way to get started is to visit a lab where the technique is done routinely. This need not take long; indeed, the basics can be learned in 1 wk. A number of companies that market *in situ* reagents and equipment also offer practical training courses in *in situ* techniques and these can be very worthwhile. You will also find that your local Medical Genetics/Cytogenetics or Clinical Genetics/Cytogenetics Unit will probably have all the expertise you need. Such units are usually attached to hospitals and universities.
2. Equipment. The only thing to recommend here is to buy the best microscope you can afford. You will not see good results with a poor microscope. Companies are very helpful and if you tell your local representative what you want to do, they are likely to be able to build the appropriate package with you. Choose your microscope and filter system very carefully.
3. Controls. Test all your probes on normal chromosomes prepared from lymphocytes. This is essential no matter what your final application is. In addition, for interphase cytogenetics, use sections from normal tissue. Pay particular attention to specificity of hybridization. Some probes such as chromosome-specific repeat-sequence probes can bind to several chromosomes if the hybridization conditions are not correct. Use commercial probes to test your reagents.

4. Commercial Probes. There are now many companies that offer a wide range of probes; a few companies are listed in **Subheading 2.3.** Commercial probes are invaluable for testing your reagents and for troubleshooting if things go wrong.
5. Alternate Ways of obtaining Probes. With the vast numbers of FISH papers written, you can always ask other researchers for probes *(6,14)*. There are probe databanks on the WorldWideWeb and some are given in the list of Web sites shown in **Note 10**. You can also develop them yourself *(13)*, or with the aid of a commercial company like Genome Systems Inc. *(22,23)*. This can be expensive, but are very efficient.
6. Probe Properties. For the quantitative assessment of gene copy number, high-efficiency probes are required. We find that P1 or cosmid clones containing your gene of interest work the best. cDNA clones are difficult to work with and virtually useless for interphase cytogenetics owing to their low sensitivity. If your lab is inexperienced in FISH, do not be tempted to start FISH with cDNA clones; use a P1 or cosmid clone. Repetitive sequence probes such as those that recognize the centromeric sequences of specific chromosomes are the easiest probes to work with and a great place to start FISH. Some probe properties are shown in **Table 1**.
7. Probe Detection. There are a number of different protocols for the detection of hybridized probe and these are summarized in **Table 2**. The choice of detection system will be dictated by your choice of probe label, (biotin or dig), and whether you are carrying out single or double hybridizations. For single hybridizations with biotin-labeled probes, we favor the avidin-detection protocol (*see* **Subheading 3.8.1.**), and for double hybridizations with biotin- and dig-labeled probes simultaneously, the avidin/anti-dig protocol (*see* **Subheading 3.8.3.**).
8. Choice of fluorochromes. **Table 3** lists the properties of a number of fluorochromes. The combination of fluorochromes you use will depend on your specific application. **Remember**, you must match the fluorochromes you use with the capabilities of your microscope. Choose your microscope and filter system very carefully. There are two common DNA counterstains, DAPI and PI. PI fluoresces red and cannot be used in conjunction with red-emitting, signal-generating systems like Texas Red, but can be used with the green-emitting, signal-generating system FITC. DAPI is a blue-emitting DNA counterstain and is compatible with both Texas Red and FITC.
9. Possible Problems. If we assume the probe is perfect, then the critical points in the procedure are specimen preparation and denaturation of the target DNA (*see* **Fig. 1**). In order for efficient hybridization to occur, the DNA in the target specimen must be made accessible (denatured). This is achieved through pepsin digestion, followed by immersion of the target in hot formamide. The critical steps are therefore length of time in pepsin, length of time in hot formamide, and the temperature of the formamide. Throughout the protocols given, suggestions have been made on these steps, but some in-house experimentation will probably be necessary. Over-denaturation can lead to a loss of target DNA and therefore a drop in signal intensity. Also over denaturation will lead to a loss of chromosome or tissue morphology, which becomes quite obvious through the microscope.

Table 1
Probe Properties

Probe Type *Unique sequences*	Insert Size	Target	Application	Characteristics	Sensitivity
P1 clones Genomic sequences	~90 kb	Genes	Mapping Interphase cytogenetics	Usually make good FISH probes	High
Cosmid clones Genomic sequences	~45 kb		Mapping Interphase cytogenetics	Usually make good FISH probes	High
Lambda Genomic sequences	~12 kb		Mapping Interphase cytogenetics	Better to use P1 or cosmid clones	Medium
cDNA clones	Wide range: 1–4 kb plus		Mapping	Not much use for interphase cytogenetics	Low
Repetitive sequences		Satellite DNA	Chromosome enumeration	Easy to use	Very high
		Telomeres	Telomere length	Very specialized	Tricky!
Chromosome Paints		Whole chromosomes	Tranlocations Chromosome identification	Easy to use	High

Table 2
Probe Detection

Hybridization	Probe label	Immunological detection
Single probe	Biotin	Avidin
	Biotin	Antibody: anti-biotin
	Digoxigenin	Antibody: anti-digoxigenin
Two probes simultaneously	Biotin/digoxigenin	Avidin/anti-digoxigenin
	Biotin/digoxigenin	Anti-biotin/anti-digoxigenin

Table 3
Properties of Fluorochromes

Fluorochrome	Max excitation wavelength (nm)	Max emission wavelength (nm)	Color of fluorescence
a) Signal Generating Systems			
Coumarin AMCA	350	450	Blue
Fluorescein FITC	495	515	Green
Cy3	550	570	Red
Rhodamine	550	575	Red
Rhodamine TRITC	575	600	Red
Texas Red	595	615	Red
Cy5	650	680	Far red
b) DNA Counterstains			
Chromomycin A3	430	570	Yellow
DAPI	355	450	Blue
Hoechst 33258	356	465	Blue
Propidium iodide (PI)	340, 530	615	Red

Chromosomes will appear fuzzy and faintly counterstained, nuclei will appear ghost-like, and central areas of DNA may even be removed from nuclei. Under-denaturation will lead to poor signal strength, with strong counterstaining of well-defined chromosomes and nuclei. From this point of view, formalin-fixed, paraffin-embedded tissue is the hardest to work with. **Table 4** shows some of the parameters we have used on a series of breast samples.

10. Useful Web Sites. There are numerous Web sites of interest to those working in molecular cytogenetics and drug resistance. Listed are a few sites that have information on probes or genetic information.
    - Online Mendelian Inheritance in Man (OMIM): http://www3.ncbi.nlm.nih.gov/Omim
    - Vysis: http://www.vysis.com

Table 4
Preparation of Paraffin Sections for FISH

Breast 51 Blocks	Denaturation Step Temp × Time		
Pepsin time (min)	75 × 5	80 × 5	90 × 5
5	4	0	0
30	0	7	0
60	1	34	2
90	0	3	0

- Hybaid:
  http://www.hybaid.co.uk
- BioMedNet:
  http://BioMedNet.com
- Oncor:
  http://www.oncor.com/new.htm
- LBNL/UCSF Molecular Cytogenetics:
  http://rmc-www.lbl.gov
- The Human Transcript Map:
  http://www.ncbi.nlm.nih.gov/SCIENCE96
- Human Genome Mapping Project (HGMP):
  http://www.hgmp.mrc.ac.uk
- Cell and Probe Banks:
  http://www.wdcm.riken.go.jp/Menu4.html
- Advanced Biotechnologies:
  http://www.adbio.co.uk
- Genome Systems Inc.:
  http://www.genomesystems.com
- Pedros Biomolecular Research Tools:
  http://www.beri.co.jp/Pedro/research_tools.html

References

1. Vogelstein, B. and Kinzler, K. (1993) The multistep nature of cancer. *Trends Genet.* **9,** 138–141.
2. Goldie, J. and Coldman, A. (1984) The genetic origin of drug resistance in neoplasms: implications for systemic therapy. *Cancer Res.* **44,** 3643–3653.
3. Harrison, D. (1995) Molecular mechanisms of drug resistance in tumors. *J. Pathol.* **175,** 7–12.
4. Dexter, D. and Leith, J. (1986) Tumor heterogeneity and drug resistance. *J. Clin. Oncol.* **4,** 244–257.
5. Deisseroth, A. and Pizzorno, G. (1997) The use of chemotherapy resistance in cancer treatment. *Cancer J. Sci. Am.* **3,** 60–69.

6. Coutts, J., Plumb, J., Brown, R., and Keith, W. (1993) Expression of topoisomerase II alpha and beta in an adenocarcinoma cell line carrying amplified topoisomerase II alpha and retinoic acid receptor alpha genes. *Br. J. Cancer* **68,** 793–800.
7. Murphy, D., Hoare, S., Going, J., Mallon, E., George, W., Kaye, S., Brown, R., Black, D., and Keith, W. (1995) Characterization of extensive genetic alterations in ductal carcinoma in situ by fluorescence in situ hybridization and molecular analysis. *J. Natl. Cancer Inst.* **87,** 1694–1704.
8. Keith, W., Douglas, F., Wishart, G., McCallum, H., George W., Kaye, S., and Brown, R. (1993) Co-amplification of erbB2, topoisomerase II alpha and retinoic acid receptor alpha genes in breast cancer and allelic loss at topoisomerase I on chromosome 20. *Eur. J. Cancer* **29A,** 1469–1475.
9. Heng, H., Spyropoulos, B., and Moens, P. (1997) FISH technology in chromosome and genome research. *Bioessays* **19,** 75–84.
10. Murphy, D., McHardy, P., Coutts, J., Mallon, E., George, W., Kaye, S., Brown, R., and Keith, W. (1995) Interphase cytogenetic analysis of erbB2 and topoII alpha co-amplification in invasive breast cancer and polysomy of chromosome 17 in ductal carcinoma in situ. *Int. J. Cancer* **64,** 18–26.
11. Sandberg, A. and Chen, Z. (1994) Cancer cytogenetics and molecular genetics: detection and therapeutic strategy. *In Vivo* **8,** 807–818.
12. van Ommen, G., Breuning, M., and Raap, A. (1995) FISH in genome research and molecular diagnostics. *Curr. Opin. Genet. Dev.* **5,** 304–308.
13. Hoare, S., Freeman, C., Coutts, J., Varley, J., James, L., and Keith, W. (1997) Identification of genetic changes associated with drug resistance by reverse in situ hybridization. *Br. J. Cancer* **75,** 275–282.
14. McLeod, H. and Keith, W. (1996) Variation in topoisomerase I gene copy number as a mechanism for intrinsic drug sensitivity. *Br. J. Cancer* **74,** 508–512.
15. Ray, M., Guan, X., Slovak, M., Trent, J., and Meltzer, P. (1994) Rapid detection, cloning and molecular cytogenetic characterization of sequences from an MRP-encoding amplicon by chromosome microdissection. *Br. J. Cancer* **70,** 85–90.
16. Slovak, M., Ho, J., Bhardwaj, G., Kurz, E., Deeley, R., and Cole, S. (1993) Localization of a novel multidrug resistance-associated gene in the HT1080/DR4 and H69AR human tumor cell lines. *Cancer Res.* **53,** 3221–3225.
17. Slovak, M., Ho, J., Cole, S., Deeley, R., Greenberger, L., de Vries, E., Broxterman, H., Scheffer, G., and Scheper, R. (1995) The LRP gene encoding a major vault protein associated with drug resistance maps proximal to MRP on chromosome 16: evidence that chromosome breakage plays a key role in MRP or LRP gene amplification. *Cancer Res.* **55,** 4214–4219.
18. Withoff, S., de Vries, E., Keith, W., Nienhuis, E., van der Graaf, W., Uges, D., and Mulder, N. (1996) Differential expression of DNA topoisomerase II alpha and -beta in P-gp and MRP-negative VM26, mAMSA and mitoxantroneresistant sublines of the human SCLC cell line GLC4. *Br. J. Cancer* **74,** 1869–1876.
19. Withoff, S., Keith, W., Knol, A., Coutts, J., Hoare, S., Mulder, N., and de Vries, E. (1996) Selection of a subpopulation with fewer DNA topoisomerase II alpha gene copies in a doxorubicin-resistant cell line panel. *Br. J. Cancer* **74,** 502–507.

20. Eijdems, E., De Haas, M., Coco-Martin, J., Ottenheim, C., Zaman, G., Dauwerse, H., Breuning, M., Twentyman, P., Borst, P., and Baas, F. (1995) Mechanisms of MRP over-expression in four human lung-cancer cell lines and analysis of the MRP amplicon. *Intl. J. Cancer* **60,** 676–684.
21. Robertson, K., Reeves, J., Smith, G., Keith, W., Ozanne, B., Cooke, T., and Stanton, P. (1996) Quantitative estimation of epidermal growth factor receptor and c-erbB-2 in human breast cancer. *Cancer Res.* **56,** 3823–3830.
22. Soder, A., Hoare, S., Muir, S., Going, J., Parkinson, E., and Keith, W. (1997) Amplification, increased dosage and in situ expression of the telomerase RNA gene in human cancer. *Oncogene* **14,** 1013–1021.
23. Soder, A., Hoare, S., Muire, S., Balmain, A., Parkinson, E., and Keith, W. (1997) Mapping of the gene for the mouse telomerase RNA component, Terc, to chromosome 3 by fluorescence in situ hybridization and mouse chromosome painting. *Genomics* **41,** 293–294.

20

Genetic Analysis of Drug Resistance by Reverse *In Situ* Hybridization

W. Nicol Keith

1. Introduction

Drug resistance is a major factor that limits the effectiveness of cancer chemotherapy, and there is considerable evidence to suggest a genetic basis for many drug-resistant phenotypes. A major drawback to many of the conventional approaches used to investigate drug-resistance mechanisms is that some prior information or guesswork on the changes that have occurred is required, thus necessitating separate reagents to screen each possible change. When analyzing genetic changes for example, screening is limited to the use of gene or region specific probes as in Southern blot or microsatellite analysis. Recently, the molecular cytogenetic techniques of reverse *in situ* hybridization (REVISH), and its more advanced relative, comparative genomic hybridization (CGH), have been developed for the rapid global detection and mapping of genetic imbalances in tumor genomes *(1–7)*. In REVISH, genomic DNA from the tumor is used as a complex probe and hybridized to normal metaphase chromosomes *(6)*. Genomic sequences amplified in the tumor are then detected as an increased intensity of signal at the normal chromosomal position from which the amplified sequences are derived *(1,6,7)*. For more accurate analysis of both loss and gain of genetic material, CGH is required; however, CGH involves complex fluorescence-comparison techniques and expert knowledge of chromosome identification *(2)*. However, both REVISH and CGH are ideal methods to detect genetic changes associated with the acquisition of drug resistance in tumors *(6,8)*.

In order to use REVISH for this purpose, a number of steps are carried out.

1. An initial reverse *in situ* hybridization is carried out using genomic DNA extracted from the test cell lines and compared to normal DNA controls. A visual

From: *Methods in Molecular Medicine, Vol. 28: Cytotoxic Drug Resistance Mechanisms*
Edited by: R. Brown and U. Böger-Brown © Humana Press Inc., Totowa, NJ

analysis of the resultant hybridization allows the key chromosomes with regional amplifications to be identified by their size and centromere position.
2. Confirmation of chromosomal identification is obtained by co-hybridizing the test cell line DNA with a whole chromosome paint and visualizing the two probes with different fluorochromes. We have found this to be an important modification to standard REVISH protocols because it allows unambiguous chromosome identification in laboratories without cytogenetic experience.
3. Precise localization of the amplified sequences is carried out using fractional length measurements (Flpter) ***(6,9,10)***.
4. Using the reference maps for Flpter measurements available through the Internet, (E.g., Resource for Molecular Cytogenetics at Lawrence Berkeley National Laboratories and the University of California, San Francisco; http://rmc-www.lbl.gov/), and also noted by Bray-Ward and colleagues ***(11)***, identify candidate loci or specific markers for the region of interest.
5. Detailed genetic analysis of candidate loci are carried out by, for example, FISH.
6. Using the information previously derived, traditional positional cloning strategies can then be applied to the newly identified region of interest.

In conclusion, REVISH is a useful approach to study genetic changes associated with drug resistance ***(6)***. A major contributing factor to the success of this approach is ease of integration of the data produced in our laboratory, with published reference maps and genome databases, thus allowing us to access both information and potential reagents. The major steps involved in REVISH are shown in **Fig. 1**. Because REVISH is a form of an *in situ* hybridization technique, all the basic techniques are described in Chapter 20 of this volume.

2. Materials

All the general materials for REVISH can be found in the preceding chapter on FISH (**Subheading 2.1.**).

2.1. Chromosome Preparation from Lymphocytes Using BrdU and Thymidine (see Note 1)

1. Chromosome medium 1A (Gibco/BRL; Gaithersburg, MD).
2. 5 mL whole blood: (Preferably male; *see* **Note 1**); collected in heparinized tube.
3. Hanks Balanced Salt Solution (HBSS).
4. Thymidine (Sigma, Chemical Co., St. Louis, MO) stock concentration at 6 mg/mL, (use at final concentration of 0.35 mg/mL). Dissolve in water, filter, and keep at –20°C.
5. Bromodeoxyuridine (BrdU) (Sigma), stock of 3 mg/mL, (use at final concentration of 0.03 mg/mL). Make in water, filter, and store –20°C.
6. Colcemid (Gibco/BRL), 10 ug/mL = 100X stock: 50 mL/tube containing 5 mL chromosome medium, final conc. 0.1 µg/mL.

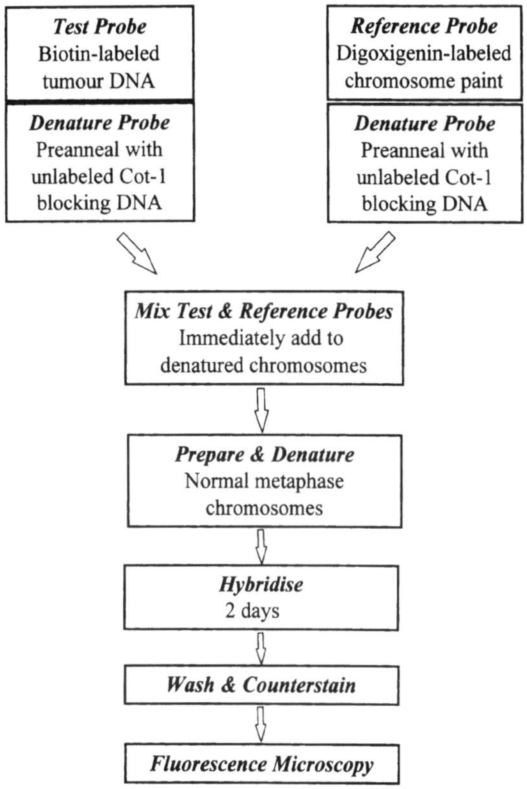

Fig. 1. Overview of REVISH.

7. Hypotonic solution: 0.075 *M* Potassium Chloride.
8. Methanol/acetic acid (3:1): Make fresh.

3. Methods

3.1. Chromosome Preparation from Lymphocytes Using BrdU and Thymidine (see Note 1)

1. Add 200 µL of whole blood to 5 mL chromosome medium.
2. Incubate for 72 h, mixing every day, at 37°C in 5% CO_2.
3. Add 294 µL of 6 mg/mL thymidine and incubate at 37°C for 15–17 h in 5% CO_2.
4. Wash 3 times in HBSS, centrifuge at 500*g* for 7 min for each wash.
5. Resuspend in 5 mL of fresh chromosome medium containing 50 µL of 3 mg/mL BrdU.
6. Incubate for 7–8 h at 37°C in 5% CO_2 in the dark.
7. Add 50 µL colcemid/tube and incubate 1–3 h.
8. Spin at 500*g* for 5 min.

9. Remove supernatant, and resuspend in 10 mL of hypotonic solution.
10. Incubate at 37°C for 10–15 min.
11. Add 2–3 mL of methanol/acetic acid (3:1).
12. Centrifuge at 500*g* for 5 min.
13. Remove supernatant. Resuspend in 10 mL methanol/acetic acid.
14. Leave at room temperature for 10–15 min.
15. Repeat **steps 12–14** at least three times.
16. Finally spin at 500*g* for 5 min and resuspend in a small volume (3–5 mL) of methanol/acetic acid, and store at –20°C.

3.2. Extraction of Genomic DNA

There are numerous protocols for the extraction of high molecular weight genomic DNA. We use commercial kits and have found the QUIAGEN range of nucleic acid isolation kits to be excellent, (QIAGEN Ltd., Dorking, UK). The kits are used according to the manufacturers protocols. The quantity and quality of the extracted DNA are checked both by absorbance measurements and by running a sample of the genomic DNA on a 0.8% agarose gel (*see* **Note 2**).

3.3. Labeling of Genomic DNA for REVISH (see Note 3)

For REVISH, we label 1.5 µg genomic DNA with biotin using the following protocol. For optimal hybridizations, the size of the biotin-labeled probes should be in the range of 500 bp–2 kb. Therefore, the nick-translation conditions require optimization prior to using the probes in hybridization experiments. The simplest way to vary the size range is to vary the length of time for which the DNA is nick-translated. We therefore recommend that the nick-translation conditions are optimized prior to starting hybridizations.

3.3.1. Incorporation of Biotin-16-dUTP by Nick Translation

1. Using Biotin-Nick Translation Mix (Boehringer Mannheim):

DNA	X µL (1.5 µg DNA)
dH_2O	(16–X µL)
Biotin-nick mix	4 µL
Final volume	20 µL

2. Mix and centrifuge briefly.
3. Incubate at 16°C for 1–4 h (usually approx 1.5 h).
4. If you are optimizing fragment size, proceed to Fragment Size Check (**Subheading 3.3.2.**).
5. If you are using probe in a hybridization, proceed to Probe Precipitation (**Subheading 3.3.3.**).

3.3.2. Fragment Size Check

The size of the biotin and dig-labeled probes should be in the range of 500 bp—2 Kb To check for this, after adding STOP buffer to the labeled probes, 7 µL of

DNA loading dye is added to the whole sample and mixed. The probes are then boiled for 3 min and put on ice for 3 min. Samples are then loaded into a 0.8% agarose gel and run with a DNA ladder. If the majority of the fragments are below 500 bp, the labeling time is reduced. If they are above 2 Kb, the labeling time is increased.

3.3.3. Probe Precipitation

1. Precipitate probe: add to the 20 µL Nick translation: 2 µL of 3 *M* NaAc, pH 8.0; 150 µL of Human cot1 DNA; and 300 µL of 100% ethanol.
2. Mix well.
3. Leave at –20°C overnight.
4. Spin down at 13rpm for 15 min in microfuge.
5. Pour off ethanol carefully.
6. Wash pellet in 100 µL 70% ethanol at 13K for 5 min.
7. Carefully pour off ethanol and dry pellet (air-dry or rotary-evaporate).
8. Resuspend in 7 µL of 50% formamide hybridization mix.
9. Mix with cut off pipet tip and leave to resuspend for 3 h.
10. Probe is now ready to be denatured.

3.4. Reverse* In Situ *Hybridization (see Note 3)

3.4.2. Preparation of Chromosome Spreads

1. Drop a volume of chromosome preparation on to a slide from a height and mark an area of spreads on the slide using a diamond pen.
2. Fix for 1 h in methanol/acetic acid (3:1) at room temperature.
3. Air-dry.
4. Incubate for 1 h in 100 µg/mL RNase in 2X SSC at 37°C. Make from frozen RNase stock.
5. Rinse 2X SSC.
6. Digest in pepsin, (0.01% in 10 m*M* HCl) solution for 10 min at 37°C. Make from frozen pepsin stock.
7. Rinse in water.
8. Fix for 10 min in Streck Tissue Fixative (STF) at room temperature. Alternatively, use 1% formaldehyde (add 4 mL of 37% formaldehyde to 146 mL phosphate-buffered solution (PBS), 50 m*M* $MgCl_2$).
9. Dehydrate 2 × 2 min 70% ethanol, 2 × 2 min 100% ethanol, and leave to air-dry.

3.4.2. Probe Denaturation: Double Hybridization of Genomic DNA and a Chromosome Paint

At this stage in the procedure you should have the following conditions:

1. Chromosomes are ready but not denatured;
2. Genomic DNA test probe is labeled with biotin, but not denatured; and
3. Commercial digoxigenin labeled chromosome paint is ready, but not denatured.

You are now ready to denature both the chromosome paint and your test genomic DNA sample. Both the paint and genomic probe require an incubation at 37°C to allow for suppression of repetitive sequences in the probe by cot1 DNA in the hybridization mix. The exact conditions for the chromosome paint denaturation and preannealing will vary with the commercial source of the paint. You will therefore want to plan the next stage to ensure that both the probes complete the preannealing step at the same time. Refer to **Fig. 1** for an overview of timing.

3.4.2.1. Denature Genomic DNA Probe

Probe is at a concentration of 1.5 µg/7 µL. This is required for each slide. Heat probe to 80°C 10 min. Place probe at 37°C for 90 min. to allow for suppression of repetitive sequences in the probe by Cot1 DNA in hybridization mix.

3.4.2.2. Denature Chromosome Paint According to Manufacturers Instructions

For Oncor biotin labeled chromosome paints:

1. Use 7 µL of paint/slide and aliquot into microfuge tube.
2. Leave at room temperature for 5 min.
3. Denature at 70°C for 10 min.
4. Spin down and incubate at 37°C for 90 min to allow for suppression of repetitive sequences in the probe by cot1 DNA in hybridization mix.

3.4.3. Denature Target Chromosomes

During the preannealing time for the probes as previously described, the chromosomes are denatured.

1. Warm 70% formamide (35 mL formamide, 15 mL 2X SSC) to temperature required.
2. Immerse the slide with chromosomes in 70% formamide for time required at 75°C for 5 min. Carry out in fume hood and use plastic coplin jars.
3. Rinse in large volume (500 mL) 70% EtOH.
4. Dehydrate in 70% EtOH for 2 min and 100% EtOH for 2 min.
5. Air-dry.

3.4.4. Hybridization

1. Mix preannealed probe and chromosome paint and add to slide.
2. Cover with a 22 × 22 coverslip and seal edges with rubber cement.
3. Hybridize for 2 d at 37°C in the dark in a humidified chamber. **IMPORTANT!** Do not let slides dry out at any stage.

3.4.5. Wash Steps

1. Remove coverslips by soaking in 2X SSC for 2 min, then peel off rubber cement.
2. Wash in 50% formamide/1X SSC for 20 min at 42°C.
3. Wash in 2X SSC for 20 min at 42°C.

3.4.6. Probe Detection Using Avidin and Antibodies for Two Colors (Fitc/Texas Red)

All detection steps carried out in humidity chambers in the dark and under parafilm coverslips. Use 100 µL of detection reagent/slide.

1. Rinse in 4X SSC, 0.05% Tween (4X SSC-T) for 3 min.
2. Block slides in 4X SSC-T/0.5% block (4X SSC-TB) for 10 min at room temperature under parafilm coverslips (in humidity chamber).
3. First layer detection: Add 100 µL to each slide of FITC-avidin DCS at 1:200 dilution in 4X SSC-TB for 45 min at room temperature.
4. Wash in 4X SSC-T for 10 min at room temperature.
5. Second layer detection: Biotinylated anti-avidin DCS 1:100 and Sheep anti-digoxigenin 1:200 in 4X SSC-TB for 1 h at room temperature.
6. Wash in 4X SSC-T for 10 min at room temperature.
7. Third layer detection: FITC-Avidin DCS at 1:200 and donkey anti-sheep Texas Red 1:300 in 4X SSC-TB for 1 h at room temperature.
8. Wash in 4X SSC-T for 20 min at room temperature.
9. Dehydrate and mount slides in *DAPI only* Antifade.

3.5. Analysis of Hybridization Sites (see Note 3)

A visual inspection of reverse *in situ* hybridizations reveals intensity changes associated with copy number alterations to sequences within the test genomic DNA *(6)*. Once the chromosomal identity has been determined by co-hybridization with chromosome paints, then hybridization signal can be characterized in more detail, if your lab is equipped with an image capture system *(6)*. A rather appealing and robust approach to mapping the FISH signals on the normal chromosomes is to define the map position of the hybridization signal as the fractional length along the chromosome in relation to the short-arm telomere (*see* **Fig. 2**), this is called the FLpter *(6–10)*. FLpter measurements are carried out on digitized images using IPLab Spectrum software (Scanalytics, Fairfax, VA) (Internet address: http://www.iplab.com/sac/software.html). Published Flpter maps are available from the Resource for Molecular Cytogenetics at Lawrence Berkeley National Laboratories and the University of California, San Francisco (Internet address: http://rmc-www.lbl.gov/) and also from Bray-Ward and colleagues *(11)*. Thus, it is quite simple to integrate your own mapping data into reference maps. This will open up the necessary reagents required to further characterize the amplicons.

4. Notes

1. Quality of chromosome preparation: The quality of the chromosome spreads are very important for REVISH. You may need to make several batches and test them to drop. In order to gain maximum information from the hybridizations, the

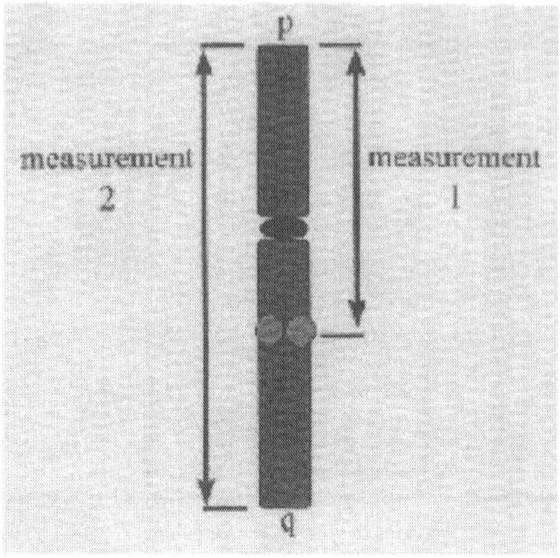

Fig. 2. Fractional length measurements, Flpter.

chromosomes spreads need to have well-separated chromosomes and nonoverlapping chromosomes. Check the spreads on a low-power light microscope before the hybridization. It is easy to drop and prepare more chromosome spreads, in comparison to re-doing a whole REVISH merely because the chromosome preparations were poor. It is also a very good idea to get a male donor for the chromosomes, because then you obtain an X and a Y chromosome to study.

2. Extraction of Genomic DNA: We find it is very important to check the DNA on a gel, because what you see is what you get, and absorbance readings can be wrong. This is particularly important if you get a DNA sample from a source outside your own lab. Run a sample with a known amount of molecular-weight markers and this will give a rough guide to its concentration. In addition, good-quality, high-molecular weight genomic DNA will not travel very far into the gel and will run as a fairly tight 'blob.' Degraded genomic DNA will appear as a smear running down the gel.
3. Labeling genomic DNA: Labeling of genomic DNA for REVISH requires approx 1.5 µg of DNA/slide which is different from FISH (*see* Chapter 19). We strongly advise that the labeling reactions are optimized for fragment size and that the probe is tested for incorporation of the hapten. Each time a test genomic DNA is labeled and a REVISH is carried out, it is vital that a normal genomic DNA control is also used. A normal DNA can be made from white blood cells. The labeled normal DNA control reverse paints the chromosomes in an even fashion, with the expected exception of blocking of repetitive sequences (owing to inclusion of cot-1 DNA), at for example centromeric sequences. Any deviation from this pattern suggests that the experiment has not worked. If uneven hybridization patterns on normal chromosomes with labeled normal genomic DNA are produced, then the most likely problem is failure to compete out repetitive sequences

with cot-1 DNA during the preannealling stage. To rectify this, increase the amount of cot-1 DNA and the time for preannealling. If hybridizations are very grainy in appearance, make sure the fragment size of the labeled probe is in the correct range.

References

1. Joos, S., Scherthan, H., Speicher, M. R., Schlegel, J., Cremer, T., and Lichter, P. (1993) Detection of amplified DNA sequences by reverse chromosome painting using genomic tumor DNA as probe. *Human Genet.* **90,** 584–589.
2. Kallioniemi, O.-P., Kallioniemi, A., Sudar, D., Rutovitz, D., Gray, J. W., Waldman, F., and Pinkel, D. (1993) Comparative genomic hybridisation: a rapid new method for detecting and mapping DNA amplification in tumors. *Seminars Cancer Biol.* **4,** 41–46.
3. Kallioniemi, A., Kallioniemi, O.-P., Sudar, D., Rutovitz, D., Gray, J. W., Waldman, F., and Pinkel, D. (1992) Comparative genomic hybridisation for molecular cytogenetic analysis of solid tumors. *Science* **258,** 818–821.
4. Houldsworth, J. and Chaganti, R. S. K. (1994) Comparative genomic hybridization: an overview. *Am. J. Pathol.* **145,** 1253–1260.
5. Van Ommen, G. J. B., Breuning, M. H., and Raap, A. K. (1995) FISH in genome research and molecular diagnostics. *Curr. Opin. Genet. Dev.* **5,** 304–308.
6. Hoare, S., Freeman, C., Coutts, J., Varley, J., James, L., and Keith, W. (1997) Identification of genetic changes associated with drug resistance by reverse in situ hybridization. *Br. J. Cancer* **75,** 275–82.
7. Lichter, P., Bentz, M., and Joos, S. (1995) Detection of chromosomal aberrations by means of molecular cytogenetics: painting of chromosomes and chromosomal subregions and comparative genomic hybridization. *Methods Enzymol.* **254,** 334–359.
8. Wasenius, V. M., Jekunen, A., Monni, O., Joensuu, H., Aebi, S., Howell, S. B. and Knuutila, S. (1997) Comparative genomic hybridization analysis of chromosomal changes occurring during development of acquired resistance to cisplatin in human ovarian carcinoma cells. *Genes Chromosomes Cancer* **18,** 286–291.
9. Lichter, P., Tang, C. C., Call, K., Hermanson, G., Evans, G. A., Housman, D., and Ward, D. C. (1990) High-resolution mapping of human chromosome 11 by in situ hybridization with cosmid clones. *Science* **247,** 64–69.
10. McLeod, H. L. and Keith, W. N. (1996) variation in topoisomerase I gene copy number as a mechanism for intrinsic drug sensitivity. *Br. J. Cancer* **74,** 508–512.
11. Bray-Ward, P., Menninger, J., Lieman, J., Desai, T., Mokady, N., Banks, A., and Ward, D. C. (1996) Integration of the cytogenetic, genetic, and physical maps of the human genome by FISH mapping of CEPH YAC clones. *Genomics* **32,** 1–14.

Index

5511848R00147

Printed in Germany
by Amazon Distribution
GmbH, Leipzig